PRAISE FOR
The First Year: Type 2 Diabetes

"If there is a better guide to living with diabetes, I've not found it."
—Professor Mark McCarthy, MD, FRCP,
Oxford Center for Diabetes, Endocrinology, and Metabolism

"It takes someone who lives with diabetes day in and day out to relate effectively to readers who have diabetes. Gretchen Becker doesn't write at you, she communicates with you. *The First Year: Type 2 Diabetes* takes you by the hand and guides you safely and securely through the challenges of living with type 2 diabetes. It will make you more competent at managing your diabetes and more confident in yourself."
—Gary Scheiner, MS, CDE,
diabetes educator and author of *Think Like a Pancreas:
A Practical Guide to Managing Diabetes with Insulin, The Ultimate
Guide to Accurate Carb Counting, Practical CGM: Improving Patient Outcomes
Through Continuous Glucose Monitoring,* and *Until There Is a Cure: The Latest and
Greatest in Diabetes Self-Care*

"With her newly revised and expanded second edition, Gretchen Becker has surpassed herself. This updated book offers the most comprehensive guide to living with and learning about type 2 diabetes available anywhere—and one that people really can't afford to live without. She tells you everything you need to know to live well, including a mix of up-to-date and down-to-earth information that you won't find anywhere else. Her book is an absolutely essential resource for anyone with diabetes."
—Sheri Colberg, PhD, FACSM,
diabetes and exercise expert and author of many books, including
Diabetic Athlete's Handbook, The 7 Step Diabetes Fitness Plan, and *Exercise and
Diabetes,* and coauthor of *The Diabetes Breakthrough* and *50 Secrets of the Longest
Living People with Diabetes*

"As a certified diabetes educator, I am forever searching for patient-friendly, comprehensive, sound, and clear information. Gretchen Becker packs the practical and science-based information and delivers it beautifully. Becker's analogies and writing style make the information come alive. I am certain that *The First Year: Type 2 Diabetes* will lead you to the best years of your life with diabetes."
—Lorena Drago, MS, RD, CDN, CDE,
certified diabetes educator, registered dietitian, and past president of the
Metropolitan New York Association of Diabetes Educators

"When I find out that a friend or colleague has been diagnosed with type 2 diabetes, I immediately recommend that they read Gretchen Becker's *The First Year: Type 2 Diabetes*. My friends have been most grateful for this suggestion. Now Becker's updated edition includes even more helpful tips and suggestions for people newly diagnosed with type 2."

—GABRIELLE KAPLAN-MAYER,
author of *Insulin Pump Therapy Demystified* and host of
www.insulinpumpdemystified.blogspot.com

"[*The First Year: Type 2 Diabetes*] walks the newly diagnosed reader through the skills he must develop and steps he should take in the first days, weeks, and months with diabetes . . . in clear, accessible language."

—DIABETES SELF-MANAGEMENT

"I was diagnosed in October and discovered your book in late November. My A1c was 10.8 when diagnosed, last week it was 5.4. I could not have done it without your tips and expertise. When I run into problems with my eating, I take your book out and it gets me back on track. I truly appreciate all you have done for other individuals with diabetes. You have simplified my life for me. Thanks so much."

—BOBBYE KIENITZ

"I had to write to say thank you for your book *The First Year: Type 2 Diabetes*. For me, it was a godsend, and I think it should be required reading for all the newly diagnosed. . . . If it hadn't been for your book, I'd still be blaming myself, feeling very much alone and at a total loss as to what to do to manage my diabetes. Surprisingly, I found the Internet of very little use. And I still very much believe it should be required reading for the newly diagnosed!"

—NS

"You provided all the info my health-care provider didn't. And after going to the diabetes classes in September, I loaned your book to my DNE. She liked it so much she's ordered a copy for herself and as a loaner. Her note said 'I cannot thank you enough! I am going to purchase for myself as a lend out and the one she wrote on Pre DM.'"

—HOLLY SHALTZ

"If you only buy one book on diabetes, buy this one."

—RHODA MARTIN

"*The First Year: Type 2 Diabetes* is fantastic. I found it extremely helpful in clearing up so much of my confusion through concise, informative, and easy to understand sections."

—STEVE MOSS

"As soon as I got my diagnosis of type 2 diabetes, I drove over to the bookstore and found *The First Year: Type 2 Diabetes*. What a godsend the book was—it helped me so much in those first frantic weeks after my diagnosis. *The First Year: Type 2 Diabetes* is a wonderful book in language that can be understood by the layperson. I felt that Gretchen was holding my hand through this whole ride."

—LINDA BETZ

"One of the first things I did when I was diagnosed was drive down to the local bookstore where I bought Gretchen Becker's book *The First Year: Type 2 Diabetes*. It was a great help and very calming for both my wife and me. Once you get an understanding of how the BG/meter/carbs systems work, you will feel better—you will be armed, informed, and ready to do battle!"

—GEORGE ABBOTT

"*The First Year: Type 2 Diabetes* has been the single best educational tool I have found. I truly believe that being diagnosed with diabetes and finding this book probably have saved my life. I tell everyone I know who has type 2 diabetes to get this book."

—SUZANNE REED, SWEDEN

"Much of the information in this book is incredibly useful for any person with diabetes, regardless of the type. It was very well written and easily understandable. It's a great reference that I'm sure I will return to again and again."

—ANDREW J. DARWIN

"I've learned more than I ever thought possible about diabetes from this book—it was and will continue to be a resource for me. In the seven weeks since I've been diagnosed, I've completely changed my diet and brought my BG levels down to the normal range. My blood pressure has also improved, along with my lipids."

—JENIFER MITCHELL

"I was recently diagnosed with type 2 diabetes and went through almost all the things Gretchen Becker wrote about. It feels like you just made a friend that is walking you through and understands how you feel about this lifetime problem."

—JONAH

"When I was diagnosed with type 2 diabetes, my doctor suggested that I take a diabetes management class, which cost over $300 and was not covered by insurance. I learned very little except how to use a glucose meter and that I should be very careful about carbs. When I found this book, many of my questions were answered, and I loved the fact that the book read like a talk with a friend instead of a lecture by a doctor."

—LAURA DUGAN

"*The First Year: Type 2 Diabetes* is walking me through the stages and I am so grateful not to feel alone, as I would have without these explanations."

—HELEN E. MILLER

"When I read something about my disease that doesn't make sense or scares me, I only have to turn to this book. Gretchen's matter-of-fact tone gives me back perspective. When I'm tempted to ignore my healthy eating plan, I remember that ultimately I am responsible for my care . . . no one else can do it."

—LORRIAN IPPOLITI

"*The First Year: Type 2 Diabetes* is right on the money, telling how it is without any sugarcoating, but with a generally positive outlook. I recommend it to my newly diagnosed patients and also to the ones that could use some guidance in getting a handle on taking care of themselves."

—RUTH BARUCH

"*The First Year: Type 2 Diabetes* stood out because many of the other books simply dealt with the biological issues, whereas this book is far more personal, based on Gretchen's own experience of dealing with the diagnosis. Each chapter mirrored my own concerns, and it seemed to answer all the questions that arose, day by day as I read on. Both my parents have read it cover to cover, and it has helped explain to them many of the problems I have had."

—DAVID HUGHES, CHESHIRE, ENGLAND

"I was so relieved to hear that it was OK for me to feel sad when I found out that I had diabetes. This book has given me the confidence to get on the path to finally taking care of myself for the first time in many years."

—ROSEANNE PACHECO

"This book has helped me deal with the diagnosis, and I have taken it to my monthly class and encouraged others to read it. It is a wonderful guide for the average person. Now that the initial shock has left, I plan to read the book again with a highlighter."

—SUE GUTHMAN

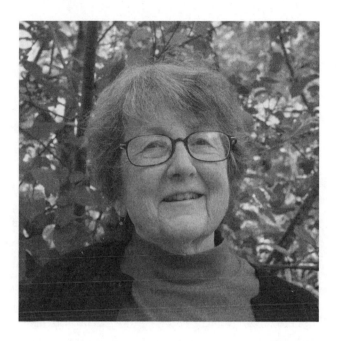

GRETCHEN BECKER, a magna cum laude and Phi Beta
Kappa graduate of Radcliffe College, is a writer and
editor specializing in medical books. She was diagnosed with type 2 diabetes in 1996 and is a long-
time participant in several diabetes email lists on
the Internet. She lives on a small farm in Halifax,
Vermont, where she also raises sheep. Becker can be
reached via email at gretchenb@myfairpoint.net or
gretchen@gretchenbecker.com.

The First Year:

Type 2 Diabetes

An Essential Guide for the Newly Diagnosed

THIRD EDITION ■ COMPLETELY REVISED AND UPDATED

Gretchen Becker

FOREWORD BY ALLISON B. GOLDFINE, MD

Da Capo
LIFE
LONG

DA CAPO LIFELONG BOOKS

A Member of the Perseus Books Group

Designed by Cynthia Young

Library of Congress Cataloging-in-Publication Data
Becker, Gretchen.
    The first year—Type 2 diabetes : an essential guide for the newly diagnosed /
Gretchen Becker ; foreword by Allison B. Goldfine, MD. — Third edition.
        pages cm
    Includes bibliographical references and index.
    ISBN 978-0-7382-1860-1 (paperback) — ISBN 978-0-7382-1861-8 (e-book)
    1. Non-insulin-dependent diabetes—Popular works.   I. Title.   II. Title: First year—type two diabetes.
    RC662.18.B43 2015
    616.4'624—dc23
    2015020979

Published by Da Capo Press
A Member of the Perseus Books Group
www.dacapopress.com

Da Capo Press books are available at special discounts for bulk purchases in the US by corporations, institutions, and other organizations. For more information, please contact the Special Markets Department at the Perseus Books Group, 2300 Chestnut Street, Suite 200, Philadelphia, PA, 19103, or call (800) 810-4145, extension 5000, or e-mail special.markets@ perseusbooks.com.

10 9 8 7 6 5 4 3 2

*To all my friends on the
Diabetes International and World mailing lists,
from whom I have learned so much.*

Contents

Foreword

by Allison B. Goldfine, MD

As a doctor, I first became attracted to taking care of patients with diabetes for two reasons. First, someone who is newly diagnosed with the condition has so much to learn about it and I enjoy teaching. Second, even though scientifically there is much we still need to learn about diabetes, there are many therapeutic options that can help people with diabetes have healthy lives. Helping people with diabetes learn to live with this disorder is extremely fulfilling work for me.

I find the two greatest challenges of diabetes are, clinically, finding the best treatment approach for each individual patient and, scientifically, realizing how much we have yet to learn. I have learned much from each of my patients, and I am continually challenged by helping them learn to manage their own diabetes. My patients range in age from eighteen to eighty, and no matter what phase of their lives my patients are going through—studying in school, getting married, having children, starting or ending jobs, or retiring—I enjoy advising them about the special considerations they need to be aware of and the accommodations they need to make to cope with diabetes.

In this book, Gretchen Becker, with whom I have had the pleasure to work over the last several years, has collected information and many valuable experiences that will assist anyone with type 2 diabetes who is adjusting to having the disease, whether newly diagnosed or now becoming interested in learning from approaches that have been effective for others.

As Gretchen discusses, the reasons why some people develop diabetes and others do not is not fully understood. There is clearly a genetic component that predisposes some people to get diabetes, yet not everyone with diabetic parents or siblings or even an identical twin develops the disorder. Similarly, many people with no family history of diabetes develop this disease. In addition, there is an environmental component in which both weight and lack of exercise play a central role. Indeed, the rapid increase in the number of people who are overweight is coinciding with a rapid increase in the number of people diagnosed with type 2 diabetes. However, not every overweight person develops diabetes, nor does every person with a sedentary lifestyle. It is not even clear if disordered insulin production or decreased insulin action (an important physiological distinction you will learn more about in this book) occurs as the very first abnormality in the development of elevated blood glucose levels. It is possible that this has been so hard to determine because it is different in different people.

It is important to understand there are two main types of diabetes (and this book further explains the two types): type 1 and type 2. Insulin is necessary for glucose (or more popularly, sugar) to get into cells. Cells use glucose for energy to function: for the heart to pump and the brain to think. People with type 1 diabetes cannot make insulin; the body identifies the pancreatic cells that make insulin as foreign and destroys them. In type 2 diabetes, the body makes insulin; in fact, most people with type 2 diabetes make more insulin than a person without diabetes. But they still cannot maintain their blood sugar levels within the normal range. They are resistant to the glucose-lowering effects of insulin. Thus, for both types of diabetes, sugar levels become elevated, and over time, elevated sugar levels can cause problems with the small and large blood vessels, causing microvascular (small vessel) and macrovascular (large vessel) disease.

In type 1 diabetes, insulin must be given by injection to sustain life, whereas treatment of type 2 diabetes centers on a few central themes to match the insulin that the body can produce to the amount required to digest food. Improved food choices and increased physical activity both decrease the body's need for insulin and improve its utilization. No drug therapy alone can work effectively in the absence of these most difficult lifestyle changes. Although it is difficult to exercise and change eating habits to lose weight, this is something that people with type 2 diabetes can do to markedly improve their health.

Diabetes treatment options have increased dramatically over the last few years. There are now medications that help the body make more insulin, there are other drugs to improve the efficiency with which insulin acts within the body, and still others that help accelerate glucose clearance through the kidneys. If these medications are not sufficient to improve the blood sugar levels of a person with diabetes, then insulin may be used to further raise levels and overcome insulin resistance. Home blood glucose monitoring provides immediate and continuous feedback to assess how therapy is working. There are also medications recently available for weight loss, and these may additionally lower blood sugar levels in patients with diabetes. Some doctors and patients also consider bariatric surgery for diabetes and weight management.

Diabetes treatment is individual. No two patients require exactly the same diet and exercise routine or mix of medications, and it is likely that two doctors may recommend different treatments in different orders for similar patients. The differences in individual needs or approaches to management can cause confusion for people with diabetes who discuss their care among themselves, or for someone seeking a second opinion. Each person with type 2 diabetes must work with his or her physician and health-care team to determine the extent of lifestyle modifications he or she is able to make and the medicinal therapy that best suits his or her lifestyle and individual disease characteristics. This complete treatment strategy must be reevaluated on an ongoing basis to determine if additional changes can or should be made.

In addition to providing routine health care, a health-care team must consider all other potential medical problems that may be associated with diabetes, either directly or indirectly, and test for them in order to initiate early preventive therapy. This includes not only eye, kidney, and foot exams, to evaluate for the risk of long-term elevations in blood glucose levels, but also blood pressure and cholesterol levels, since the treatment of hypertension and cholesterol are as important to protecting the heart as maintaining glucose levels as near to normal as possible.

In this book, Gretchen covers all of these subjects in detail. She presents the material in a manner that is clear to the person without years of medical training, something that many health-care professionals find difficult to do. She offers many practical suggestions and an array of approaches to coping with diabetes on a daily basis that come from her years of living with the condition and from the experiences of her acquaintances. Her advice is sound and presented with humor. Her book is a most valuable companion for any person first learning about living with diabetes and overwhelmed by the idea of making daily lifestyle changes.

ALLISON B. GOLDFINE, MD, is an associate professor at Harvard Medical School and an investigator at the Joslin Diabetes Center in Boston. Her research work focuses on understanding insulin resistance and its role in the development of type 2 diabetes and complications. She lives outside Boston with her husband and three daughters.

Preface

Almost twenty years have passed since I was diagnosed with type 2 diabetes in 1996, but it seems like yesterday. Time flies when you're having fun.

Because of the diabetes, my life is definitely different. It's *better*. Yes, you read that right: my life is better. Having diabetes forced me to take better care of myself. I lost weight. I get more exercise. I eat better food, and I eat less of it, so I haven't regained the weight I lost after the diagnosis. Except for looking almost twenty years older than I did in 1996, I have no complications.

In the previous edition of this book, I mentioned that I hadn't decided what I wanted to do when I grew up. I still haven't decided. But one thing I do know is that I don't want to spend my remaining years handicapped with diabetes complications.

When I was diagnosed, I read a devastating statement in some medical book that the average survival time after a diagnosis of type 2 diabetes was eight years. That, and the possibility of complications, made me take this disease seriously. According to those authors, I should be dead now. I much prefer my current state.

If I'd been given the advice that was all too common at that time, namely, "You have diabetes. Watch your sugar," I might have gone on as I had been, simply eating a little less dessert, and I would probably be in much worse shape today—if I were alive at all. With time, I came to realize that the dire prediction of that medical book was probably based on old data from an era in which the diagnostic criteria for determining elevated blood sugar levels were higher, which meant that many people were diagnosed at late stages of the disease. In earlier times, treatment was limited to one or two drugs. Many people with type 2 diabetes still do *not* take it seriously and do not do much to change their way of life. I did.

Since that time, there have been a lot of exciting changes in the world of type 2 diabetes treatment. The blood sugar levels that are considered normal have been lowered so that people are being diagnosed at earlier stages of the disease, when they have a much greater chance of getting good control and avoiding complications.

Standards for acceptable diabetes control have also improved, and the goal for many patients today is to have normal blood sugar levels. Many new drugs have become available, and physicians can now mix and match until they get a drug combination that helps patients reach their blood sugar goals.

However, one thing in diabetes treatment has not changed at all, which is that the patient must participate in the treatment. You can't simply sit back passively and let a physician perform an operation or prescribe a miracle drug that will cure you. You must take control, learn all you can about this disease, and find out which diet and which kinds of exercise work best for you. Then you have to stick to that diet and exercise regimen.

This takes effort, but it can also be rewarding because you have some control over your future health. The first step to taking control is becoming informed. I hope this book will help you to do just that.

Introduction

Diabetes, perhaps more than any other chronic disease, must be managed in large part by the patient, because everything you do affects your blood sugar levels. Most especially, every morsel of food you eat has a major effect. Exercise, or its lack, also plays an important role.

Other life situations can affect blood sugar levels as well. These include both physical stress, such as getting the flu, and emotional stress, such as losing a job. Medications can also make your blood sugar go either up or down.

Physicians and nurses can guide you in your quest for normal blood sugar levels, but they cannot be at your side twenty-four hours a day. You may not see them for weeks or even months at a time. Thus to gain good control, you must take charge and learn to do a large part of the management of your diabetes yourself. In order to make wise daily decisions about the myriad factors that can affect your blood sugar levels, you need knowledge.

Diabetes is an immensely complex disease that affects every system in the body. To make things even more complex, type 2 diabetes comes in many forms. A treatment that works wonderfully for someone else may not work at all for you.

Your doctor, and even a complete "health-care team," cannot control your diabetes without your help. Learning how diabetes works and then working with your doctor to figure out which of the many treatments available today will be best for you is extremely important if you want to obtain normal blood sugar levels, and this is the best way you can reduce your chances of ever developing complications from this disease.

You have a lot to learn, and no one expects you to learn everything at once. It takes time before you can absorb it all. I know. I have type 2 diabetes myself.

What happened to me

The first sign—I realized later—that something was wrong with me was in late summer 1995, when I noticed the blackfly bites I'd scratched in May when working on my sheep farm in Vermont had still not healed. That fall, some strange pink algae persisted in growing in my toilet, despite numerous cleanings with chlorine bleach. I get my water from a spring, so I concluded there was a new type of algae in my water supply. I didn't feel sick, so I didn't worry about it.

The following January, I noticed I was thirsty a lot and attributed this to the fact that I used a lot of salt. Later I noticed I seemed to need to visit the bathroom a lot and attributed that to all the coffee I drank while I earned a so-called living copyediting medical books.

I got more and more myopic and attributed that to the fifty to sixty hours a week I spent trying to edit a manuscript an ophthalmologist had sent to a publisher single-spaced, in tiny type. I figured he was trying to drum up business (and had succeeded in my case).

I started craving sweets. One day in April, I realized I was rushing through my dinner, not enjoying it as I usually did, so I could get to the big glass of fruit juice I usually drank at the end. The next day I visited a friend, who offered me a cup of coffee. "What I'd really like is a glass of water," I said. "I don't understand why I'm thirsty all the time." She suggested I be tested for diabetes.

So I rushed home, where I had some of those tablets people used to use to test for sugar in urine. My mother had been diagnosed with diabetes some years before, so I'd kept them on hand to do periodic checks. Previously they had always stayed blue, meaning no sugar. This time, they turned deep brown.

Going to the doctor's office simply confirmed what I already knew. I had diabetes. The blood sugar test the nurse did gave a reading of 303, four hours after my last meal. "Is that bad?" I asked, totally uninformed about what a normal blood sugar reading should be.

Later the nurse said, "You're not terribly overweight, so we don't know if we'll have to put you on insulin or not," which didn't cheer me up a lot.

I'd never been seriously ill, so I was stunned. Now I not only had a disease but also had an incurable one. I'd never be able to eat normally again. Maybe I'd have to take shots. I'd have huge medical bills because I didn't have good medical insurance. I didn't know how I'd cope.

But I wanted to know more. So I bought books about diabetes. Then I explored the Internet and found David Mendosa's website that linked to almost every page available on the net. I signed up for several email mailing lists and read other people's accounts of their experiences, started asking them questions, and learned and learned. Now I would like to share some of this information with others.

How to use this book

Because I know what a shock it is to receive a diagnosis of diabetes and how much there is to learn, I have tried to break down the information into small bits that you can absorb slowly, starting with the most essential things you should know right away and then gradually moving on to the more subtle aspects of dealing with this disease. Sometimes I outline the bare essentials of a complex topic like diet in an early chapter and then later discuss it in more detail.

Ideally, you would get this book the day you are diagnosed, but it may take days or weeks before you find it or are ready to read about this disease. Whenever you get the book—or open it—start with Day 1 and work your way through it at your own pace.

The book is modeled after the classic approach for creating a fine oil finish on a piece of furniture, in which you oil the wood every day for a week, every week for a month, and every month for a year. After that, you only need to touch it up every now and then.

So too, when you are diagnosed, there is so much to learn that you need to spend a little time every day learning about this disease. Then, as dealing with it becomes part of your regular routine, you can spend a little less time until eventually you'll only need to "touch up" your knowledge every now and then.

Each day or week or month in this book is divided into a Living and a Learning section. The Living sections deal with the problems of living with this chronic disease. I hope the Living sections will help you to understand that you are not alone; that the emotional upheavals you'll probably go through are normal; that living with diabetes is sometimes hard, but it's possible to lead a rewarding life nevertheless; and that once you come to terms with having diabetes and get your blood sugar under control, you may find you feel better, have more energy, and enjoy your food more than you ever have before.

The Learning sections explain some of the science of diabetes. Some of you may be more comfortable reading about science than others. If you've always liked science and technology, I hope you will appreciate the depth of the discussions in the later Learning chapters. There is material there you won't find in other popular books about diabetes.

Even if you are a technophobe, I hope you will read the Learning sections in Days 1 through 7, at least, because they include important information that you really should know, as well as the summaries at the ends of each section. Skimming the subheads in each chapter should also give you a general idea of what the chapter says. Later, as you get more comfortable with the science of diabetes, you can go back and read the rest of the Learning sections, or you can consult them for reference when you have a question about some aspect of diabetes. Terms in **boldface** are defined in the glossary at the end of the book.

I will not prescribe

I am not a doctor, and I will not prescribe for you. I will not tell you which treatment I think is best or how much medication or vitamins you should take. Diabetes research is going on at a furious pace. New diabetes drugs and paraphernalia are appearing every year, and opinions on the effectiveness of vitamins and supplements sometimes seem to change from newscast to newscast. A medication or vitamin recommendation that seems best today might seem wrong in a couple of years.

Thus instead of giving you a lot of specifics that will soon be outdated, I've tried to give you enough background information about how diabetes, current drugs, and current meters work so that you can understand what you are reading when you encounter new treatments, medications, and supplies. As your knowledge about diabetes evolves, I hope what you learn from this book will enable you to keep up with the new advances so you can work with your doctor to ensure that your own individual treatment plan evolves as well.

Because there are different philosophies about how to treat type 2 diabetes, rather than prescribing what you *should* do, I have tried to describe different approaches so you and your doctor can decide together which philosophy might be right for you.

Like many people, I started off on the American Diabetes Association exchange diet, and I lost thirty pounds. However, I was hungry twenty-four hours a day, and my blood sugar levels continued to be above normal. So I gradually cut back on my carbohydrate intake and ended up on a low-carbohydrate diet. On this diet I stopped losing weight, but I also stopped being hungry all the time. My blood sugar levels are mostly in or close to the normal range, and the weight I lost, I've managed to keep off for almost twenty years, plus another few pounds lost slowly in recent years.

I hope my own experiences haven't biased my discussions toward this dietary approach; what works for me might not work for you. There are no studies comparing the long-term effects of the various diabetic diets, so your choices must be based on conjecture about how a particular diet will affect you in the long term, as well as your own experience with its short-term effects.

Where the focus is

This book is aimed at people going through their first year with type 2 diabetes. I focus on preventing diabetes complications instead of details of how to treat them. If you can use the knowledge in this book to maintain near-normal blood sugar levels, I hope you will never get major complications. If you already have early signs of them, I hope you can reverse them with good control.

I have assumed that you are an intelligent person who wants to take an active part in your treatment rather than just accepting your doctor's prescription without understanding the reasons behind it. I have also assumed you have already received—or will very soon receive—from your doctor or a nurse the very basic instructions or pamphlets usually given to patients just diagnosed with type 2 diabetes. Rather than simply parroting what you'll get from these professionals or pamphlets, I focus on some of the things you probably *won't* be told, some of the emotional upheavals you'll undoubtedly go through and some of the challenges you'll face in those first few weeks after receiving the diagnosis. Later, when I hope your emotions have become more stable, I go back and review some of the basic things you were probably told in those first meetings with your doctor, just to make sure you've absorbed them all.

If for some reason you did not receive any of the basic instructions after your diagnosis, you might want to go right to Month 2 and read through the "diabetes ABCs." Then you can go back and review them later, when your emotions have settled down.

Throughout this book I emphasize the need to use a home meter to learn what your blood sugar levels are. In fact, I mention testing so often you may begin to think I have stock in a test strip company. I don't. I just care about your health.

I have quoted comments from real people who are living with type 2 diabetes, although their names may have been changed to preserve their privacy. As you read these comments, keep in mind that what works for one person may not work for you. But sometimes reading about what someone else has gone through strikes a chord and makes you realize that your own feelings and reactions are normal. I hope it helps.

Keep on learning

By the end of your first year with diabetes, I hope you will understand where you can go to continue this learning process, as well as share your knowledge with others, and how to evaluate the announcements of diabetes news in the popular press.

If you have access to the Internet, the excellent section by Internet diabetes expert David Mendosa will provide you with a guide to using that immense resource to increase your knowledge about diabetes, learn about advances in treatment as they occur, and share experiences with other people living with diabetes.

Diabetes is a chronic genetic disease that today is incurable. The good news is that it can be controlled. With knowledge and care, most people with type 2 diabetes can live near-normal lives for many years. It has been said that the best way to live a long life is to get a chronic disease because it makes you take care of yourself. Many people who take charge of their type 2 diabetes find this to be true. They lose weight, start exercising, eat healthy foods, and feel healthier and more energetic than they have in years. I certainly do.

This is not to say that a diagnosis of type 2 diabetes means unmitigated joy. There are obvious sacrifices involved, especially isolation from sharing "normal" food with friends and family, and some people do suffer handicapping side effects. So I am sorry that you have become a member of the "Type 2 Diabetes Club," but I welcome you to our worldwide community. Remember, you now have diabetic "brothers and sisters" all over the world who understand what you are going through. You are not alone.

The First Year

Type 2 Diabetes

living

It's Not
Your Fault

You've just been diagnosed with type 2 diabetes. If you're like most people, you're probably in a state of shock. When you got your diagnosis, your doctor probably told you a lot of things about diets and drugs and insulin and glucose and carbohydrates and blood tests and avoiding this and doing that, and you probably came out of the office with your head spinning, not remembering much of what the doctor said.

Don't worry, you're not alone. Most people feel that way.

If no one in your family ever had diabetes, and especially if you're thin and thought diabetes only happened to fat people, you're probably especially puzzled. "What did I do wrong? Why is this happening to me?"

Sometimes a diagnosis comes like a thunderbolt on a sunny day. Sophie C. consulted a doctor about a toenail fungus, and he drew some blood for routine tests. "Next day the phone rang, and my doctor informed me quite bluntly that I was diabetic," she said. "Talk about a slap in the face! I was scared out of my mind. There must be some mistake here. I wasn't blind; my feet weren't gangrenous. No family history of the disease, no warning signs (that I knew of at the time), not a clue."

Or maybe you were expecting a diagnosis someday. You've got relatives with diabetes: your grandmother had diabetes and died from gangrene in her foot. Your father got it when he was sixty-five and died from a heart attack a few years later. If you're also overweight, maybe you figured someday you'd get diabetes yourself. But you probably figured "someday" would be far in the future, when you were old. Not today. Not now. "I'm not ready yet."

Whether you expected it or not, a diabetes diagnosis is a shock.

Getting diabetes is not your fault

There's so much to learn about diabetes, but you can't learn it all at once. Trying to accept the diagnosis is enough for your first day. Here's what you should remember as you deal with this: getting diabetes is not your fault.

A lot of people may tell you that if only you'd eaten less sugar, or eaten less fat, or exercised more, or eaten more fiber, or smoked less, or done none of the things that 95 percent of the American population does, you wouldn't have gotten diabetes. Especially if you're overweight, because most people with type 2 diabetes have a problem with weight, people will suggest that it's your fault that you got diabetes because you let yourself get fat.

There is no question that type 2 diabetes is *associated with* obesity. Therefore, most people assume that the excess weight *causes* the diabetes. But here's something to think about: it's possible that diabetes causes obesity.

You need the genes

In order to get diabetes, you need to have diabetes genes. One of the causes of your diabetes is a poor choice of ancestors. People without those genes can spend their lives lying around eating chips and watching TV and they'll probably get fat. But they won't get diabetes.

Having the genes, however, isn't enough to give you the disease. Even if you have diabetes genes, if you live in an environment where you don't get a lot to eat and you do hard physical labor all day, you still probably won't get diabetes. Some people think the diabetes genes are **thrifty genes** that make your body use its food more efficiently, meaning that you can gain more weight with less food. In times of famine, this comes in handy, and when food was extremely scarce, your ancestors probably fared better and had more children than other families who didn't have those genes.

But when your family moved to a different country or into a different type of lifestyle where food was plentiful and machines did all the work, those diabetes genes weren't so handy after all. When food is limited, it doesn't matter how hungry you are. You can't eat enough. When food is readily available, having a good appetite can be a disaster.

Diabetes may cause hunger

Having diabetes genes may affect the appetite. Alex E. described the time someone brought some scrumptious pastries to work. A thin person walked in, looked at the pastries, and said, "Oh my, those look good. I wish I were hungry so I could try one." Alex was flabbergasted. He was hungry all the time and thought everyone else was too. Only after he learned to control his blood sugar levels did his hunger abate, and he learned what normal hunger is like.

Some people find that they get ravenously hungry when their blood sugar is fluctuating rapidly. You may have had poor blood sugar control for years before you were diagnosed with diabetes. This means that after every meal, your blood sugar went abnormally high. Then it came down again. This may have triggered intense hunger, which would make you eat again. Then the roller coaster would repeat. No wonder you put on a little weight.

"All my life I was hungry! The more 'healthy' I ate, listening to all the diet gurus, the more hungry I became," said Linda C.

You can't change your genes

So it may have been those diabetes genes that made you hungry. The hunger made you eat. The thrifty genes were especially efficient in turning that food into fat. And the fat made it harder for you to exercise. So you had another snack instead.

I've probably already told you more about diabetes than you wanted to know right away. But for now, just remember this. To get diabetes, you need to have diabetes genes. There's nothing you can do to change your genes.

Your diabetes is not your fault.

IN A SENTENCE:

■ *Diabetes is not your fault.*

What Is
Diabetes?

Diabetes is an incredibly complicated disease that comes in many flavors. Later, we'll discuss some of those exotic flavors. But for now, we'll stick with the two basic groups, called **type 1** and **type 2 diabetes**.

Type 1 is autoimmune

Type 1 diabetes, which used to be called *juvenile diabetes*, or **insulin-dependent diabetes mellitus (IDDM)**, is usually, but not always, diagnosed in children and young adults. It is an **autoimmune disease**, meaning that for some reason, the immune system has mistaken its own **pancreas** for foreign tissue and destroys the pancreatic cells that produce **insulin**, which is a **hormone**. As a result, people with type 1 diabetes produce almost no insulin and must take daily insulin injections.

Type 2 means insulin resistance

Type 2 diabetes, which is what you have, used to be called *adult-* or *maturity-onset diabetes*, or **non-insulin-dependent diabetes mellitus (NIDDM)**, sometimes popularly called *old-age diabetes*, because it is usually, but not always, diagnosed in older people. Today, more and more younger people, even children, are being found to have type 2 diabetes. Because this book is about type 2 diabetes, whenever I say just *diabetes*, unless I specify otherwise, I am referring to the type 2 variety.

Type 2 diabetes is probably *not* an autoimmune disease, and you probably don't have less insulin than normal. In fact, you may have *more* insulin than normal. The problem is something called **insulin resistance (IR)**.

Insulin lets glucose into cells

Before we discuss IR, let's go back and try to understand what insulin does. Like a car that needs energy to run and uses gasoline as an energy source, your body also needs energy to function and uses a sugar called **glucose**. When you eat food, the body converts much of that food into glucose. The glucose is taken up by the brain and the muscles so that you can think well and run fast, both useful characteristics if you're trying to avoid being eaten by a saber-toothed tiger or snag a taxi in New York.

The brain doesn't need insulin to take up that glucose, but the muscles do. In the presence of insulin, the muscles produce what are called **glucose transporters** —which you can think of as little boats that carry glucose passengers—to ferry the glucose across the cell membrane into the cell. Without enough insulin, the cell doesn't produce enough transporters, so a lot of the glucose can't get into your muscle cells. The glucose just builds up in the bloodstream and causes all kinds of problems.

If you're thin, you may be one of the minority of people with type 2 diabetes who for some unknown reason simply don't produce enough insulin. In this case, your IR may be normal.

If you're overweight, it's more likely that you're producing plenty of insulin, but you've got IR. For some unknown reason, the insulin just doesn't work very well. The body (which is generally much smarter than we are) recognizes this and produces more insulin to compensate for the IR. But after many years, the cells in the pancreas that produce the insulin (called **beta cells**) can't keep up with the demand and eventually get "exhausted," not able to produce all the insulin you need. Then your blood sugar (**blood glucose**) level rises, and that's usually when you're diagnosed with diabetes.

The soda machine analogy

If you like analogies, think of muscle cells as soda machines. If you want a soda, you put money (insulin) into the soda machine and a can of soda (glucose transporters) comes out.

Throckmorton is a single father who just got fired from his job. He's thirsty and he finds a functioning soda machine, but he simply has no money to put into the machine, so he can't get any soda. Throckmorton is like the thin person with type 2 who just isn't producing enough insulin (money), even though the glucose-transporter factory (the soda machine) is working well.

Rhoda, on the other hand, is wealthy. She has all the money she needs, because she prints her own money on a machine in her basement. She's thirsty, finds a soda machine, puts in some money, and discovers that the machine is broken; no soda comes out. But Rhoda is in luck for today. She discovers that if she puts in fifty dollars, she can get a soda out of the machine. Getting money is no problem for her, so she keeps using the soda machine because it's near where she works.

Rhoda is like the overweight person with IR. She can produce plenty of money (insulin), but the machine (her glucose-transporter factory) is broken. For a while, things work all right for Rhoda. When she needs a soda, she just prints more money.

Then one day, Rhoda's money-printing machine (her insulin-producing beta cells) starts wearing out. Every day, she's got less and less money (insulin). Finally, she doesn't have enough money for even one soda. Now she's like the person with IR whose beta cells are exhausted.

Focus on the basics

No one yet understands exactly how all these processes work, but scientists are working hard on the problem. Later, we'll discuss some of the details. For now, it's enough just to understand the basics: Diabetes is a disease of insulin deficiency, in either quantity (the beta cells don't produce enough) *or* effectiveness (you've got plenty of insulin, but it can't work very well). As a result, your blood glucose levels are too high.

There are many ways to treat type 2 diabetes. For now, trust your medical team to make the best choice for you and don't worry about all the whats and whys. You've probably gone for many months, maybe even years, with high blood glucose levels, but with no treatment at all. Now, almost any treatment will improve your situation. You've got a lot to learn in the days ahead, so concentrate on becoming informed and let your medical team lead the way.

IN A SENTENCE:

■ *Diabetes means you don't have enough (in quantity or effectiveness) insulin to keep your blood glucose levels in the normal range.*

Is It All
a Mistake?

I suspect most people with diabetes have the same fantasies.

In the first fantasy, you're sitting at the kitchen table surrounded by diabetes paraphernalia and lists of food choices called *exchanges* that you got from the nurse. You're trying to understand what insulin resistance is, and you can't remember if your doctor said you had too much of it or too little. You're wondering if you'll have to take shots.

Then the telephone rings.

"Hello? Is this Mr. Bigappetite? This is Dr. Birdwhistle's receptionist. There's been a mistake here at the lab. They mixed up your lab results with Mr. Bigape E. Tight's. Your blood sugars were fine. You don't have diabetes after all."

Unfortunately, that fantasy is not likely to come true. Your diabetes is real. And it's not like the flu or a bad case of bronchitis. It doesn't go away. Someday in the future, they'll discover how to cure diabetes. But that day isn't here yet. Your diabetes is going to be with you for a long, long time.

You want it to go away

Diabetes doesn't show. You don't have any obvious outward signs like a high fever or black warts on your nose or joints that scream when you move. Many people feel perfectly healthy once they've gotten their blood glucose levels under control. So it's easy to fantasize that your diabetes might have gone away. In this fantasy, you're checking out your groceries at the supermarket. You smile as you see a copy of the latest *National Enquirer*, with your picture on the front. The cover story says, "Middle-aged diabetic miraculously cured."

There is a picture of you, eating a chocolate fudge sundae. "It was the oddest thing," you are quoted as saying. "After dinner last night, I had a bite of this strange Tibetan candy, and the next day my blood sugar stayed normal no matter what I ate. Then this morning, I discovered I'd lost five pounds." Doctors confirmed your recovery. "We can only say it's a miracle," says Dr. Charge A. Lott.

This second fantasy never comes true either. Unfortunately, your diabetes is here to stay.

You can be diagnosed with or without symptoms

You may have been diagnosed because you weren't feeling well. Many people feel fatigued when their blood glucose level is high. High blood glucose levels can cause constant thirst and frequent urination. It can cause recurrent yeast infections. It can also cause problems with the lens of your eyes so that you have to change the prescription for your glasses too often. Some of you may have had elevated blood glucose levels for five or ten years before you were diagnosed. If that is the case, you may have had more severe symptoms, such as sores that wouldn't heal, numbness or tingling in your arms or legs, problems with your kidneys, or damage to the retinas of your eyes. You may even have had a heart attack before you were diagnosed.

If you've had any of these symptoms of diabetes, it may be easier for you to believe that you do, in fact, have this disease, especially when the symptoms disappear, or at least stop getting worse, after you get your blood glucose levels under control.

But you may have been diagnosed on the basis of a random blood glucose test during a physical exam or screening at a health fair when you were feeling perfectly fine. Then someone pricked your finger and tried to tell you that you've got diabetes.

How can you believe that when you're feeling so good? Surely it must have been a mistake. No one in your family has diabetes. You've always eaten "healthy." So OK, you don't run the Boston Marathon every year, and you don't lift weights every day. But you're reasonably fit and reasonably active. You thought diabetes only happened to overweight people who never went far from the TV remote. How could this happen to you?

It must be a mistake. Maybe the machine was broken. Maybe that nice woman doing the test didn't get enough instruction in how to use it. Or maybe it was just because you had some candy before you took the test and probably when you eat regular food again everything will be back to normal. Right? Unfortunately, wrong is the right answer here.

Acceptance is difficult

Accepting that you have diabetes is difficult for anyone, even if you had obvious symptoms when you were diagnosed. One day, you're just like everyone else. Then suddenly everything is changed. You're different. Simple things that you've always taken for granted are now suddenly forbidden to you—probably forever.

How do you deal with this sudden curtain falling down on the world as you knew it? The easiest way is to deny it. They think you're going to stop eating almost everything that tastes good? No way.

Taking oral medication is easy. But changing your entire way of living is more difficult. "I went through the various phases of being unable to imagine giving up my favorite foods, or feeling cheated that certain foods would be taken from me, or that I had a right to these foods and it was unfair for this disease to treat me this way, and even a little, 'I'm strong, these high blood glucoses won't hurt me,'" said Edd A.

But acceptance leads to control

Accepting your diagnosis as soon as possible is absolutely the best thing you can do for your control of this disease, because there's both bad news and good news about type 2 diabetes. Diabetes is incurable. That's the bad news. The good news is that diabetes is controllable. And the most important agent in that control is you.

Of course, it's not easy. Acceptance takes time. But once you are able to accept the fact that you really do have type 2 diabetes, a condition that won't ever go away, you can start taking control of your disease. In many cases, you will eventually feel healthier and more energetic than you ever have before.

That first step may be one of the hardest to take, and it normally takes a while to fully accept this new way of life. The *National Enquirer* fantasy will probably be with you for years to come. But acceptance is the key. Acceptance allows you to dump all the unnecessary baggage of pretending and blaming and resenting and wasting your energy looking for medical mistakes or miracle cures.

You know that diabetes is not your fault. It's simply one of those bad breaks. You've got it, and it's not going to go away. Now you can focus on learning more about this complicated disease so that you can control it well and lead a happy, rewarding life.

IN A SENTENCE:

■ *Accepting that you have diabetes is the first step toward controlling it.*

Measuring Your Blood Glucose Levels

The best thing you can do for your diabetes is to get a blood glucose meter. Right away. Now. There are many different kinds of meters and subtle differences among them that I'll discuss later. But for now it doesn't really matter what kind of meter you get. What matters is that you get a meter and that you *use it*.

A simple meter may be best to start

If your meter and strips will be covered by your health insurance, you may be limited to the brand they'll pay for. Otherwise, if money is not a problem, get whatever is available locally. You can trade up later and keep your first meter as a spare.

If money is tight, look around a little for a good deal on a meter. Manufacturers make their money from the test strips you need to use with them. Each meter takes a different kind of strip. So, like the old razor companies that gave away razors so you'd have to buy their blades, manufacturers usually offer huge discounts on their meters. Most brands of strips cost about the same, but check before you buy the meter. In the long run, you'll be paying a lot more for the strips than for the meter.

You can often get a meter almost free through manufacturer rebates or from your doctor or diabetes educator. If you can't find a cheap meter that way, ask your diabetic friends. Many people have several meters and would be happy to loan or give you one they're not using anymore. Make sure to clean it—especially the finger pricker—thoroughly before you use it to avoid any chances of picking up a blood-borne disease.

If money is a serious problem, you can buy strips that you read by comparing the color to the colors on a chart, although such strips are not used much anymore because it's so easy to get a free meter if you watch for sales. They're not as accurate as the meters, but they're better than nothing. You can save a little money by cutting each strip in half lengthwise. Make sure you cut them quickly and return the unused half to the original container. You can never do that with strips you insert in a meter.

Some meters offer fancy extras. If you're a gadget freak, you'll want to check these out right away. If you're visually impaired, look for a meter with a large display. There are also talking meters that give the results in either English or Spanish as well as little gizmos that help you aim the drop of blood onto the strip when you can't see it very well.

Otherwise, a simple meter is just as good, especially to start with. The important thing at this point is not the bells and whistles in the meter. The important thing is to get a meter, learn how to test, and do it every day.

Every meter operates slightly differently, so of course you'll need to read the instruction manual for your own particular meter before you actually do a test. Or your doctor or nurse or diabetes educator may show you how to use it.

Pricking your fingers is a minor annoyance

Some aspects of testing are pretty much the same no matter which meter you have. Testing your blood glucose (which from now on I'll call **BG**) requires you first to obtain some blood. This means that you must puncture your skin. Ouch. Yes, it does hurt a little. It's the least painful if you prick the sides of the fingertips, where there are fewer nerves than at the tips. And yes it does take a few days before you stop worrying about the pain. I remember the first time I tested my blood. I knew that all I had to do was press this little button on my finger pricker and it would do all the work for me. I did a few dry runs pricking imaginary fingers in the air. Then I put the pricker on my finger and . . . and . . . finally I closed my eyes and clicked, and ouch, a little hurt, and then it was done.

It doesn't take long to realize that pricking your fingers is one of the minor annoyances of having diabetes. When you're starting out, it's the anticipation that hurts the most. And certain types of finger prickers hurt more than others. The best kinds are the ones that you can adjust for different depths. At the lowest setting, you hardly feel a thing.

Blood is usually easy to get

But wait. Let's go back a minute. Before you stick your finger, wash your hands in warm water. This not only reduces the number of germs on your fingers, but it also ensures that you don't have any traces of sugar on your fingers that might interfere with the test, and it's also easier to get blood from warm hands. Then dry your hands thoroughly. Extra moisture on the skin could dilute the blood and give a wrong result. Don't use **alcohol**. It doesn't sterilize, and if you don't get it all off, the alcohol might interact with the test materials and cause false results.

After you've pricked your finger, wait a second or two, and then gently squeeze out a little blood and let it drop onto the test strip or let the strip suck it up, depending on the type of strip you're using. If you're visually impaired or your hands shake and you have difficulty getting the blood on the right place, you can use special devices that help your aim. Your meter will start working, and in less than a minute, you will know what your BG level is. This may seem like a lot of work, but compared with the "good old days" when people had to add chemicals to test tubes containing urine samples, which then told them what their BG levels had been several hours ago, this is a marvelous invention.

The best place to stick your fingers is on the sides of the tips, close to the nail (but not too close, or the blood will run all over the nail and won't drop onto the strip). Some people test on the backs of the fingers, between the joints. That doesn't work for me. It hurts more and I don't get much blood, but it might work for you.

Many people rotate their fingers, using a different finger every day, so each finger has several days to heal before being used again. This is a sensible method, but I find that my ring finger and little finger are the easiest to get blood from, and I tend to use them day after day.

The instructions to your meter will tell you to make sure to use a fresh **lancet** every time you test, but many people use the same lancet for days, weeks, or even months without changing. It seems that people usually build up immunity to the germs on their own skin, and infections from used lancets are rare. For the same reason, it's not absolutely essential to wash your hands before lancing your fingers, but if you're near a washroom, it certainly doesn't hurt and reduces the chances of contaminating the blood sample with something on your fingers that might affect the test. Of course, to avoid getting infected with hepatitis, AIDS, or other viruses, you should *never* use a lancet that has been used by anyone else.

Use a few tricks when the blood won't flow

Sometimes blood is easier to get than other times. Anything that increases your circulation, such as exercise or a hot bath, makes the blood run out more easily. That's a good time to use your "bad" fingers—the ones that don't bleed as well. Sometimes you may have difficulty squeezing a drop of blood out, especially if your hands are cold. If this happens, try warming your hands up in hot water. If that's not enough, try swinging your arms to push the blood out into the fingertips. Then, after you've pricked a finger, hold your hand well below your heart, the lower the better, and relax your hand for a few seconds before you try to squeeze some blood out. Don't worry. You'll get the hang of it pretty quickly.

Although "milking" the finger by grasping it at the base and squeezing toward the tip can help, it's best to avoid getting blood this way if you don't have to as it can force nonblood fluids (called **interstitial fluid**) into the drop, and this sometimes affects the results. If all else fails, try putting a rubber band on your finger like a tourniquet to build up pressure at the tip. Needless to say, you'll want to take it off as soon as possible. Some phlebotomists say you shouldn't do this, as constricting blood flow could produce falsely low results. Keep this in mind and do it only as a last resort.

Test as often as you can

Once you've learned how to measure your BG level, you'll want to do it (OK, you *should* do it) as often as you possibly can. This is especially important early on, when you're learning how your body reacts to various things like the foods you eat and the exercise you get. We're all different, and we all live under different circumstances. No book and no doctor and no diabetes educator can tell you exactly how your particular body is going to react to your particular diabetes treatment plan. Only by testing as often as you can will you be able to learn about your own particular physiology.

If your BG strips are paid for by your insurance, you may be limited in the number you can have. In this case, if you have sufficient income, you might consider buying extra strips on your own. In the long run, it will be a worthwhile investment. BG testing strips are cheaper than diabetic complications.

The best times to test depend on your situation

When should you test? Most people like to test as soon as they arise in the morning. This is called a **fasting test**, and it sometimes gives a very approximate indication of how good your control was on the previous day. Other common times to test are one and two hours after a meal, which tells you how high your BG level goes when you eat particular foods; before the next meal, which tells you whether the BG rise that usually follows a meal has come down to the starting point before the next meal; before and after exercise; at bedtime; and any time you feel that something is wrong.

This sounds as if you have to test yourself almost ten times a day. If you can afford it, you could learn a lot by testing this often. But many people can't. Either you can't afford that many strips or you just don't have the time for that many tests. **Continuous glucose monitors** that test BG levels every few minutes have been developed and are becoming available, but they are expensive.

When the number of strips is limited, you can rotate the testing times to get additional information. For instance, on Monday, test fasting and before-lunch levels. On Tuesday, test fasting and after-supper levels. On Wednesday, test before and after exercise. If your diet and exercise patterns are pretty regular, eventually you'll get a sense of how various factors affect your BG levels.

Here's some good news. After a year or so of this intensive testing, you'll get a very good sense of how your body reacts to various influences, and unless you are taking insulin, you won't have to test as often. I often don't test at all for days, and then I use the saved-up strips to do a detailed test of some new food or exercise pattern.

Advanced meters are being developed

New meters seem to be coming out almost every month. More and more allow you to get blood from less sensitive parts of your body (such as the arms) as well as the fingers. However, when BG levels are changing rapidly, readings from meters used on the arm lag behind readings taken from fingertip blood, especially when the arm is not rubbed first to bring blood to the surface. Furthermore, some people find that arm tests result in little bruises.

Continuous glucose monitors (CGMs) use implanted sensors. With these, you can see unexpected highs and lows that a person measuring only a few times a day wouldn't detect. The CGMs are not cheap, and insurance won't always cover them, especially if you have type 2, but if you can afford one, you can learn a lot by using it.

Another continuous meter beams the BG readings to a handheld sensor and stores the readings for future analysis. Others are in the works.

CGMs are also being integrated with insulin pumps. The technology in this field is moving so fast that whatever is available at this writing may well be outdated next year. You can keep abreast of developments by consulting diabetes magazines (see Month 12) and online sites.

Because most people don't really enjoy punching holes in their fingers and the market is huge, companies are working fast and furiously to develop *noninvasive meters* that will allow BG testing without drawing blood. Creative ideas include using a sensor implanted in a contact lens; measuring thermal radiation from the ears; various types of spectroscopy; and ultrasound. Many interesting technologies never reach the marketplace.

Some meters on the market today test **ketones** (see Day 5) as well as BG levels. A few will test for **lipids** (see the box in Month 6), ketones, and glucose, with more tests planned for the future.

But don't wait for all the new gadgets. The important time to do a lot of testing is now, as soon as you can. The sooner you get into the habit of knowing what your BG level is, the sooner you will begin to learn how to control this major inconvenience called *diabetes*.

IN A SENTENCE:

■ *Testing your blood glucose levels regularly is the best way to learn how to control your diabetes.*

How Do I Tell My Friends and Colleagues?

Several days after your diagnosis, you probably still haven't accepted this new way of life emotionally. Accepting a chronic disease is a lot like accepting the death of a good friend. It takes a lot of time. In this case, the good friend is someone you've known all your life: your former nondiabetic self. Before you can fully accept your new condition, you need to take some time to mourn your loss.

But as you go through the slow process of acceptance, you need to deal with the other people in your life. Your closest friends and relatives have probably already heard about your diagnosis. But what about your casual friends? Should you tell them? If so, how? Should you tell your colleagues at work? Will it affect your job security if you do?

Some people tell everyone

Of course we're all different and have different life situations. Some people are very up front about their condition. I try to tell everyone. Well, maybe not everyone. I don't walk down the street snagging total strangers by the collar and informing them that I have type 2 diabetes. But if it's relevant—for example, if someone invites me to dinner and I want to make sure they know in advance that I won't be able to eat certain foods because of my condition, not because I hate their cooking—then I tell them. This comes in very handy if I do, in fact, hate their cooking.

As a freelance writer and editor, I told my primary client because I wanted the client to understand that I could no longer spend fifty or sixty hours a week at a computer terminal; I needed some time to exercise every day. Because clients don't supply medical insurance and a freelancer bills only for the time spent working, they got less of my time but didn't have to pay me as much. My disclosure had little effect on our working relationship. Not everyone has the freedom to be so forthright in a business situation.

Some don't want to tell

Some people find it difficult to communicate their condition with the rest of the world. Katherine G., who was diagnosed on the basis of a random blood test when she was feeling perfectly fine, said, "When I was diagnosed, I went through all the stages of emotions. First I was sure there had been a mistake with the blood test. Then I tried to keep anyone from finding out and asked Frank not to mention it to any of the offspring. I had guilt feelings. What had I done wrong? I got angry and wanted to smack every overweight person I saw. I refused to attend meetings where all those diabetics talked about their problems, since I didn't belong with that group. I didn't want anyone seeing me go into the diabetic center. I wouldn't use the local library to get books about diabetes, so I went to the library in another town. I worried that I'd passed on the genes to my children and grandchildren. I had nightmares about being blind, in a wheelchair because I had no feet, and being wheeled in to use a dialysis machine."

It may be especially difficult to accept a diagnosis of a chronic disease if you've always been the strong one in the family, the one who coped when things got rough, the healthy one who took care of other people when they got sick. Now all of a sudden someone tells you that you're the "sick" one, even if you're feeling perfectly OK. If you tell the rest of the family what's going on, will you lose your long-standing role in the family? Is your life going to totally change?

Many men are raised to think that men should always be strong and soldier on no matter how much they hurt. They may see illness as a type of unmanly weakness and want to deal with it by pretending it doesn't exist. If this describes you, you naturally wouldn't find it easy to broadcast your new vulnerability to the world.

Whether to tell your employer depends on the circumstances

Deciding whether to tell people at work that you have a chronic disease is even more difficult than telling family and friends. If you are taking diabetes drugs or insulin that might make your blood glucose (BG) levels go too low (see Week 3 and Month 5), it would be wise to let someone at work know this so that person would understand if you suddenly started acting differently or needed to interrupt work in order to have a snack. If you operate dangerous machinery and are taking medication that could make your BG levels go so low that you could pass out and hurt other people, then of course you have a moral obligation to inform your employer. And if asked outright if you are diabetic, it's not wise to lie.

If there's no reason your employer needs to know about your diabetes, you may feel a "don't ask, don't tell" approach makes sense. You may worry that letting your employer know that you have an expensive chronic disease will jeopardize your career. The employer may worry that the company's health insurer will raise its rates when it discovers that someone with diabetes is on the payroll or worry that you will take a lot of sick days. Or your employer may think all people with diabetes spend a lot of time away from their work giving themselves shots.

It's illegal to discriminate against people with diseases like diabetes. But we all know that unscrupulous employers can get around the laws by inventing excuses to lay you off or to make your life so unpleasant that you decide to resign. If you're the only breadwinner in the family, deciding whether or not to tell your employer about your diabetes is not an easy decision.

The "diabetes police" can be annoying

Although the consequences of telling your friends might not be as serious, they can also cause problems. For example, people who know about your diabetes may assume the role of "diabetes police." Most people think that people with diabetes can't eat any sugar, but that other foods, including bread and potatoes, are fine. So they'll watch you like a hawk. After watching you slug down a plate of potato salad sandwiches on buttered white bread without comment, if you reach for a tiny cookie, they'll say, "Are you allowed to eat that?" as if you weren't able to take care of yourself.

Sometimes the diabetes police take an even more active role. A friend told me about Loretta, who had type 1 diabetes and "had an insulin reaction, stopped at the country store, grabbed a candy bar and began munching it down, muttering to the clerk that she was diabetic and was having a reaction. The clerk leaped on her and grabbed the candy bar away, screaming, 'Diabetics aren't supposed to have sugar!'"

People deal with the diabetes police in different ways. Some simply ignore them. Some explain. My favorite is the woman who turns to the policeperson and says, "That's odd. You don't *look* like my mother."

If you don't tell your friends and coworkers that you're diabetic, you won't need to worry about the diabetes police. But then when sugary treats are served at office breaks and social gatherings, you'll have to either risk your health by eating things that aren't good for you or risk hurting your friends' feelings by turning down their delicious offerings.

If you're overweight, you can always say you're on a diet—which of course you are—and simply refuse to give in when everyone says, "Oh come on, one bite won't hurt you." They may all hate you for your strong willpower, but at least you won't let the food hurt you. If you're thin, that excuse won't help.

As someone once said, "I always tell the truth, because that way I don't need to remember what I said." It's always easier to be truthful. But if you're worried about keeping your job, it may not always be possible to take the easy route.

There is no one right way to decide when to tell your friends and colleagues that you have diabetes. Like the disease itself, this decision is complex and different for each of us. You have to take charge and make the decision that is best for you.

IN A SENTENCE:

■ *How to tell friends and colleagues about your diabetes is as individual as you are.*

How Does Food Affect My Blood Sugar?

When most people think of diabetes, they think of **sugar**. People with diabetes can't eat sugar; anything else is OK. I'm not surprised by this narrow view of diabetes because it's what I thought before I was diagnosed with the disease.

The sad truth is that almost every type of food you put in your mouth will affect your blood glucose (BG) levels one way or another, and it's important to understand how.

There are three types of food

There are basically three major classes of food: fat, protein, and carbohydrate. You probably know quite well what **fat** is. It's that greasy stuff that tastes so good and seems to leap directly from the plate onto your thighs or stomach. To be more specific, fat includes solid fats like butter, stick margarine, and vegetable shortening; oils like olive oil; and hybrids like squeezable margarine.

Fat is composed of long, water-insoluble molecules called **fatty acids** attached to a small molecule called **glycerol** (known as *glycerin* in pharmaceutical preparations). Glycerol is shaped like the letter E, and when three fatty acids are attached to glycerol (one on each arm of the E), the resulting fat is called a **triglyceride** (sometimes called *triacylglycerol*; it means the same thing). This is one of the blood lipids that is usually measured when you have a **lipid panel** done. Fat contains 9 calories per gram (cal/g).

Protein foods are mostly meat and fish, eggs, and cheese. Most meats and cheeses also contain a lot of fat, so if you want to limit your fat intake, you'll have to limit your intake of fatty meats and most cheeses as well.

Proteins are composed of long chains of **amino acids** strung together like Christmas tree lights and then molded into three-dimensional shapes. Proteins are made up of many different kinds of amino acids. Protein contains 4 cal/g.

Carbohydrate foods include both starchy foods, such as bread, rice, beans, and potatoes, and sugars (see the box Understanding Sugars, Other Sweeteners, and Bulking Agents), such as **sucrose** (table sugar), **lactose** (milk sugar), and **fructose** (a sugar found in honey and fruits).

The starchy foods contain **polysaccharides**, which are composed of long chains of sugars, and when you digest polysaccharides, they are broken down into the sugars they contain. Some people call polysaccharides *complex carbohydrates*, but this term can be misleading (see Month 10). Sometimes the chains form a lot of branches, and the degree of branching can affect how quickly they are digested. Sugars, like amino acids, come in many types, and the types of sugars in the carbohydrates can also affect how quickly they will raise your BG levels. Carbohydrate contains 4 cal/g.

Fiber is the portion of carbohydrate that humans are unable to digest. Much of the fiber is *cellulose*, a main component of plant cell walls. Ruminants such as cows and sheep can eat grass, and bacteria in their rumen—one of their four stomachs—digest the cellulose for them. Having only one stomach, we are unable to digest cellulose, and much of the fiber passes right through us. Some of the fiber in humans can be digested by bacteria in the *colon* that convert the fiber to fatty acids and gas, a phenomenon often observed when a person eats a lot of beans. Fiber contains very few calories; the number depends on how much of the fiber the colonic bacteria are able to digest.

Most foods are mixed

Many foods contain a combination of food types. For instance, beans, rice, and grains contain a lot of carbohydrate, but they contain protein as well. Eggs, nuts, and tofu have a lot of high-quality protein, but they also contain fat. Even lean meats may contain several grams of fat per serving.

Cream contains a lot of fat, but it has some protein and carbohydrate as well. Fruits and vegetables are mostly carbohydrate, but vegetables also contain some protein and fat, and even fruits contain trace amounts.

Today, knowing the exact composition of the food you eat is pretty simple. Food labels tell you how much of each type of constituent is in most of the food you buy. Nutritional tables are available in books or, if you have Internet access, on numerous sites on the Internet (see For Further Reading).

If you do have a computer or a smart phone, there are numerous nutritional software packages that not only will determine how much of each constituent is in the various foods you use but also will keep track of the total amounts you've had each day and alert you if you've had too much or too little of a nutrient that is important to your diet.

Carbohydrate has the greatest effect

The food that has the greatest effect on BG levels is carbohydrate. This is true whether you have diabetes or not. The BG levels of people without diabetes also rise after they eat a carbohydrate-containing meal. The difference is that their BG levels only go up a little, maybe 30 **mg/dL** (**milligrams per deciliter**—the units with which Americans usually express BG levels; see Table 1 on page 34 for conversion to European units) after a meal containing a lot of carbohydrate. Then their pancreas secretes just the right amount of insulin, and their BG levels come down quickly.

The BG levels of people with diabetes increase a lot more than that. Some people might see their BG levels increase 100 or even 200 or more mg/dL after eating a lot of carbohydrate. The pancreas tries to put out enough insulin, but it can't. Or it secretes a lot of insulin, but because of insulin resistance (IR), the **effective insulin** (meaning the amount that it's equivalent to because of IR) is insufficient.

Without enough effective insulin, your BG levels not only go up higher but also take longer to come down. It is this long-term increased BG level that causes diabetic complications, and that is what you want to control with your diabetes treatment.

Fiber is important too

Fiber has a large effect on how fast the carbohydrate raises your BG levels. There are two types of fiber, soluble and insoluble. **Insoluble fiber** is a lot like sawdust. It doesn't dissolve in water and pretty much just goes right through you, absorbing water and adding a lot of bulk. Insoluble fiber, although it has a healthy effect on elimination, is thought not to make much difference to how quickly your BG level goes up after a carbohydrate meal.

Soluble fiber forms a gummy solution that slows down the speed of digestion of carbohydrate. It has a big effect on how quickly a carbohydrate meal will raise your BG levels. It is also thought to decrease **cholesterol** levels (see the box in Month 6). Soluble fiber eaten at one meal can even decrease the rate at which your BG level increases at a later meal. Soluble fiber is a very good food for people with type 2 diabetes, and many of the folk remedies for the disease, such as fenugreek, guar gum, prickly pear (nopal), barley, and aloe, are very high in soluble fiber. Soluble fiber is also found in oat bran, flaxseed, and many fruits.

Fiber is considered a carbohydrate, but unlike other carbohydrates, it isn't broken down into sugars in the human small intestine. Thus when you want to know how much **effective carbohydrate**—the amount that your body will convert to sugar—a food contains, you should subtract the fiber on a food label (from North America, Africa, or Asia) from the total carbohydrate. This will give you the amount of carbohydrate that will make your BG level go up. Thus a hypothetical ice cream flavor called Garlic Ripple with Sawdust Chunks might contain 34 grams of total carbohydrate but 14 grams of fiber, so the effective carbohydrate would be only 20 grams.

Some other countries have different rules for their food labels. In Europe and Oceania, for instance, the fiber has already been subtracted. So if the Europeans sold Garlic Ripple with Sawdust Chunks, their labels would list 20 grams of carbohydrate and 14 grams of fiber. It is important to remember this when you are reading food labels on imported food.

Protein and fat have smaller effects

Protein also affects your BG levels. This is because some of the protein we eat, usually estimated at 40 to 60 percent, is converted to glucose in the liver. This conversion takes time, so not only will a pure protein meal cause a lower increase in your BG levels, but the increase will also be much longer after eating, usually four to six hours. Some people with type 2 diabetes still produce enough insulin to cover slowly released sugars. If so, you might not see any increase in your BG levels at all after a small protein meal.

Fats eaten by themselves won't cause an increase in your BG levels. But who wants to eat a meal consisting of chunks of butter swimming in olive oil with cocoa butter for dessert? Eaten with other foods, however, fats have an effect on your BG level.

First, fats decrease the rate at which the stomach empties. This means that if you eat carbohydrate, which might make the BG level peak in sixty minutes if you ate it alone (see Figure 5 in Month 9), but add some fat, the BG level might peak at ninety minutes instead.

Some people find that eating a little fat with carbohydrate not only delays the peak but makes it lower. Their BG level never goes as high when they add the fat. Other people say that just a little bit of fat makes their BG levels go much higher, perhaps by increasing IR. Sometimes this effect can still be seen with a higher fasting level the next day. Because different people react differently to fat, the best way to find out how fat affects your BG levels is (alas) to prick your fingers a few extra times after you've eaten fatty meals to see if the fat makes your BG go up or go down.

Alcohol reduces blood glucose levels— sometimes too much

Alcohol is neither a fat, a protein, nor a carbohydrate, but it does contain 7 cal/g. If you're following an **exchange diet** (see Day 4), alcohol is usually counted as a fat.

People used to say that anyone with diabetes should never drink alcohol. This is because alcohol can lower BG levels, and if you are taking insulin or **sulfonylureas** (see Week 3 and Month 5), which can make your BG levels go too low, the alcohol can increase the effect and paralyze the mechanisms that normally bring the BG levels back to normal.

However, if you are not taking these drugs, small amounts of alcohol, such as a small glass of red wine with a meal, may help moderate the BG-raising effects of the meal as well as possibly having heart-protecting actions. Note that the important word here is *small*. Excessive drinking is not a good idea when you have diabetes of any kind.

Knowledge is power

In Month 9, I discuss in more detail how you can get actual numerical values for your after-dinner BG tests. You probably don't want to get that fancy right away. For now, you should just know that all these foods interact and will affect your BG levels after a meal, and as usual, the best way to find out how your favorite foods affect your own BG levels is to test, test, and test again.

All this finger pricking and testing of foods may sound depressing. Granted, it's inconvenient, and it does hurt a little bit. But the rewards are immense. Knowing from the beginning just how you react to the various foods you eat is the best way you can keep your BG levels as close to normal as possible and avoid any of the complications that occur in people whose BG levels are uncontrolled.

Trust me. Your BG levels matter. Take charge, test, and learn. Knowledge is the best weapon you have against diabetes.

Understanding Sugars, Other Sweeteners, and Bulking Agents

Here is a list of most of the sweeteners you will encounter. Refer to this list whenever you see an unfamiliar name on a list of ingredients and wonder what it is.

- **Sugars.** The names of **sugars** end in *ose*, but not everything ending in *ose* is a sugar (for example, cellulose, which is insoluble fiber). They include single sugar units called **monosaccharides**. The most common of these are *glucose*, *fructose*, and **galactose**. They also include sugars made of two sugar units, or **disaccharides**. These include *sucrose*, or common table sugar (made of glucose and fructose); *lactose*, or milk sugar (made of glucose and galactose); and *maltose* (made of two glucose units).

  Most sugars contain 4 cal/g (16 kilojoules per gram in the European system of units), the same as **starch**. They are carbohydrates, and the calories should be counted in your diet plan.

  Fructose, a natural sugar found in fruits and vegetables, is **metabolized** (broken down) slightly differently from glucose and doesn't raise BG levels as quickly. However, it has the same number of calories, and it tends to increase triglyceride levels more, especially if eaten in excess.

  Sucrose, also a natural sugar found in fruits and vegetables, contains half glucose and half fructose. Hence table sugar won't actually raise your BG levels quite as fast as starch, which contains 100 percent glucose.

  Agave syrup is mostly fructose.

  Carob powder, a chocolate substitute, contains 75 percent sucrose, plus glucose and fructose.

- **Other names.** Often the word *sugar* is not mentioned in a list of ingredients, but sugar-containing syrups are. These include *honey, corn syrup, high-fructose corn syrup, rice syrup, molasses, treacle, sorghum, turbinado, starch syrup, malt extract,* and *maple syrup.* You can assume these will affect your BG levels the same as sugars. Processed starches such as *cornstarch, potato starch, wheat starch,* and *tapioca starch* will also raise your BG levels at least as fast as sugar.

- **Fructooligosaccharides.** The fructooligosaccharides are short chains of fructose found in onions and asparagus. *Yacon syrup* is mostly fructooligosaccharides with some fructose and sucrose. Because fructooligosaccharides are not broken down in the small intestine, they are eaten by bacteria in the colon, where they are supposed to stimulate the growth of favorable bacteria.

(continues)

(continued) **Understanding Sugars,
Other Sweeteners, and Bulking Agents**

Longer chains of fructose are called *inulin*, which is found in Jerusalem artichokes. Inulin has often been recommended as a good food for people with diabetes because, like the fructooligosaccharides, it isn't broken down in the intestines and doesn't raise BG levels. Many people confuse the words *inulin* and *insulin* and will tell you to eat Jerusalem artichokes because they're full of insulin. Even if they were, the insulin would be destroyed in the stomach.

- **Dextrose.** Dextrose is just another word for glucose. So too, *levulose* is an older term for fructose. (These terms come from the fact that solutions of these sugars rotate polarized light in a particular direction. When you break down sucrose into a 50:50 mixture of glucose and fructose, the mixture is sometimes called *invert sugar*, because the direction that a solution rotates polarized light is inverted in the process.) Another name for glucose is *grape sugar* because grapes contain a lot of glucose.

- **Bulking agents.** Many artificial powdered sweeteners are so intensely sweet that you only need tiny amounts, and it would be difficult to measure such small amounts. Hence the manufacturers add *bulking agents*. One such agent is glucose (usually listed as *dextrose*). You may think it odd that sugar substitutes contain glucose, but the amounts are relatively small, usually less than 1 gram. If your diet includes a lot of carbohydrate, this amount is negligible. However, if you're on a **low-carbohydrate diet**, it may be significant, and you should use liquid or tablet sweeteners instead. Some tablets also contain bulking agents, so check the labels.

  Another common bulking agent is *maltodextrin*. This is simply starch (a polysaccharide made of glucose) that has been partly broken down into smaller units but not completely broken down into glucose. However, it will raise your BG levels about the same as glucose or starch and has the same number of calories (4 cal/g). It does not taste sweet. *Polydextrose* (see later) is also a common bulking agent.

  The "measure-for-measure" sweeteners that let you substitute one teaspoon of the sweetener for a teaspoon of sugar usually have the most bulking agents. Liquid sweeteners don't need bulking agents but contain preservatives.

- **Sugar alcohols.** When you treat sugars with hydrogen, you can reduce their aldehyde or ketone groups to alcohol groups. If you don't remember from chemistry courses what this means, don't worry about it. It's not important.

What is important is that when you do this, the resulting **sugar alcohols** are *metabolized* (broken down and converted to energy) slightly differently than the sugars, so they don't raise your BG levels quite as fast and have fewer calories. They are not intoxicating, like ethyl alcohol, the formal name for booze.

The names of many sugar alcohols end with *itol*. Common ones are **sorbitol** (or *glucitol*), *xylitol*, *mannitol*, and *lactitol*, made from *glucose, xylose, mannose*, and *lactose*, respectively. Polysaccharides containing a lot of sugar alcohols are called *polyols*.

The number of calories and the amount the sugar alcohols raise your BG levels vary with the different ones. Most of them are considered to have from 2 to 3 cal/g according to Food and Drug Administration (FDA) standards, but some of them (for example, sorbitol) have as many calories as sugars (4 cal/g). With European labeling standards, they're all listed as the same (10 kilojoules per gram).

The sugar alcohol **maltitol**, which consists of half glucose and half sorbitol, raises BG levels about as much as table sugar. Maltitol is a common sweetener in "sugar-free" candies. The sugar alcohol *erythritol* has the least effect on BG levels and the fewest calories. Erythritol does not have a laxative effect.

Some sugar alcohols have names that don't tip you off to what they are. These include isomalt, polydextrose, and HSH, all carbohydrates that have been treated to produce some sugar alcohols.

Isomalt is a combination of glucose-sorbitol and glucose-mannitol. It is used as a sweetener and bulking agent and works synergistically (meaning the two agents acting together have a greater effect than the sum of their effects when used alone) with aspartame and acesulfame K (see later). It has about 2 cal/g.

Polydextrose is made by reacting glucose and sorbitol in the presence of citric acid. It contains a complex mixture of glucose units connected by bonds that aren't broken down easily by human digestive **enzymes**, so it has fewer calories (1 cal/g) than other carbohydrates. It is not sweet and is used as a bulking agent.

Hydrogenated starch hydrolysate, or *HSH*, is another carbohydrate alcohol. It's made by partially breaking down starch and then adding hydrogen to make various monosaccharides, disaccharides, and polysaccharides containing sugar alcohols. The different ones have different degrees of sweetness. HSH has about 3 cal/g.

When carbohydrates aren't broken down in the small intestine, they keep moving through your digestive tract, and as they do, they draw in water. For this reason they can act as laxatives if you eat a lot of them. Bacteria in the

(continues)

Understanding Sugars,
Other Sweeteners, and Bulking Agents

colon can break down some carbohydrates that human digestive enzymes can't, and the result is gas. Most of the sugar alcohols result in gas and diarrhea if you eat too much of them. Some sugar alcohols occur naturally in fruits, especially plums—which is why prunes are a traditional laxative.

■ **Other sugar substitutes.** Sweeteners available in stores include the following. They are used in such tiny amounts that the calories are negligible.

Acesulfame K (Sunette, Sweet One, Sweet N Safe) is not metabolized and has no calories. It acts synergistically with *aspartame* and *cyclamate* but not with *saccharin*. It is heat stable.

Aspartame (Equal, NutraSweet, NatraTaste, Insta Sweet) is made from two amino acids linked together. It is primarily metabolized like other amino acids. Aspartame is synergistic with other sweeteners, especially acesulfame K, but it is not stable to heating and is not suitable for cooking. Some people do not tolerate aspartame well and say their BG levels go up when they use it. There is a lot of controversy about its safety, especially in hot climates, but the FDA says it's safe.

Neotame is made from the same ingredients as aspartame but is sweeter, and less of it is absorbed by the intestine. Advantame, like neotame, consists of aspartame linked to another molecule, in this case vanillin. It was FDA approved in 2014.

Cyclamate is available in Canada but not in the United States, where it was banned in 1969 after some studies suggested it might be carcinogenic. It's often combined with saccharin.

Saccharin (Sugar Twin, Sweet'N Low, Necta Sweet) is one of the oldest artificial sweeteners used (since 1879). Early studies showed that high levels caused bladder cancer in rodents, and some countries have restrictions on its use. However, people with diabetes who have used it for years don't seem to have more bladder cancer than other people, and more recent studies have suggested that the sweetener is not dangerous at the amounts usually eaten. In December 2000, the FDA removed the requirement for a warning label on saccharin products.

Unprocessed stevia is not FDA approved as a sweetener, but it tastes sweet and is sold as a supplement in health-food stores. It comes from the leaves of a South American plant, and you can buy ground-up stevia leaves, which are green, or highly purified stevia extract, which is so intensely sweet that you have to use tiny amounts. In 2008, the main sweet compound in stevia, called *rebaudioside A*, or *reb A*, was FDA approved as *generally recognized as safe* (GRAS). This means it can be added to foods without further approval. Some people get a licorice-like aftertaste when they use stevia. Others do not. This may depend on the batch, as the taste can vary with the extraction method. If you don't like the taste of one brand, try another. Unlike regular sugar, stevia extracts have expiration dates, suggesting that the sweet compounds may break down with time. As with other sweeteners, packets of stevia contain bulking agents.

Reports indicate that stevia improves glucose tolerance—your ability to keep your BG levels down when you eat glucose—but the tiny amounts used to sweeten probably wouldn't have an effect.

Monk fruit, or *lo han guo*, is a Chinese fruit. As with stevia, an extract of lo han guo has been FDA approved as GRAS. Nectresse, a commercial sweetener containing monk fruit, was discontinued in 2014 because of low sales.

Sucralose (Splenda) consists of sucrose in which some alcohol groups have been replaced by chlorine atoms. It is stable when heated and can be used for cooking.

Tagatose is a monosaccharide found in plant gums and in small amounts in yogurt. It is approved as a sweetener in Australia and New Zealand and in 2001 received a GRAS designation by the FDA. It is said to have the bulking and browning properties of sucrose. However, it is not yet available to consumers except in mixtures, and in 2006, the board of directors of a company producing it put the product on hold, saying they couldn't identify a large enough market to continue investing in it.

Some sweeteners contain mixtures, for example, Truvia and ZSweet. The composition of these tends to change as new ingredients are approved, so your best bet is to read the ingredient list. Some contain "natural flavorings" or "fruit extracts" without saying what they are.

■ **Bitterness.** Many of the artificial sweeteners have a bitter aftertaste when you use too much of them. One way to minimize this problem is to use smaller amounts of several different sweeteners together.

TABLE 1
CONVERTING GLUCOSE VALUES BETWEEN MG/DL AND MMOL/L

To convert units exactly, divide mg/dL by 18.016, or multiply mmol/L by 18.016. To approximate, simply use 18 as the conversion. The following table has done some of these conversions, rounded off.

MG/DL	MMOL/L	MMOL/L	MG/DL
30	1.7	2	36
50	2.8	3	54
70	3.9	4	72
80	4.4	5	90
90	5.0	6	108
100	5.6	7	126
120	6.7	8	144
126	7.0	9	162
130	7.2	10	180
140	7.8	11	198
150	8.3	12	216
160	8.9	13	234
170	9.4	14	252
180	10.0	15	270
190	10.6	16	288
200	11.1	18	324
250	13.9	20	360
300	16.7	22	396
400	22.2	25	450
500	27.8	30	540
600	33.3	35	631

IN A SENTENCE:

▪ *Foods contain protein, fat, and carbohydrate, and carbohydrate has the greatest effect on your blood glucose levels.*

Networking with Others

By now you may have begun to accept the fact that you really do have diabetes, and it's time for you to connect with other people who are in the same boat.

If you have access to the Internet, one of the best things you can to is to join one of the many Internet groups that are now available. If you do not have Internet access either at home or at your local library, you will probably benefit from joining a local diabetes support group.

Start with the Mendosa site

In Month 12, Internet diabetes expert David Mendosa will guide you through diabetes resources on the Internet. The best place to start is the newbie page on his site: www.mendosa. com/advice.htm. David understands the problems of type 2 diabetes; he has diabetes himself. When he was first diagnosed, he learned so much from the Internet that he wanted to share his knowledge with others and created at his own expense what many feel is the best diabetes home page available today.

I like David's webpages because he focuses on information instead of fancy graphics or animated advertisements. He also provides short reviews of the sites he has links to, which helps you decide which ones to visit.

Most of you already have computers and smart phones and are familiar with navigating the web. If you don't and can't buy a computer, check your local library's resources. Most have computers for public use, with high-speed Internet access. If money is a problem, look into getting a second-hand computer. Technology progresses so fast in the computer field that today's computers are often considered old hat before the ink on the check is dry, and fast-lane people who need to be on the cutting edge of technology often sell perfectly good used computers at good prices.

Major websites offer vast resources

There are several major ways you can use the Internet to get information about diabetes. The first is through the World Wide Web. Once you have access to the web, you can use David Mendosa's home page to link to all kinds of diabetes information including the American Diabetes Association (**ADA**) pages; the Joslin Diabetes Center in Boston—one of the best diabetes treatment and research centers in the world; alternative medicine treatments; vitamin sources; PubMed, the National Library of Medicine's free database of summaries of professional journal articles; and teaching resources in endocrinology, biochemistry, and general medicine.

As you browse the Internet, you should keep in mind that there's a lot of incorrect information along with the good on the Internet—for example, snake-oil salespeople may try to sell you mysterious wonder cures at high prices. But this is no different from information available in print or on television. You wouldn't accept a report of alien invaders in a supermarket tabloid or an infomercial on a new weight-loss cream that is supposed to melt your stomach flab and make you rich and healthy while you eat chocolate sundaes and cheddar hot dogs. So too, you must evaluate the source of anything you find on the Internet.

Newsgroups provide support

Another resource is the Internet *newsgroups*. Newsgroups are like bulletin boards. People post messages, and if you sign up for a particular newsgroup—such as misc.health.diabetes or alt.support.diabetes—you can then see the titles of all the messages people have recently posted to the board. If one of the messages sounds interesting, you can click on it to download and read it. If you wish, you can reply to the message, and everyone else will be able to see the title of your reply and read it if they wish.

Email lists are more private

The third resource is the *email list*. With an email list, you subscribe to the list, and all the messages that everyone writes are sent directly to you, as part of your daily email download. If you reply to a message, your reply is sent to everyone on the list. The email lists are often more private and less vitriolic than the newsgroups because administrators may screen the subscribers and remove spammers—people who send the Internet equivalent of junk mail—or people who don't follow the rules of the list. Some lists are *moderated*, meaning someone reads every message before it is posted to make sure the list rules are followed.

Some of the email lists have *archives* that you can search for information that was posted before you joined. Other lists prefer not to keep archives, which means your comments won't be available for the whole world to read forevermore. David Mendosa's website has a vast list of these email lists, where you can look for one that may appeal to you.

The email lists provide information that is often even more valuable. You can ask questions, and other people who have lived with diabetes longer than you have are often able to provide interesting answers. Even if you don't ask questions yourself, other people often ask about things you were wondering about, and you can benefit from the answers.

Often the discussion centers around the inconveniences—or worse— of living with diabetes, and there's nothing like learning how other people cope with common problems to give you ideas about how to deal with the same problems in your own life. Just reading descriptions of how different people react to various foods, medications, or types of exercise gives you a sense of how variable people's responses can be. What works for me might not work for you. On the lists we call it **YMMV** (Your Mileage May Vary).

One benefit of the lists is the instant feedback you can get. Someone with a serious problem might get a response within minutes. And people care about each other. On one list, a woman who had been depressed once posted a note asking how much insulin you'd need to inject to commit suicide. In less than thirty minutes, another list member managed to find out where she lived and sent an ambulance to her house in case she had actually tried such a thing. It turned out the action saved her life.

Another advantage of lists is the ability to vent. Everyone gets down in the dumps every now and then, or maybe angry at the health-care system, or at the family who doesn't understand, or whatever. Being able to vent and finding out that other people often feel the same way can be very therapeutic.

A fascinating aspect of these lists is their international membership. One list I'm on has had active members not only from the United States and Canada, but also from England, Romania, India, Australia, Scandinavia, Central America, Brazil, Belgium, Israel, and South Africa. One learns not only about diabetes but also about different approaches and recipes from different places in the world.

Online social networking sites are popular

Today, the trend is away from email lists, which come into your mailbox without action on your part, to online Facebook-type sites. A few popular ones are TuDiabetes (www.tudiabetes.org), which had more than 35,000 members in 2015, Diabetes Forum (www.diabetesforum.com), with close to 25,000, Diabetes Daily (www.diabetesdaily.com), which had 110,000, and dLife (www.dlife.com), which also has a TV program, with 1.2 million members. There are many more.

In this case you go to the site and see what's new, or you can search for information that might have been posted earlier. These sites offer similar things, including blogs, forums, diabetes news, chats, recipes, special interest groups, and so forth, but they're presented in different ways. Some are stronger on news and features and others on patient forums and blogs. On some sites you can sign up to get email notification weekly or monthly when there are new featured articles.

Many sites also have Twitter feeds.

Most manufacturers of diabetes supplies also have sites, and many groups, including the American Diabetes Association, are on Facebook. I tend to be cynical about pages run by commercial enterprises that want to sell you something, but you may find some such sites useful. Look around and find a site that works for you. Mendosa's site has a roundup of useful sites as of 2010 (www.mendosa.com/genl.htm). Websites come and go, so no list can include everything as of this moment, but you may find something interesting that is still viable.

The advantage of the big sites with thousands of members is that you have access to a tremendous amount of information from people who have had diabetes for decades. They are usually more than willing to help you with yours. The disadvantage is that the amount of information can seem overwhelming, and the newest posts can scroll off the home page in minutes, although you can still find them by clicking on "view all" or something similar.

Through their forums, the social networking sites offer the same advantages as the email lists, including the possibility of instant feedback and the opportunity to vent. One difference is that on some sites, anyone can read the posts even without joining, so the messages are less private than email lists that you have to join and that are sometimes moderated.

Networking apps are available

There are apps that will let you network on your smart phone, although not yet as many as other diabetes apps. The number of apps is growing rapidly, however, and you should soon be able to choose from a large selection.

Chat rooms offer instant feedback

Another form of personal communication on the Internet is the *chat room*. In this case, you are communicating with people in "real time," meaning that as you type, your message is posted for everyone to read. It also means you don't see the messages that were posted when Fido insisted that you take him for a walk, and you have to spend a lot of time sitting in front of the screen waiting for someone else to type an answer. If several people are chatting at once, it can get confusing. I'm too impatient to use this form of communication, but many people enjoy it.

Support groups offer personal contact

Internet websites, newsgroups, email lists, and chat rooms are great conveniences when you don't have transportation to get to public meetings or are shy about going to them and just want to read what other people are saying about diabetes on the various lists (reading without posting is called *lurking*, but it's not considered rude). But you might also enjoy the social aspects of support groups given by your local hospital or other health-care center. If your area doesn't have one, you might think about organizing one yourself.

Usually such groups have a public speaker, such as a physician, nurse, **dietician**, or **certified diabetes educator (CDE)**, to talk on some aspect of diabetes, and then members can get together to chat and eat diabetes-friendly snacks.

Such support groups offer most of the benefits of online lists except for the instant feedback. Members may become good friends and can communicate by telephone, but it's obviously more difficult to ask a question of more than one member at a time except at the meetings themselves.

Magazines can also help

If you just want to read about other people with diabetes, you can subscribe to a diabetes magazine (see Month 12). However, in today's world more and more information is available online and less and less in print.

Networking speeds up learning

Whether you choose to network online or at a local support group, such networking will in most cases speed up your learning about this complex disease, give you advice about where to go for more information, offer recipe suggestions no matter what diet approach you are taking, keep you in touch with the latest advances in diabetes research, and, perhaps best of all, give you new friends who really understand what you're going through as you adjust to this new way of life.

IN A SENTENCE:

▪ *Networking with other people who have diabetes is one of the best ways to come to terms with the disease.*

What Is a
Diabetic Diet?

No one likes to diet. It's especially difficult in a society that seems to be focused on food. We expect to eat Often, Abundantly, and Fast, which in a sense makes us all OAFs. Many of us have been duped by advertisers to think that we need to nibble on candies, chips, and sodas all day and then wolf down "supersized" restaurant meals or gargantuan pizzas before we settle in for an evening in front of the TV.

Even "from scratch" organic health-food restaurants often serve portions that are too large, and social gatherings may focus more on the gourmet food that is served than on interesting conversations with dinner companions.

In such a land of abundant food and a constant barrage of media messages urging us to eat even more, it's difficult for anyone to try to limit calories. When you have thrifty genes that are ever so efficient at turning every extra calorie on the plate into fat on the stomach—and often give you an unusually large appetite to boot—this is even more difficult. But unfortunately, that's what you've got to do. **Limiting the amount you eat is one of the most important things you can do to control your type 2 diabetes.**

Controlling what you eat helps control your diabetes

That's the bad news. But wait! There's more! The good news is that carefully controlling what you eat will help you slim down and have a lot more energy. Many people say that after they started controlling their blood glucose (BG) levels through diet, they felt better than they'd felt in years. Many also find that when they get their BG levels under control, their formerly mammoth appetites become human sized again.

Controlling what you eat may also allow you to remain on very low dosages of diabetes drugs or very minimal amounts of insulin, or off drugs and insulin altogether, for many years. In addition, research has shown that limiting food intake may increase your lifespan. It's not easy to do, but making the effort today will probably give you more tomorrows.

Diabetic diets differ

When you were diagnosed, your doctor or a dietician may have handed you a copy of a "diabetic diet." (Some people try to avoid the loaded word *diet* and refer to *food plans* instead. I don't like euphemisms. Diabetes isn't a "suboptimal blood glucose control condition," it's a disease. And as far as I'm concerned, a specific eating plan is a diet. Why try to sugarcoat it? We're not dummies.) Or perhaps you've been scheduled to meet with a dietician, who may show you some rubber food to give you an idea of portion sizes and then write out a diet that is appropriate for you. (Actually, the rubber food is a good idea. After looking carefully at a lot of worn rubber hamburgers and orange juice, I wasn't sure I ever wanted to eat again.)

When comparing notes with someone else who has diabetes, or reading one of the many diabetes diet books on the market, you may discover that the diet you've been given is quite different from the diet someone else with diabetes is following. What's going on here?

The fact is, people have been arguing about the best diet for diabetes for centuries (see Appendix 2), and they still can't agree. That is, they can't agree on the best composition of the diabetic diet. Unfortunately, one thing most people agree on is that type 2 diabetes is greatly helped by limiting the number of calories in your food.

No one ever said this disease was going to be easy.

Almost all the diabetic diet "experts" agree that lean meats and fish, green leafy vegetables, and other low-calorie, high-fiber vegetables such as cucumbers, broccoli, cauliflower, peppers, asparagus, and cabbage are good foods to eat. Raw or undercooked is usually better for your BG levels than overcooked.

Then the various diet proponents begin to, well, I'll call it "disagree," although the mention of a suitable diabetic diet often brings forth heated debates.

So there are several approaches to diabetic diets, and different people are successful with different approaches.

Low-carbohydrate diet helps with both weight loss and glucose control

The **low-carbohydrate diet** severely limits the intake of any kind of carbohydrate, either starch or sugar, but allows larger portions of both protein and fat. For many years, a high-fat, low-carbohydrate diet was the standard way to treat diabetes. It worked. People who followed this diet were able to keep their BG levels down, and before insulin was discovered, it kept many people with type 2 diabetes alive.

The problem was that people with both types of diabetes are at higher risk of heart disease than people without diabetes. And because studies had shown that high-fat, high-carbohydrate diets increased the risk of heart disease, it was assumed that high-fat, low-carbohydrate diets would have the same effect. Thus it was decided to give people with type 1 diabetes less fat and more carbohydrate and also more insulin to handle the additional carbohydrate load. Later, the **high-carbohydrate diet** was recommended for people with type 2 diabetes as well—even for those who were trying to control with diet alone.

Today, there is evidence that total dietary fats don't increase heart attack risks, but the relation between various types of fat and cardiovascular problems is still controversial

Now some people believe that the original low-carbohydrate diet may be best for people with diabetes after all. Dr. Richard Bernstein, the author of the *Diabetes Solution*, who has type 1 diabetes himself, is the main proponent of the benefits of this diet for people with diabetes. The *Atkins* and *Protein Power* diets are also low-carbohydrate diets but are designed primarily for people who want to lose weight, not specifically for people with diabetes. Thus their emphasis is more on the total amount of carbohydrate in the diet that will make you lose weight rather than whether or not that particular carbohydrate will raise your BG level.

There's not total agreement on how a low-carbohydrate diet is defined. Some people go to the extreme of the Atkins induction diet, which allows only 20 grams of carbohydrate a day. Other people call diets with up to 130 grams of carbohydrate "low carbohydrate." Because the average American eats between 230 and 330 grams of carbohydrate a day, the 130 grams are, indeed, lower than average, but they're not low enough to control **post-prandial** (after-eating) BG levels except in people who are still able to produce a lot of insulin.

Critics of these diets claim that their high fat content will increase the risks of heart disease, but many people on these diets see their lipid profiles improve. Almost all see a reduction in their BG levels, especially after meals, and recent research has suggested that postprandial BG levels are more important than **preprandial** (before-eating) BG levels in determining overall BG control.

Many people find that their appetite is reduced on a low-carbohydrate diet, so if having a raging appetite has been your main problem, this diet would be a good choice.

Some people do find that their cholesterol levels increase on high-fat, low-carbohydrate diets. For such people, several modifications of the low-carbohydrate diet exist. The *Ezrin diet* (*The Type 2 Diabetes Diet Book*) is a low-fat, low-carbohydrate diet designed for weight loss. Another modification of the low-carbohydrate diet, the *Four Corners Diet* (formerly the *GO-Diet*), emphasizes **monounsaturated fats** and low-glycemic-index, high-fiber foods, thus combining the benefits of a high-fiber diet with the benefits of a low-carbohydrate diet. Very low carbohydrate diets can cause constipation, sometimes severe, and fiber helps prevent this.

Some people consider the low-carbohydrate diet the "default diet," meaning that unless there are strong reasons not to do so, you should start with this type of diet. Then if, for whatever reason, it doesn't work for you, you can try another approach. Others say no one can stick to a low-carbohydrate diet for very long. I've been on one for about seventeen years and don't plan to change. I consider that pretty long. Trends in diabetes diets swing from high carb to low carb, so who knows what the preferred diet in 2075 will be, but for now, a low-carbohydrate diet works for many.

High-carbohydrate, high-fiber diet follows USDA recommendations

At the other end of the spectrum is the very low fat, **high-carbohydrate, high-fiber diet**, sometimes called the *HCF diet*. The HCF diet limits fat and emphasizes carbohydrates that are the least processed and contain a lot of fiber (about 40 or 50 grams a day), for example, whole grains instead of white flour; brown rice, beans, or lentils instead of white rice; and starchy vegetables like corn and potatoes, in addition to the green vegetables mentioned earlier. Some people have difficulty dealing with the large amount of fiber in this diet.

The HCF diet is in accordance with the US Department of Agriculture (USDA) guidelines, which many dieticians also recommend. The current USDA recommendations are formalized in **MyPlate**, in which fruits, vegetables, grains, and protein should each occupy about a quarter of your plate, and dairy is also included. MyPlate recommends low-fat products but doesn't recommend as much carbohydrate as the HCF diet and isn't as strict about avoiding some **processed carbohydrates**. Note that MyPlate is designed for healthy eating in general, not specifically for diabetes. The HCF diet contains about 20 percent protein, 70 percent carbohydrate, and 10 percent fat.

Carbohydrates are broken down in the intestine to produce sugars, mostly glucose, and a lot of glucose is what people with diabetes can't handle. So it may seem odd to prescribe what is essentially a high-sugar diet to a person who can't deal with sugar. Why would anyone want to do that?

There are several reasons behind this diet. First, a high fat intake may increase insulin resistance (IR), and a high carbohydrate intake may reduce IR. So if IR is your main problem, this diet may help. In addition, people with diabetes are at greatly increased risk of **cardiovascular** disease, and in the general population (including people without diabetes), a low fat intake has in the past been associated statistically with a reduced risk of cardiovascular disease, although this association is now being questioned.

The HCF diet usually makes your BG go higher after meals, but some people feel this is less important than its beneficial effects. Of the popular diet books, *The Starch Solution (McDougall diet)*, *Forks over Knives*, and *Eat More, Weigh Less (Ornish diet)*, which all promote vegetarian diets, and *Eat to Live (Pritikin diet)* and *Choose to Lose* would be in this category.

Low-glycemic-index diet focuses on blood glucose increases

The third approach is the **low-glycemic-index diet**. This diet is similar to the high-carbohydrate, high-fiber diet in that it recommends low-fat, high-carbohydrate foods, but it allows a little more fat and limits the carbohydrates even more than the other high-carbohydrate diets, emphasizing those carbohydrates that have what is called a *low glycemic index*.

The **glycemic index** is a measure of how quickly foods raise your BG level. You might be surprised at some of the results. For instance, potatoes (which used to be called *complex carbohydrates* and were thought not to raise BG levels very fast) in fact have a higher glycemic index than table sugar. The *glycemic load* takes into account both the glycemic index and the *amount* of carbohydrate in the meal. Of the popular diet books, the *New Glucose Revolution for Diabetes* and the *Sugar Busters!* diets are in this category. Each of these diets specifies a slightly different percentage of nutrients.

Exchange diets allow a little of everything

The fourth approach is what used to be called the **ADA** (American Diabetes Association) **diet**. In recent years, the ADA has modified its position somewhat and now agrees that one diet isn't best for every patient, so I'll refer to this as the *exchange diet* instead.

The exchange diet is designed for a person who doesn't want or is unable to undergo a total change of food choices. Almost any food is permitted on the exchange diet, as long as the portion sizes and the number of portions per day are controlled. Each food is assigned to a category such as a fat, protein, starch, milk, fruit, or vegetable group, and you are assigned a certain number of the various exchanges for each meal. For example, on a 1,500-calorie exchange diet, you might be allowed two starch exchanges for lunch (in addition to meat, milk, fruit, vegetable, and fat exchanges). One starch exchange would consist of one slice of bread or one-third cup of rice or a small potato. Each starch exchange is *approximately* equal to 15 grams of carbohydrate.

Like the previous diets, this one is relatively low in fat and relatively high in carbohydrate. But any kinds of carbohydrate can be used, including white bread, breakfast cereals, and orange juice—all foods with high-glycemic-index values.

Nevertheless, because the number of calories is controlled on the exchange diets, many people are able to control their BG levels while continuing to eat (in small portions) their favorite foods at home or in restaurants. Many "diabetic cookbooks" and "diabetic foods" take this approach and tally the number of exchanges found in each portion, which is a convenience for the person without a lot of time to devote to preparing special food.

The ADA exchange diet used to contain about 55 to 60 percent carbohydrate, 10 to 20 percent protein, and less than 30 percent fat, but that can now be individualized. Newer recommendations are 10 to 20 percent protein, with the rest of the calories distributed between carbohydrate and fat, emphasizing monounsaturated fat (see the box in Month 6), depending on your needs. The popular *Zone diet* is actually a type of exchange diet in which exchanges are called *blocks*, and there is less carbohydrate (40 percent) and more protein (30 percent) than in the ADA exchange diet.

Carbohydrate counting works well when you use insulin

A variation of the exchange diet is called **carbohydrate counting**. With this approach, you are allowed a certain number of grams of carbohydrate for each meal. As with the exchange diets, you are not limited in what type of carbohydrate you choose to eat. You use tables to calculate the amount of carbohydrate in each food, but you don't need to keep track of the amount of protein and fat. So instead of being assigned two starch exchanges, one fruit exchange, and one milk exchange, you might be assigned to 57 grams of carbohydrate for lunch, and you would calculate how much carbohydrate there was in each food you chose.

This method is more accurate than the exchange method when you're trying to match your insulin shots to the carbohydrate you eat, so it is especially suited to people who are using insulin to control their BG levels. But because carbohydrate counting doesn't keep track of the amount of protein and fat you eat, it probably won't help you lose weight and would not be the best way to start if you are overweight when you are diagnosed.

Other diets are always being developed

Because most Americans would like to weigh less, new diets are constantly being developed. Some are designed primarily for healthy eating for everyone, and others are designed for weight loss.

The *Mediterranean diet* is popular with many health-care professionals because it's not an extreme diet. Although not everyone in the Mediterranean area eats this way, the Mediterranean diet emphasizes whole foods, including fruits, vegetables, beans, nuts, olive oil, seafood, chicken, seeds, and whole grains. It's definitely healthier than the standard American diet.

The *Paleo diet* is based on the theory that we are healthiest when we eat the same food that our ancestors ate ten thousand years ago, when they were hunter-gatherers. This means no processed foods, no grains, no legumes, and no dairy foods. You're allowed eggs and nuts and grass-fed meats. Like the Mediterranean diet, the Paleo diet emphasizes whole foods. And depending how you interpret the diet, you could lose weight and control your BG levels. For many people, giving up grains means a pretty low carb diet. But you're allowed fruit on a Paleo diet, and if you ate a ton of sugary fruits, your BG levels would go up.

Intermittent fasting means that you alternate eating normally with fasting. Different people fast for different lengths of time. As a result of the fasting, your overall weekly calorie count is lower, and some people find this is a good way to lose weight. It does take time to adapt to the fasting.

However, because when you're not fasting, you're allowed to eat whatever you want, it wouldn't be a good way to control BG levels, unless you used this approach along with another diet during nonfasting times. If just losing weight will control your BG levels and you really don't want to give up any foods, then intermittent fasting might make sense for you.

Find the best diet for you

I discuss more of the pros and cons of the various diet approaches in Months 10 and 11. For now, what you should understand is that dietary recommendations for people with type 2 diabetes are highly controversial. What you eventually need to do is to find the diet that works best for *you*.

To start, the best approach is to try the diet that your doctor or your dietician recommends. Follow it carefully for a few weeks or months and test your BG levels when you get up in the morning and after eating various meals.

Then, when you've had time to absorb more information about diets and when you've seen how your own BG levels respond to the diet you're on, take stock (see Month 7). If your BG and lipid levels are well controlled on this diet and you're content with the food choices that you have, stick with it. It's a good diet for you.

If not, you might try another approach. As I mentioned before, type 2 diabetes is an incredibly complex disease, and we all have different life situations, economic situations, taste preferences, and weight-loss needs. What works best for someone else may not work best for you.

The important thing for now is to accept the hard fact that you're going to have to be on some kind of diet (OK, call it a "meal plan" or a "nutritional minimization attack strategy" or an "OOO" [OAF-overcoming orientation] if you prefer) for a long time.

If you can find a diet plan that works for you and follow it rigorously—well, most of the time, none of us are perfect—you will have accomplished one of the most difficult things you can do to control your diabetes. Diet (alas) is the key to control.

IN A SENTENCE:

■ *There is no single "diabetic diet," and you need to find what works for you.*

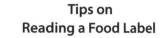

Tips on
Reading a Food Label

Most food labels indicate the total calories and the amounts of the three basic food classes (*protein, fat,* and *carbohydrate*) as well as the percentage of your daily needs that a serving size should provide. Here are a few tips to make your reading of food labels more accurate. If this is more complex than you want to deal with right now, come back to it later when you've had more experience calculating your daily nutritional needs.

- Sometimes the classes are broken down into subclasses; for example, total fat may be broken down into **saturated fat, trans fat, polyunsaturated fat**, and *monounsaturated fat* (see the box in Month 6). Sometimes not all the subclasses are listed.

  To estimate the amounts, first add the grams of the subclasses. If the total grams of the subclasses don't equal the grams of the class, then something isn't listed. For example, if a label says you have 10 grams of total carbohydrate, including 5 grams of fiber, 2 grams of sugars, and 1 gram of sugar alcohols, then there are 2 grams of something else. This is probably starch. Many labels list only total fat and saturated and trans fat. You can assume the rest includes monounsaturated and polyunsaturated fat, but you can't tell how much of each.

- Multiply the grams of total carbohydrate and total protein by four, and then multiply the grams of total fat by nine. Add them together. If this doesn't equal the total number of calories, something is probably missing.

  Note that the numbers listed on the labels are usually rounded off. So if the food contained 8.4 grams of carbohydrate and 2.4 grams of protein, these would be listed as 8 grams of carbohydrate and 2 grams of protein, which you would calculate as 10 x 4 = 40 calories. But in fact the calories would be 10.8 x 4 = 43.2 calories. So small differences may be the result of rounding.

  If you get a lot more calories than are listed on the label, this might be because the manufacturers don't have to include calories from the insoluble fiber. They do have to include calories from the soluble fiber (4 cal/g). You have no way of knowing how much of each is included.

  If you get a lot fewer calories than are listed on the label, this could mean that the food contains something not listed on the label. For example, some of the "low-carb" bars now being marketed don't list carbohydrates such as glycerol and other sugar alcohols (see Day 3, page 30) that they claim don't raise your BG levels.

(continues)

(continued)   **Tips on Reading a Food Label**

As an example, one such bar lists 2 grams of carbohydrate, 22 grams of protein, and 8 grams of fat. This would represent $(24 \times 4) + (8 \times 9) = 168$ calories. But the label lists 230 calories. This means 62 calories are not accounted for and must represent unreported carbohydrate. At 4 cal/g, this would be an extra 15.5 grams of glycerol and other sugar alcohols, both of which can be converted to glucose, albeit slowly, in the "2 grams of carbohydrate" bar.

- American manufacturers calculate the carbohydrate content by the "difference" method. This means they determine how much protein and fat it contains and assume that everything else is carbohydrate. In most cases this is pretty accurate. Sometimes it isn't.

  For example, yogurt is usually considered to have about 11 grams of carbohydrate per cup. But the bacteria that turn milk into yogurt do so by converting a lot of the milk sugar (lactose) into *lactic acid*. Using the difference method, the lactic acid is calculated as a carbohydrate, but it doesn't raise your BG levels. Thus according to the authors of *The Four Corners Diet*, you can subtract 8 grams of carbohydrate per cup from the amounts listed on the yogurt food labels.

- Manufacturers don't have to report small amounts of ingredients: less than five calories or less than 0.5 gram of carbohydrate, protein, or fat per serving can be reported as zero. As long as you eat only the amounts shown as serving sizes, this is not a big problem. But if you eat a lot more, it can be misleading.

  For example, a carton of cream might say it contains 0 grams of carbohydrate, because the serving size (one tablespoon) contains only 0.41 gram. But if you ate a whole cup (sixteen tablespoons), it would contain 6.6 grams of carbohydrate, which could be significant for someone on a low-carbohydrate diet.

  When you see 0 grams of something on a label and you're going to be using large amounts, the best way to check is to look at the amounts in standard nutrition tables (see For Further Reading).

- Pay special attention to the listed portion size. The label on Food A says it has 10 grams of carbohydrate, and the label on Food B says it has 20 grams of carbohydrate. But the portion size on Food A is a half cup and the portion size on Food B is a whole cup. So both foods actually contain the same amount of carbohydrate when you use the same portion size.

- When looking at the DV (daily value) percentages, note that they are based on a 2,000-calorie diet. If you need more or fewer calories than that, your needs may differ.

- In 2014 the FDA proposed a few changes to food labels, including more realistic serving sizes and listing of added sugars. If the changes are approved, manufacturers will have several years before the new regulations are enforced.

It's Time to Get Moving

Next to controlling your food intake, getting exercise is probably the best thing you can do to control your diabetes. Unlike medications, exercise is "all natural" and has no side effects.

Exercise really works

Exercise will usually make your blood glucose (BG) levels go down and will continue to help control them for hours after you stop the exercise. Exercise will also help to build up your muscles, and muscles are the tissues that use the most glucose and hence are most important in keeping your BG levels from going too high.

If you've always loved exercise, you're in luck. Keep it up. If not, here's another reason to start moving. Studies have shown that after you've lost weight, no matter how, the best way to keep that weight off is to continue a regular exercise program.

Many people with type 2 diabetes don't want to hear this information. Especially if you're overweight, your idea of the ultimate pleasure in life is probably not to strap ice picks on your shoes and climb up the side of the Empire State Building instead of taking the elevator, no matter how much electricity it saves.

However, exercise really does work, and if there is any way you can get more of it, you'll ultimately be glad that you did. My idea of the perfect exercise has always been strolling through the aisles of a bookstore, or pulling open the door to a refrigerator. But since my diagnosis, I find that when I exercise regularly, my muscles want to be used. One day, I was watching a movie in which a bunch of peasants were throwing huge mounds of hay onto an even huger hayrick. "That looks like fun," I thought. I was astounded at my reaction. My muscles used to complain that turning the pages of a book was too much hard work. Now they wanted to sling pitchforks of hay.

The trick to getting into the habit of getting exercise without passing out from fulminating boredom is to find some way of moving more that is fun for you.

It doesn't have to be vigorous

Exercise doesn't need to be vigorous to benefit you in some way. You don't need to think that you'll have to spend the next twenty-five years running the Boston Marathon while carrying one-hundred-pound barbells or leaping over sawhorses with one bound. Just walking can help.

You may be middle-aged or elderly, maybe with painful arthritis, severe obesity, or previous strokes that have left you unable even to walk. You still may be able to get some exercise. If you can't stand up, maybe you can swing your arms. Painful joint diseases make exercise more difficult; in that case a **physical therapist** may be able to help you find some movement that doesn't hurt but works some of your muscles.

The important thing at the beginning is just to do a little more exercise than you're accustomed to doing. Then gradually increase it until you're getting in about thirty minutes to an hour of moving every day.

If you prefer organized exercise routines with lots of company, there are myriad aerobics classes at gyms, Y's, and adult education programs. If you prefer to move your, er, sumptuous body in private, there are a multitude of books and videotapes on exercise that will give you specific exercise movements that you can do alone or with one or two close friends. But exercise doesn't need to be regimented. You don't need to say, "Now I'm going to exercise," and then run through a dull set of specific movements. You can often sneak exercise into your daily routine. Instead of parking as close to the mall as possible, park as far away as you can. Instead of taking the elevator to the second floor, walk up instead. When that becomes too easy, walk up two floors. You're saving energy and slowing down global warming as well as helping your own health. Instead of using the cart to carry your packages to the car, see if you can carry them in your arms instead.

Walking is especially good exercise because it doesn't require any special equipment and it doesn't cause damage to the joints as hard running can. The trick here is to turn the daily walk into something that is fun, something that you look forward to.

I live in a small town with many scenic back roads, and I've set a goal of walking every single road in town. I note where I left off, and the next day I drive to the place I stopped and start from there. In this way, I've found fascinating places I never knew existed, and I've also gotten in a lot of exercise time.

If you work in a city, you could eat a quick lunch and then take the rest of your lunch hour to explore neighborhoods near where you work, if that's safe. Or you could park a mile or so from your office and walk the rest of the way. Or you could park somewhere on your way home and explore those neighborhoods.

Make your exercise interesting

Walking with friends usually makes the activity more enjoyable. Anything you can do to make your exercise seem like an interesting social occasion instead of a dreaded exercise routine will increase the probability that you'll do it. And actually doing a little bit of exercise is much more therapeutic than sitting in a recliner planning on doing a lot of exercise tomorrow.

Another trick for making the exercise interesting is to listen to recorded books. I don't usually do this when I'm walking the back roads in town, because just exploring the woods is interesting enough. But I also lift weights, and this is, let's face it, dull. That's when I put on the recorded books. I don't allow myself to listen to the books except when I'm lifting the weights, which means I sometimes actually (no really, I mean it) look forward to the time when I can get out the weights.

There are obviously days when it's too cold or too hot or too rainy or whatever to enjoy walking outside. Some people then walk in a mall. You can also obviously work out in a gym. Or you can get your own exercise equipment for use on such days.

Some people find exercise bicycles a good solution, but a lot of the bicycles end up being used as coat racks. A treadmill might be a better choice. With either of these machines, you can watch TV or listen to recorded books, or music if you prefer, or even read a book or magazine as you exercise.

Yee Wan R., who listens to books as she walks on a treadmill, said one book she chose was so interesting that she ended up walking for three hours because "I didn't want to put the book down."

Aerobic and anaerobic exercise are both good

There are two main types of exercise that will help your diabetes. The first is **aerobic exercise**, which is running or walking fast, the kind that gets your heart rate up. This type of exercise is good for your cardiovascular system. And because diabetes is associated with cardiovascular problems, this is a good thing.

The other type of exercise is **anaerobic exercise**, lifting weights, which is the kind of exercise that makes your muscles stronger. Men will see an increase in the size of their muscles with this type of exercise. Women will find that their muscles are stronger and slightly larger but needn't worry that they'll end up looking like Charlotta Atlas. Our physiology is different, and without all that bothersome testosterone, we don't bulk up like the men do.

Anaerobic exercise is especially good when you have diabetes because muscle tissue uses the most glucose. So the more muscles you have, the easier it will be for you to lower your BG levels when they get high. A nice side effect is that anaerobic exercise will turn some of your fat into muscle, so you will feel and look thinner as well, even at the same weight.

Here's how Edd A. described his results with weight lifting: "I was very determined to be thin, so I dieted a great many years. And it got me nowhere. A few times, I actually got thin. But it always came back. I'm probably fatter now from all the dieting than I would have been if I'd never wasted my time. I can't say I enjoyed being fat, but I'd become reconciled to it. I decided I would waddle through life as proudly as I could.

"Well, the weight lifting has put a new spin on all this for me. In the several months since I began, I've lost five inches around the waist. I've lost about thirty pounds. Five inches of fat should weigh more than thirty pounds, so the difference seems to be more muscles on my frame.

"Since I stopped dieting, I've lost my obsession with food. When I dieted, I thought about food all the time. Now I don't struggle with food twenty-four hours a day. I don't have to muster my willpower."

Weight lifting increases blood pressure

One caution: lifting weights can cause an increase in your blood pressure. So if you have high blood pressure, glaucoma, **retinopathy** (see Month 10), kidney disease, or other medical conditions that can be aggravated by such pressure increases, you should not try lifting weights without checking with your doctor first. Such caution is also warranted for anyone who hasn't been off the couch for years and suddenly embarks on an exercise program of any kind, but it's especially important for potential lifters of weights.

For women thinking of trying the weights, I recommend the book *Strong Women Stay Young* by Miriam Nelson. One nice thing about this book is that it's aimed at middle-aged women trying to get stronger, not young things trying to bulk up, so the exercises seem realistic, something we could all really do.

Nelson has done research showing that even people in their nineties can increase their muscle mass with the regular lifting of weights. She recommends working with the weights only thirty minutes two or three times a week, which isn't a lot of time.

Even this small investment of time brings results. One thing I like about weight lifting is that you're not supposed to do it two days in a row. The idea is that the exercise causes small tears in the muscle tissue, and you need a day or so for those tears to repair and for the new muscle to grow. It's so nice to have a good excuse not to exercise every day.

Another thing I like is that as you get stronger, you increase the weight of what you are lifting, but you don't need to increase the time. That's not true of many other kinds of exercise. Once you can do ten sit-ups, you're supposed to do fifteen. When you can do fifteen, you do twenty-five. It's as if you're always being punished for your success by having to spend even more time doing the dull routine.

Find something that is fun

Whether you do weights or walking or waving your arms to catchy music or swimming or contra dancing or skiing or roller skating or climbing mountains or even leaping tall sawhorses at a single bound, the most important thing is to find something that you enjoy doing, so you'll do it.

When you start out being more active, you may think you won't be able to stick with it for long. Maybe you've failed in the past. But the combination of getting your BG levels under control and moving a lot more makes most people feel better than they've felt in many years. Try it, one day at a time. You may get addicted.

IN A SENTENCE:

■ *Moving more is one of the most important things you can do to control your diabetes.*

Understanding Lab Tests for Diabetes

Understanding your diabetes means learning how to interpret the results of the many lab tests you will have. Some of these tests are specialized, and you may not have them done right away, or at all. So don't feel you need to learn, or even read, everything in this section right away. Later, if you have a new test, you can come back and read about it here.

Blood glucose levels are basic tests

Some of you were diagnosed with diabetes because your blood glucose (BG) levels had gotten quite high and you were exhibiting typical diabetic symptoms: constant thirst, frequent urination, recurrent yeast infections, and even weight loss.

Others may have had mildly elevated BG levels that were ignored for years, either because physicians saw the small elevations but had the old-fashioned notion that **borderline diabetes** wasn't important or because you just never had standard lab tests and didn't know your BG levels were high.

No matter which category you fit into, the measurement of your BG level was undoubtedly critical in the diagnosis of your disease. The BG test is a straightforward lab test to understand. It's what you can do yourself using your own BG meter.

It tells you what concentration of glucose is in your blood at the time the blood was drawn.

For diagnosis, your BG level is usually measured after a six- to fourteen-hour fast (meaning no food or beverages except water for six to fourteen hours before the blood is drawn) to give a level called (not surprisingly) the *fasting level*. The current cutoff point for a diagnosis of diabetes is a fasting level of 126 mg/dL (milligrams per deciliter) in the current American system of units (often written without the units) or 7 millimols per liter (mmol/L, sometimes written mM) in the Canadian, Australian, and European systems (see Table 1 on page 34 in Day 3 for conversion chart). I use the American system throughout this book. Many people feel that this cutoff point, which was only recently lowered from 140 mg/dL, should be lowered even further so that people could be diagnosed sooner, when it is easier to control the disease and before they have had a chance to develop any debilitating side effects. (Note that for reasons I will describe later, the values that you get when you use your BG meter may be lower than the lab values.) Don't try to learn all these units right now. I mention them only for reference. If you come across the European units in your reading and wonder what they mean, you can come back here and check. To convert from the American to the European system, divide the mg/dL by 18; to convert from the European system to the American, multiply by 18.

Another test is a *random BG test*, which is a BG measurement taken under nonfasting conditions. In this case a reading of at least 200 mg/dL is considered a good indication of diabetes. Most physicians would then recommend a fasting test to confirm the diagnosis.

A 2015 study showed that a random BG test greater than 100 mg/dL was a stronger predictor of diabetes risk than body mass index.

Hemoglobin A1c measures long-term control

Another test you may take is called the **glycohemoglobin test**. This test is based on the amount of glucose that is attached to the **hemoglobin** in your blood. A more specialized test, called the **hemoglobin A1c test**, often just the **A1c**, tests for the **A1c** subfraction (see later).

Everyone has glucose in the blood. You need it to produce the energy that runs your body. With time, some of this glucose becomes attached to the hemoglobin (the red pigment in your **red blood cells** that carries oxygen from the lungs to the tissues). The amount of glucose that becomes attached to the hemoglobin depends on how much glucose you have in your blood, so people with diabetes who have elevated BG levels also have higher levels of **glycated** (glucose-containing) **hemoglobin**, or *glycohemoglobin* for short. Just to make things more complicated for you, some people use the term *glycosylated hemoglobin* instead. It means essentially the same thing, and you'll see both terms used when you read about diabetes. Different sources define *glycation* and *glycosylation* in different ways that would be of interest primarily to biochemists. For our purposes, they're the same, and I'll use *glycated* because it's easier to spell.

Chemists can separate the glycohemoglobin from the rest of the hemoglobin and express it as a percentage of the total. There are several different ways to measure glycated hemoglobin. In the past, results were often reported simply as *glycohemoglobin*. Normal values for this older test, not much used today, were about 6 to 7.5 percent. Someone with poorly controlled diabetes might have a glycohemoglobin level of 16 percent or even more. As the diabetes is brought under control, the glycohemoglobin level should come down toward normal.

Once glucose gets attached to a hemoglobin molecule, it essentially stays there for the lifetime of the red blood cell that contains the hemoglobin molecule. Most red blood cells live for about 120 days, and then they are broken down by the body and replaced by new cells with new hemoglobin molecules that have no glucose attached. So the glycohemoglobin level gives an estimate of the average glucose level since about three months ago, especially in the past few weeks, as I'll discuss in Appendix 1.

The A1c test tells you the same thing as the glycohemoglobin test, but it is even more specialized. Chemists can separate hemoglobin into various fractions, called *hemoglobin A* (for adult), *hemoglobin F* (for fetal), *hemoglobin S* (for sickle cell), and so forth. In addition to the major adult fraction hemoglobin A, there are minor fractions called *hemoglobin A1* and *A2*, and the A1 fraction can be further separated into A1a, A1b, and A1c. It turns out that the A1c fraction is the one that contains most of the glucose and hence most accurately represents the average level of BG for the past month or so.

When labs report results simply as *glycohemoglobin*, they are usually reporting the level of hemoglobin A1 (A1a +A1b + A1c). But the word *glycohemoglobin* means "hemoglobin with a sugar attached," so some people use it to refer to both the A1 and the A1c tests. If your results don't specify A1c, try to find out which test you had.

Today, almost all labs report their results as an A1c level. For the A1c, results are usually about 1 percentage point lower than the results of the A1 test, with a normal range usually given as about 4 to 6 percent. So if you had an A1 result of 7.6 percent and then had an A1c result of 6.6 percent, it would mean your control was about the same, just that you'd had a different test. (Some labs outside the United States may report these values as 0.06 instead of 6 percent. It means the same thing. And the results are often expressed without the percent sign: 6 means 6 percent.) Although the "normal" range for the A1c is usually given as 4 to 6 percent, some people consider a true normal A1c to be in the 4s. A person with an A1c of 5.8 or 5.9 is likely to be headed toward diabetes.

With both the plain vanilla glycohemoglobin test and the more specialized A1c, there are different methods to separate out the hemoglobin fractions, and they give slightly different results, so each result must be compared with the *normal range for that particular laboratory*, not the number viewed in isolation. In a lab that had a normal range of 4 to 6, an A1c of 6.5 would indicate good control but well above normal. The same A1c would be considered normal in a lab with a normal range of 4.5 to 6.6.

Thus you should never simply accept a number as a result of a glycohemoglobin or A1c test. **Always insist on knowing the normal range for your lab.** And don't be discouraged just because someone else has a lower test result than you do. Their laboratory might have a different normal range.

Labs today may also report the **estimated average glucose (eAG)** level. This means they use the A1c to calculate what they estimate to be your average BG level during the period covered by the A1c. Different groups use slightly different formulas to calculate the eAG, and you can find tools to calculate your eAG on the Internet.

If you are in Australia or the United Kingdom, your lab may report the A1c with different units, mmol/mol (millimols of A1c per mol of total hemoglobin). This is called the IFCC (International Federation of Clinical Chemistry) system. If you need to convert the numbers, the National Glycohemoglobin Standardization Program website has a conversion tool (www.ngsp.org/convert1.asp).

I discuss various factors that affect the glycohemoglobin and A1c tests in Appendix 1. For now, you should just understand that this test gives an estimate of the average BG level over the past few weeks or months. Although it is not usually considered diagnostic of diabetes by itself, it gives a good indication of how much your BG levels have been elevated and for how long. If your BG levels were elevated for months before you were diagnosed, your A1c will be high when you are diagnosed. People with type 1 diabetes, which can manifest quite quickly, may have normal A1c levels when they're diagnosed.

Fructosamine measures a shorter time period

Like the A1c, the **fructosamine test** measures the average level of glucose in your blood over an extended period of time, but the measured time period is shorter.

Instead of measuring the sugar attached to hemoglobin, the fructosamine test measures the amount of sugar attached to other proteins in the blood, primarily **albumin**. These proteins don't live as long as hemoglobin, so the test measures the average BG level over the past two weeks.

There are different tests for fructosamine, and different labs use different units in reporting the results, so again, make sure you find out what the normal range is at the lab you are using. This test is not routinely done, and a home meter that measured fructosamine has been discontinued.

Anhydroglucitol measures even shorter time periods

The compound 1,5-anhydroglucitol (AG) is normally present in **plasma** in stable amounts. But its concentration decreases when BG levels are high. The test for this compound measures BG levels over a short period of time, about forty-eight hours to two weeks.

This test has been used clinically in Japan for some years, and a company has started marketing it in the United States under the name Glycomark. Time will tell if this test becomes commonly used. Some physicians may not be familiar with it.

Note that unlike most other tests, the AG test results in a higher number with a lower BG level.

All the tests have limitations

As described in more detail in Appendix 1, all the tests for BG control have limitations. The A1c test assumes that your red blood cells live 120 days. If they don't, or if you have an unusual hemoglobin, the results may not be accurate. The fructosamine test assumes you have a normal amount of the protein albumin in your blood. The AG test assumes your renal threshold for glucose is normal (see discussion of urine tests later in this section), but the threshold often changes with age and other conditions.

In an ideal world, we'd all have all these tests regularly. In the real world, your doctor is most likely to use the A1c test, at least in the near future, and use one of the other tests only if the A1c results don't seem to agree with your home BG testing.

Glucose tolerance test is used for gestational diabetes

Occasionally, and especially when physicians are diagnosing **gestational diabetes**, the kind that is precipitated by the stress of pregnancy and then usually goes away after the baby is born, you may be given what is called a **glucose tolerance test (GTT)**.

In this test your fasting BG level is measured and then you are given a huge dose of glucose solution and your BG levels are measured every so often for several hours. This is because some people in the early stages of diabetes are able to keep their fasting BG levels in the normal range, but they can't keep them normal after meals. This intermediate state between normal BG control and overt diabetes is called **prediabetes** (formerly **impaired glucose tolerance**).

In most cases, however, by the time you or your doctor has begun to suspect that you might be diabetic, your disease has progressed beyond this point, and most doctors no longer do the GTT except in special circumstances, for example, testing for gestational diabetes.

Urine tests are also useful

Glucose in urine means diabetes. Sometimes your diabetes may be diagnosed on the basis of a routine urine test. This is because your kidneys are very clever, and when the BG level gets too high, usually about 180 mg/dL, the kidneys start extracting the extra glucose from the blood and excreting it in the urine, which becomes sweet. In ancient times, people noticed that the urine of some people attracted more flies than usual because of the extra sugar. And even in the recent past, dyers of indigo cloth who fermented the plant in a urine solution preferred the urine of diabetic people in their vats because the extra sugar resulted in a faster fermentation.

In fact, this is the reason for the name *diabetes mellitus* (sometimes abbreviated DM). The word *mellitus* means "honey sweetened" and distinguishes it from a form of diabetes called *diabetes insipidus*, in which the urine is extremely dilute and not particularly sweet. This form of diabetes is much less common and has a different cause than diabetes mellitus. Even today some people refer to diabetes mellitus as "sugar diabetes."

There are **dipsticks** that measure the glucose level of your urine. You dip the stick into a little urine and it changes color depending on the level of the glucose in the urine. If you enjoy messing around with chemistry sets, you can also buy tablets that you mix with a diluted sample of urine. The solution fizzes and then changes color if there's sugar in the urine, and you match the color of the solution with a chart provided with the kit.

In the bad old days, people with diabetes had no way of measuring their BG levels except for these tedious urine tests. But because it takes the kidneys a while to extract glucose from the blood, and because the bladder may then store the urine for several hours, urine tests can only measure how high your BG level was several hours before and are not useful in daily treatment now that we have ready access to BG meters.

Also, because the BG level has to exceed about 180 mg/dL before you begin to "spill" glucose into the urine (and sometimes the threshold can even exceed 180 mg/dL), urine tests are not a good method for detecting the minor BG elevations that are seen in the early stages of the disease. Nevertheless, they are cheap and painless ways to screen large populations for diabetes.

Ketones in urine mean you're burning fat. Another urine test you may have had is the test for *ketones*. Normally, cells use glucose as their main fuel. However, when glucose is scarce, the cells burn fat instead. Such a glucose scarcity may occur in starvation, if you are on a low-carbohydrate diet, or in the absence of effective insulin, that is, too little insulin or too much insulin resistance (IR). In the latter case, there may be plenty of glucose in the blood, but it can't get into the cells because the insulin doesn't work (in the analogy in Day 1, the soda machine is broken), so you don't have enough glucose transporters. Thus as far as the inside of the cell is concerned, there's a scarcity of glucose.

When the body is burning a lot of fat, it also produces products of fat breakdown called *ketone bodies,* often called just *ketones*. Some cells can use these ketones for energy, but there are usually more of them in the bloodstream than the cells can use, so the extra ketones—like the extra glucose in the blood when the BG level is high—are excreted in the urine. When the levels get extremely high, some of the ketones are converted to sweet-smelling substances that give the breath a fruity smell like banana.

Even small amounts of insulin can slow down the formation of ketones, and most people with type 2 diabetes still produce enough insulin to stop the production of a lot of ketones. So people with type 1 diabetes are more apt to spill ketones into the urine than people with type 2. Thus finding a lot of ketones on diagnosis might suggest to the doctor that you were type 1 and not type 2. However, because other factors such as eating very little carbohydrate or eating a lot of fat can also stimulate the metabolism of fat and the formation of ketones, finding ketones in the urine does not necessarily mean that you do not have type 2 diabetes.

Like the glucose dipsticks, ketone dipsticks can be used to test your urine for ketones at home. You can also buy double-duty dipsticks that test for both sugar and ketones on one strip. There are meters that will give a numerical value for blood ketone levels, just like a BG meter. And there is a gizmo called *Ketonix* that will estimate ketones from your breath. But this doesn't give a number, and the relation between ketones in your breath and those in blood and urine is not exact.

Protein in urine means your kidneys are damaged. Healthy kidneys keep protein out of the urine (see Month 10 for a more detailed discussion of kidney function). When your kidneys are damaged, they begin to let blood proteins leak into your urine.

The most accurate test for this is what is called a *twenty-four-hour microalbumin test*. In this test, you collect all your urine for twenty-four hours, and the urine is then tested for the presence of the protein *albumin*. This test allows the doctor to quantify exactly how much albumin you are excreting every day.

There are also simpler but less accurate tests. A standard dipstick test will detect a lot of protein in the urine, but by the time this amount of protein is detected, the kidney damage has progressed to the point that it's not apt to be reversed. A special dipstick will detect microalbumin levels. A test for albumin in a random sample of urine (not a twenty-four-hour collection) will detect smaller amounts of protein (earlier stage of kidney damage) than the standard dipstick but is not as accurate as the twenty-four-hour test.

Strenuous exercise can increase the protein level in your urine, so one positive test is not conclusive for kidney disease.

Kidney function can also be estimated by testing for other substances. One of these is called *creatinine*. It is a normal waste product of your muscles, and thus its level in your blood is proportional to your total muscle mass. A muscular man has more creatinine than a small woman.

The creatinine is normally removed by the kidneys. When your kidneys are damaged, the creatinine isn't removed, the creatinine level in your blood increases, and the level in your urine decreases. So sometimes you are tested for creatinine levels in both your blood and a twenty-four-hour urine sample and your *creatinine clearance rate* is determined.

The creatinine clearance rate can be estimated using only the serum creatinine level and a formula that corrects for your weight (larger people produce more creatinine), your age (even normal kidneys decline in function with age), your sex (men have higher levels than women), and your race (blacks have higher levels than whites). If you have a computer and Internet access, you can find online calculators that will estimate your creatinine clearance rate. Open your favorite search engine and search on "creatinine clearance rate calculator."

Another test for microalbuminuria measures the amount of both albumin and creatinine in the urine. Depending on how much liquid you've been drinking, your urine can be very dilute (clear and pale yellow) or very concentrated (very dark yellow). If you excrete a constant *amount* of a substance like creatinine, the *concentration* of that substance will change when the urine is more or less concentrated.

Hence, a high concentration of albumin in the urine could mean that your kidney function is impaired, or it could simply mean that you are dehydrated and your urine is very concentrated.

The *amount* of creatinine you excrete tends to be constant throughout the day, so it can be used as a measure of how concentrated the urine is. Calculating the ratio of albumin to the amount of creatinine in your urine is a way to get a more accurate estimation of the amount of albumin you're spilling in your urine every day and is almost as accurate as the twenty-four-hour microalbumin test.

Another substance that can estimate kidney function is the level of urea in your blood, expressed as *blood urea nitrogen (BUN)*. Urea is a waste product from the normal turnover of protein in your body. Like creatinine, BUN is usually removed by the kidneys, and blood levels increase when your kidneys are damaged. However, BUN levels also increase when your liver is breaking down a lot of protein and can be elevated when you are dehydrated; are on a high-protein diet; are starving or your insulin levels are low, which causes your body to break down its muscle proteins for energy; have fever; have internal bleeding; or are on some drugs. BUN levels can be low with liver disease, a low-protein diet, or excessive urination.

Thus doctors often measure several different markers of kidney problems before concluding that your kidneys are damaged.

C-peptide test tells how much insulin you're making

A test that is not often ordered as a routine part of diabetes diagnosis is called the **C-peptide test**. This test can help determine whether you have type 1 or type 2 diabetes and approximately how much IR you have.

The simple explanation of this test is that it gives an idea of how much insulin you are producing. This is because when insulin is synthesized in your pancreas, it is produced as a large protein called *proinsulin*. Before it is secreted into the bloodstream, it is snipped into two smaller protein molecules called *insulin* and *C-peptide* (C stands for "connecting"). For every molecule of insulin that you produce, you also produce one molecule of C-peptide. Insulin doesn't last long in your blood because it's quickly taken up by the liver. The C-peptide hangs around longer. Also, insulin tests are not accurate in anyone who is injecting insulin. For these reasons, the C-peptide test is used as an indirect way of finding out how much insulin your pancreas is producing.

As with the A1c test, the normal C-peptide ranges differ slightly from laboratory to laboratory, and different labs may use different units to express the results. At one laboratory they range from 0.5 to 1.5 picomols per liter (pmol/L). If you tested 0.3 pmol/L at this lab, it would mean you weren't producing a lot of insulin and probably had type 1 diabetes. If you tested 4 pmol/L, it would mean you had a lot of IR (you needed to produce extra insulin to achieve the same effect as someone without IR could achieve with insulin levels in the normal range; in the analogy in Day 1, you would need to put extra money into the soda machine to get out the same amount of soda).

Some physicians don't order C-peptide tests because they would treat the disease the same regardless of the results. If your doctor doesn't mention the test, ask about it. I'll discuss the reasons for wanting to know your C-peptide results in Week 4. For now, you should just be aware that such a test exists.

Anti-islet cell antibodies tell if you have type 1 diabetes

If your doctor thinks there's a possibility that you might, in fact, have type 1 diabetes, there are a few specialized tests that you might have done. In most cases, type 1 diabetes is what is called an *autoimmune disease*. Normally, the immune system of the body attacks any foreign invaders but leaves its own cells alone. Sometimes, for example in rheumatoid arthritis, rheumatic fever, and type 1 diabetes, something goes wrong and the immune system starts destroying the cells of its own body.

In the case of type 1 diabetes, the immune system attacks the *beta cells* in the pancreas that produce insulin, eventually destroying them almost completely. Scientists are beginning to learn which particular molecules in the pancreas are the targets for the immune system, and they can test for the **autoantibodies** (**antibodies** against an organism's own tissues) that produce this damage.

As a group, these antibodies are called *anti-islet cell antibodies*, because the beta cells are one type of cell found in structures called the *islets of Langerhans* in the pancreas, or **islet cells** for short. Many of the tests for these antibodies are done only in research centers. There are several antibodies that can be tested for. The most common one is called *anti-GAD* (glutamic acid decarboxylase). Don't worry about what the name means. The important thing is to understand what the test results mean. A person with type 2 diabetes almost never tests positive for anti-GAD antibodies. People with type 1 diabetes test positive for the anti-GAD antibodies about 80 percent of the time. So a negative test means you *probably* don't have type 1 diabetes but doesn't prove it. A positive test means you *probably* have type 1 diabetes but again is not proof.

As type 1 diabetes progresses and most of the beta cells are destroyed, the anti-GAD antibodies often disappear. So if it is done at all, an anti-GAD test should be done as soon as possible after diabetes is suspected.

Other tests may be important too

Your doctor may also order a battery of other tests, for example, tests for *cholesterol* and other *lipid* levels (see Month 6) or tests for thyroid function. These tests aren't specific for diabetes but they provide important information about your general health.

When you have any of the lab tests described here, refer back to this section to see what they mean. If you have questions, make sure your doctor explains. Worrying about a slightly abnormal lab test is stressful, and there may be a simple explanation for an out-of-range test.

IN A SENTENCE:

▪ *Learning how to interpret your lab tests is an important step toward taking charge of your diabetes.*

Will Diabetes
Disable Me?

Most people have heard about some of the serious complications that can result from years of high blood glucose (BG)
levels. The main complications are what I think of as the
Three O'Pathy Sisters—**neuropathy** (damage to the nerves),
nephropathy (damage to the kidneys), and **retinopathy**
(damage to the retina of the eye)—and their backup band
led by Arthur O. Sclerosis—**atherosclerosis**, which can
lead to heart attacks, strokes, and open wounds on the feet
and legs.

The Three O'Pathy Sisters are often grouped together as
microvascular complications, meaning they result from damage to small blood vessels. The results of atherosclerosis are
usually referred to as **macrovascular** complications, meaning
that they involve the larger blood vessels in the body.

Unfortunately, these complications are no joke; they are
real and serious. You should be aware of their symptoms, make
sure you are tested for their presence, and, most important,
*keep your BG levels as close to normal as possible so these com-
plications never occur.*

Landmark study showed that good control matters

People used to think that complications of diabetes were inevitable, that it didn't make much difference whether you kept your BG levels near normal or not. In fact, some health-care professionals preferred that their patients kept their BG levels elevated above normal, because doing so reduced the chances of low BG levels that can cause people to pass out.

Then in 1993, a ten-year study of "normal" versus "tight" BG control in 1,441 relatively young people with type 1 diabetes was reported. Normal control was what health-care professionals had been recommending for their patients: hemoglobin A1c values averaging 8.9, where normal was anything under 6. Tight control meant aiming for lower BG levels by injecting insulin more often; these patients had A1c values averaging 7.2, still above the normal limits.

This trial, called the **Diabetes Control and Complications Trial**, usually referred to as the **DCCT**, showed beyond a doubt that people with tight control of their BG levels had significantly fewer microvascular complications (decreases ranging from 35 to 76 percent) than those on the normal treatment regimens that allowed their BG levels to go higher.

Later, in Japan, a similar effect was shown in 110 people with type 2 diabetes. And in 1998, the results of a twenty-year study in England (the **UK Prospective Diabetes Study**, or **UKPDS**) showed that microvascular complication rates in more than five thousand people with type 2 diabetes decreased when BG levels were kept lower. Lowering blood pressure to 144/82 also reduced both micro- and macrovascular complication rates.

After the DCCT was concluded, researchers conducted a follow-up study of the participants, called the Epidemiology of Diabetes Interventions and Complications (EDIC). The results were surprising. At the conclusion of the DCCT, those in the "conventional treatment" group were taught how to get better control, and eventually both groups ended up with very similar A1c's, close to 8.

Despite the eventual similarity in A1c's, however, the original "tight control" group continued to have significantly lower rates of all microvascular complications, as they had during the DCCT. They also had lower rates of atherosclerosis (see Month 6). Cardiovascular complications (heart attacks and strokes) could not be measured in the DCCT because the participants were relatively young and the number of cardiovascular events was too low to analyze.

Thus the mean of 6.5 years of good diabetes control was able to lower all complication rates even 10 years after the DCCT was concluded.

If those studies don't convince you, recent studies have shown that **even in people who don't have diabetes, the lower the average BG levels, the lower the rates of cardiovascular events** (heart attacks and strokes).

What all these studies mean is that yes, these complications exist. If you let your BG levels stay high for a long period of time, it is very likely you will develop some or all of these complications (Table 2). The good news is that these frightening complications are not inevitable. **Keeping your BG levels normal may mean that you will never develop any complications at all.**

TABLE 2
PERCENTAGE CUMULATIVE RISK OF FIRST-TIME
THREE-STEP PROGRESSION OF RETINOPATHY

| | A1c | | | | | | |
Yr	6	7	8	9	10	11	12
2	1.25	1.28	1.72	2.58	3.16	4.54	6.22
3	1.33	1.69	3.15	4.70	7.18	11.52	16.54
4	1.41	2.09	4.11	6.69	11.26	18.14	26.82
5	1.49	2.52	5.25	9.19	16.37	27.03	40.57
6	1.58	3.05	6.64	12.30	22.68	38.53	57.67
7	1.66	3.64	8.47	16.19	30.80	52.87	76.48
8	1.76	4.14	10.42	21.22	41.07	69.14	91.33
9	1.85	4.61	12.87	27.98	53.36	85.26	100.00
10	1.95	5.33	15.99	35.79	67.08	96.50	
11	2.04	6.24	19.37	44.57	81.10	100.00	
12	2.15	7.14	23.44	54.86	92.6		
13	2.25	8.15	28.17	66.12	100.00		
14	2.36	9.28	33.63	77.73			
15	2.47	10.53	39.85	88.69			

Calculated by the late Ron Sebol on the basis of published graphs.

Fern H., who has been working incredibly hard to keep her BG levels in the normal range, has had diabetes for almost five years and has no signs of complications at all. She described her friend Dewitt, "the Bowling Club guy who was diagnosed at the same time I was. He's in terrible shape. Neuropathy, retinopathy, and now his hair is falling out. He's the one who wouldn't give up his sausage pizza or desserts for anything. He'll have a piece of every dessert at the VFW Christmas Party even if he has to hobble to the dessert table."

The sacrifices are worth it

Keeping your BG levels down will not be easy. I know. I've been there. But I think the sacrifices are worth it.

If you're tempted to eat a big slice of thick chocolate cake with super-sweet icing, ask yourself, "Which is more important to me? About thirty seconds of pleasure from this sweet dessert or having good enough vision in ten years so that I can see my first grandchild celebrate her first birthday?"

If the guys are going out for pizza and beer and you know pizza and beer make your BG levels go sky-high, ask yourself, "Which would I rather do? Have pizza and beer with the guys or order grilled chicken so I won't have to spend the day in the dialysis center when my son is getting his PhD from Harvard?"

As Sophie C. said, "I still miss my old habits of eating massive quantities of whatever tasted good, but not as much as I would miss spending time with my husband instead of pushing up daisies!"

Could any piece of cheesecake taste so good that it's worth the risk of having a stroke in a few years? Well, OK, yes, there are times it probably might. No one is perfect. Being diabetic doesn't mean you have to totally give up all these treats forever. The trick is to **remember the stakes and limit the damage** from the occasional dietary indiscretions.

How many times have you been on a diet, blown the diet with a small lapse, and then figured, "Oh, what the heck. I had one taste of blueberry pie so I've blown the diet. Might as well eat the whole thing, with whipped cream. Tomorrow I'll be really, really good."

That logic doesn't work when you're diabetic. **Smaller indiscretions mean smaller increases in BG levels.** If the temptation is overwhelming, there's no need to eat a whole pie. Have a taste instead.

It's too bad to have to use a negative motivation—fear—to stick with your program. But let's face it: fear is a powerful motivator. You have probably been trying other motivations for getting into better shape for years, and they haven't worked. Now you've got diabetes. This is different. This is serious. It's not a question of starting on a healthy diet next week, or maybe next month, or three months from now when Christmas is over. We have the evidence now. The longer your BG stays high, the greater the chance that you will develop some complications.

You may have had diabetes without knowing it

One thing to remember is that it usually takes about ten years of high BG levels before the complications begin to manifest themselves. "Oh, good," you may think. "No need to start on my new healthy lifestyle right away."

Unfortunately, you may have had high BG levels, especially after meals, for many years before being diagnosed. One reason for this is that the blood tests that are often done during regular physical exams usually measure only fasting BG levels, not how high they go after meals. Many people who develop type 2 diabetes have years of normal fasting BG levels and high BG levels after carbohydrate-containing meals, or *prediabetes* (formerly called *impaired glucose tolerance*).

Another reason is that some doctors who were trained in the old days, when it was felt that slightly elevated BG levels were no big deal, may have noticed your fasting BG levels going up every year but didn't bother to tell you because they thought your diabetes wasn't "serious" enough to be treated, or that because of employer prejudices and potential insurance problems, you wouldn't want to be labeled *diabetic* before such a label was absolutely necessary.

Some doctors used to tell their early type 2 patients that they had "a touch of diabetes" or say, "Your blood sugar is a little high; you should watch your sugar" and left it at that. Or they might have said, "You have a little diabetes. Here, take this pill and that will fix it," so you went home and took your pill and kept on eating what you'd always eaten and exercising as much as you'd always exercised, meaning as little as possible.

Also, not everyone has regular physical exams with lab tests, either for financial reasons or because they simply don't like going to see a doctor.

For whatever reason, because of this delay in treatment, you may have developed early diabetic complications even before you were officially diagnosed. This is even scarier than worrying about something that might happen to you in five or ten years.

Early complications can often be reversed

The good news is that bringing your BG levels close to normal can actually reverse some of the microvascular complications of diabetes such as tingling or pain in the feet or early signs of kidney disease. Obviously, if you've already had a heart attack or a stroke, controlling your BG levels can't reverse that fact, but it can lessen the chance that it will occur again.

If you can keep your BG levels as close to normal as possible, the chances that you will be disabled from the complications of diabetes are small. They are, however, real. There are no guarantees. There is no threshold BG level below which you can be assured of never getting complications. A tendency to having complications seems to be genetic, and some ethnic groups have higher complications rates than others (see Month 10). Even a 1 percent risk is small but real. You should never forget the dangers of high BG levels, but you should also not be frightened.

You may remember a diabetic grandmother who was blind and in a wheelchair when she died, and this memory may frighten you so much that you can't focus on learning how to take charge of your own diabetes. Or maybe, remembering her, you think her fate is inevitable, and it's so hopeless you might as well give up trying to control your BG levels and just enjoy life for the few years you've got left.

Keep in mind that things have changed a lot since your grandmother, or your father, or your great-uncle had diabetes. They probably had their BG levels measured once a year, if that, and tried to "watch their sugar" but otherwise ate pretty much as they always had.

Technology for people with diabetes has changed a lot in the past years, and it will change even more in the future. Treatment options have also expanded several-fold. Only a decade or so ago, doctors had a choice of either insulin or one type of drug for their patients with type 2 diabetes. There are so many treatment options for type 2 diabetes available today that if you are willing to stick to whatever treatment works best for you, the probability that you will be disabled is very small.

It's not easy, but the results are worth the effort.

IN A SENTENCE:

▪ *Keeping your blood glucose levels as close to the normal range as possible reduces the chances that you will ever develop diabetic complications.*

Frequently
Asked Questions

Most people have the same questions when starting out. These are the ones that are asked most frequently.

What are normal blood glucose levels?

Normal fasting blood glucose (BG) levels are usually considered to be between about 70 and 100 mg/dL (milligrams per deciliter). After meals, nondiabetic people can peak as high as 140 mg/dL, although lower increases from about 80 to about 110 or 120 are more common. The amount of the increase depends on the type of food eaten and each person's physiological response. After a small meal that didn't contain a lot of processed carbohydrate, the BG level might stay below 100. After cotton candy on an empty stomach, it might go up to 140. BG levels in people without diabetes usually return to their starting levels within a few hours.

"I cannot get my BG over 120 mg/dL no matter what I eat, or when I test," said Jim D. "And it is at that high for only a few minutes, before plunging. Even getting it over 100 is rare, and takes a *lot* of sugar. Any slower carb, and I will not leave the 90s, no matter what the quantity."

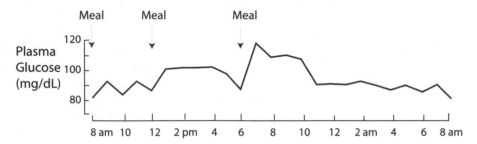

FIGURE 1. Blood glucose (BG) levels in a nondiabetic person over a twenty-four-hour period. Notice how the increase in BG levels and the time it takes to return to the starting point vary with different meals, larger meals having higher peaks that take longer to come down again. This nondiabetic person took almost five hours to come down to 90 mg/dL after lunch and supper.

The peak BG level also depends on how low the BG level is when a person eats. A person who starts with a BG level of 70 mg/dL can increase 30 points and end up around 100. Someone who started at 99 (near the top of the normal fasting level) would obviously end up higher with the same 30-point increase.

Figure 1 shows how the BG level of a nondiabetic person might vary throughout the day. People who have tested their friends with their home meters say that some never go over 90 mg/dL, even after huge carbohydrate-containing meals. Children tend to have smaller BG excursions than older people.

I was told to test two hours after the meal. Does that mean two hours after I start eating or after I finish eating?

If you gulp your whole meal in five minutes, it doesn't make much difference. Most people take a little longer, and if you always spend the same amount of time on a meal, it doesn't matter much either, as long as you're consistent. What you're looking for here is some way of comparing your control from one day to the next, so you don't want to test two hours after starting a meal on Monday and two hours after finishing a meal on Tuesday.

Because most people spend different amounts of time eating from day to day, it's easier to calculate the time after you *started* to eat. If you're told to keep your BG level under a certain value "after meals," this usually means two hours after the meal has started.

My vision is blurry. Does this mean I'm going to lose my sight?

Most people have heard that diabetes sometimes causes blindness, and it does. This blindness is called *retinopathy* and involves the retina of the eye. I'll discuss it in more detail in Month 10. It usually, although not always, occurs after many years of high BG levels.

There is another effect of BG levels on the eyes, however, and this effect is temporary. When the BG levels in your blood are high, the increased *osmotic pressure* causes the fluid levels in the lens of the eye to change. Changes in the fluid levels change the refractive index of the lens, and this causes visual changes, usually increased myopia (nearsightedness).

If your diabetes has been progressing very slowly for many years, your eyes may have been changing very slowly as well, and you may not have noticed the changes. Or it may have happened fairly quickly, causing you to complain of "blurry" vision and having your glasses changed frequently.

Once your diabetes is diagnosed and your BG levels start falling, the fluid levels in your eyes start to change again, and you start becoming more farsighted (hyperopic). Then if you can finally stabilize your BG levels at near-normal levels, the eyes will adjust to that level, and your vision will revert to what it should have been in the first place.

If your BG levels continue to roller-coaster from high to low during the day, you may continue to see fluctuating vision during the course of the day. Some people find that their vision changes about twelve hours after an episode of high BG levels. This is another reason to try to normalize your BG levels as much as possible; it's no fun when you can't see well.

If you do have vision changes after you're diagnosed, don't rush to the eye doctor for new glasses. There's no point in wasting money on a new pair of glasses that won't last.

When I was diagnosed with BG levels in the 400s, I had become quite myopic, meaning I could see quite well up close, but I needed glasses to distinguish a sheep in my pasture from a white rock. After I brought my BG levels down toward normal, I became farsighted. I could now see the mountains across the road quite well without glasses, but I couldn't see a person sitting at the other side of the kitchen table without wearing what used to be my reading glasses. This period of farsightedness seemed to peak at about two weeks, and then I started to revert to my "normal" state of slight myopia.

Just remember that these changes are usually temporary and are not damaging to your eyes. You are not going blind.

The real problem is how to see well enough to do things like driving and working for the month or so while these changes are going on. I bought a pair of cheap discount store glasses that I took out of their frames and pasted over my distance glasses with cellophane tape, because I needed the astigmatism correction in my prescription glasses. It looked a bit odd, but I'm not vain about my appearance, and it worked for me.

In a work situation in which you need to look fashionable, maybe a pair of cheap glasses alone might work for you. If your vision changes are not great, you might be able to get along with your old glasses, or with no glasses at all. You might also contact the groups who collect used glasses to donate to charity and see if they would loan or rent you a pair that would work well enough to get by.

Why is my blood sugar higher in the morning than when I went to bed?

This comes as a big surprise to almost everyone. I remember the first time it happened to me. I measured my BG level before going to bed. It had come down from a high number earlier in the day, and without eating all night I figured it would be even lower the next morning, just as one expects to weigh less in the morning if one hasn't eaten anything since dinner. It's logical, right?

The next morning, I eagerly got up, zapped my finger, put the blood on the strip, and waited. The reading was twenty points higher than it had been the evening before. Huh? I was puzzled. Was my meter broken? It turns out this is a common phenomenon that is referred to formally by those who are not intimately acquainted with it as the **dawn phenomenon**. Those who know it only too well often call it the **dawn effect**.

Maintaining your BG level in a rather narrow range is a very complicated process that involves various hormones that interact with various organs in the body. The two big players are *insulin* and **glucagon**, and it's the ratio of these two important protein hormones that determines whether your BG levels will go up or down. Insulin makes the BG level go down so that you don't go high (when everything is working perfectly, which it isn't when you have diabetes), and glucagon makes the BG level go up so that you don't go too low and pass out. When I say "you don't go too high or low," what I mean, of course, is "your BG level doesn't go too high or low."

The rising BG levels after a meal make the pancreas produce insulin, which brings the BG level down again. As you sleep at night without eating, the falling BG levels make the pancreas produce glucagon, which brings the BG level back up again.

But sometime in the early morning hours, levels of other hormones such as **cortisol** and **growth hormone** begin to increase. Some of these hormones, called *insulin antagonists*, or **counterregulatory hormones**, seem to make the insulin less effective. Some people also think that the liver clears the blood of more insulin in the morning. For our purposes, the mechanism doesn't really matter. The important thing is the net result: a sort of temporary morning insulin resistance.

In nondiabetic people, who also have a dawn effect, this might make the BG level increase slightly, which might help the person wake up and have enough energy to get started with the day's work. If the BG level went up too much, a nondiabetic person would quickly secrete a burst of insulin to bring it back down.

If you have diabetes, however, and produce less insulin than usual to begin with, you can't quickly secrete more insulin if the BG level goes too high, so the BG levels are often considerably higher in the morning, and eating carbohydrate for breakfast seems to increase the BG level even more than it does later in the day.

Some people find that they have a real "dawn" effect, meaning that the BG level begins to rise around 3 or 4 A.M. and keeps going up all day until they have something to eat. (Yes, they *did* set the alarm for the wee hours to test for this.) But the continuing rise is not universal. Others find that if they don't eat anything at all, the BG level will increase in the morning for a few hours and then come back down again.

Some people find that the dawn effect is really more like a "getting up effect." In other words, if they measure at 5 or 6 A.M. and then go back to bed and measure again when they get up at 8 or 9 or even 11 A.M., the readings will be exactly the same. But once they get up and start moving around, no matter what the time, the BG level starts going up.

Some have wondered if "morning people" who leap out of bed eager to get going have a real dawn effect that gives them the extra energy to wake up quickly and "night people" who sit comatose for a long time before they are able to face the day have a "waking up effect." I don't know that anyone has ever studied this.

Remember the term YMMV (Your Mileage May Vary). We are all different and often react in different ways. If your dawn effect doesn't follow the textbook pattern, don't worry about it. Just understand that some kind of dawn effect is normal, and keep testing until you understand how yours usually works. Then you can design your menu choices around your particular dawn effect.

Many books on diabetes discuss another supposed cause of increased BG levels in the morning. This is the *Somogyi phenomenon*. The Somogyi phenomenon is a rebound from episodes of low BG levels; the body overcompensates, and if the lows occur during the night, the morning readings are too high. The way to distinguish this from the dawn effect is to measure your BG level at 3 A.M. If it's low and the morning BG reading is high, you might have the Somogyi phenomenon.

However, some people are now beginning to question the importance of the Somogyi phenomenon in causing high morning BG levels. If it does happen, it occurs mostly in people with type 1 diabetes, and even then, not very often. I mention it only because you'll come across the term if you read about diabetes, and you might wonder what it is.

Will exercise always make my blood glucose levels go down?

The effects of exercise on BG levels are confusing. In the long run, exercise is extremely important in helping you control your diabetes. But sometimes exercise makes your BG levels increase temporarily.

When you start to exercise, your body senses that you are going to need more energy than usual. So if your BG level is normal or slightly low, the liver will quickly pump more glucose into the blood to send to the muscles, and the BG level will temporarily rise.

In a nondiabetic person, the increased BG level will trigger a fast release of insulin, and the muscles will quickly take up the glucose, so the BG level won't go up very much. But if you're diabetic, you can't release a lot of insulin or the insulin won't be as effective, so your BG level may go up a lot when you start to exercise.

However, if your BG level is high when you start to exercise, your liver will sense that you probably won't need a lot more glucose than is already there, and it won't pump any more glucose into the blood. In addition, when you exercise, whatever insulin you have in your system becomes more effective. So if you start exercising with a high BG level, you'll also have a high insulin level, and you'll usually find that exercise brings your BG level down faster than usual.

If you start exercising when you have almost no insulin in your system, for example, first thing in the morning, that tiny bit of insulin can't do much even if it is more effective. Twice zero is still zero. So exercise first thing in the morning may make your BG level go up.

One trick that works with some people is to eat a little bit of carbohydrate before you exercise. About thirty or forty-five minutes before your workout seems to be best. This has two effects. First, it makes your BG level go up so the liver doesn't worry about not having enough glucose to send to the muscles and doesn't pump more into the blood. Second, the increased BG level stimulates the production of at least some insulin. The exercise makes the insulin more effective, and this helps to bring the BG level down.

Even if this method doesn't work for you in the short run, the exercise will help you in the long run, as the muscles will continue to take up glucose for hours after you have done your exercise. In addition, exercise makes more muscle, and muscle is what burns a lot of the glucose in your blood.

I'll discuss exercise in more detail in Month 8. For now, just understand that it's not unusual to see your BG level increase after an exercise session.

IN A SENTENCE:

■ *Most people have the same questions at first, so don't ever think your questions aren't worth asking.*

living

Breaking Bread

In almost every culture in the world, sharing food with other people is a way of bonding. Serving food to guests, even strangers, is sometimes considered an obligatory part of the social exchange. Not to accept it is considered rude.

Every celebration has special foods, often specially rich and sweet ones. They not only taste good, but eating them reminds us of similar celebrations in past years, connecting us with our youth and with those who are no longer here to share those special foods with us.

When you are on a strict diet that doesn't permit most of the special celebratory foods and even restricts the most common everyday fare, you face an immense challenge. How can you maintain your social connections without compromising your diabetes care?

As with so much of diabetes control, the answer is, it's not easy, but it's possible.

Eating at home is the first challenge

The first challenge is dealing with eating at home. You may live alone, in which case it's relatively simple to toss out all those

tempting cream-filled pastries and candies that you are no longer supposed to eat. Revising all your favorite recipes to use only the foods on
your diet is not easy, but it is probably easier than it is for someone who
has to eat a hunk of lettuce seasoned with lemon juice while the rest of
the family chows down on aromatic pizza or fry bread, smacking their lips
and commenting on how wonderful it all tastes.

Having to eat with nondiabetic family members is especially difficult at
first. "I have to leave the room every time Chet eats an orange," said Barbara F., who had just started a low-carbohydrate diet that didn't include
fruit. "I want it so much, and the smell drives me crazy."

If you're not the cook in your family, you'll have to educate the cook as
well as yourself. Ideally, the whole family will help you stick to your diet
plan by joining you in your new, healthier way of eating. But life is often
not ideal, and family members may not be willing to make such changes
in their diet for another family member. "Why should I give up mashed
potatoes and gravy just because Dad is sick?"

Cooking for others might mean constant temptation

If you *are* the cook, the temptations may be even greater. On the one
hand, you will have more control over what foods you serve to the family.
You may be able to wean them gradually away from the least healthy
foods, serving less and less of them and slowly substituting more and
more of the healthier things that you can eat. They may not even notice
the changes if they are gradual. Or they may discover that they actually
prefer some of those nicely spiced high-fiber vegetable dishes you're
learning to serve instead of mashed starch with thickened grease sauce.
Maybe some nondiabetic family members will lose some weight without
realizing what's going on. You may even help prevent them from developing diabetes in the future.

On the other hand, if your family simply refuses to eat "rabbit food" and
insists on macaroni and cheese or breaded deep-fat-fried pork balls in cream
gravy followed by fudge brownies every night, you'll have to fix all this forbidden stuff and smell it and feel it and lick the edges of the batter bowl
without realizing what you're doing because that's what you've always done.
It means facing temptation, and being reminded of your deprivations, at
least three times a day for 365 days a year. This is not an easy thing to do,
and it's one reason networking with other people who are going through the
same thing and sharing tips for overcoming these temptations is beneficial.

Take-out food is often not healthy

If everyone in the family works and you've always relied on take-out food, you've got another difficult problem. Most take-out food is high in processed carbohydrate and saturated fat, two things that are bad for diabetes control no matter what kind of a diet you're on. In this case, you'll have to either look for take-out places that serve at least one dish that works with your diet or else make up your own individual meals on the weekend, freezing them for future use.

You may be tempted by supermarket low-fat frozen dinners that are supposed to be "heart healthy." Read the ingredients carefully. Many of these dinners do have less fat than other convenience foods, but they usually substitute those fat calories with highly processed carbohydrates that raise your blood glucose (BG) levels quickly. Quite often the calorie and fat count are low because the portions are tiny, and they often leave you hungry. You're better off eating larger portions of dishes made with home-prepared fresh vegetables that are full of fiber and will fill you up.

Institutional food may not offer choices

If you live in an assisted-living facility or a nursing home where a dietician decides what a "diabetic diet" should be, you may not have much control over what you eat. It would still be good if you could learn as much as you can about how various foods affect *you*. If their diabetic menu isn't working for you, see if the dietician will work with you to come up with better choices.

Eating out means new challenges

Eating at home is difficult enough. Eating out is even more difficult because you are surrounded by enticing sights and smells and specialties of the house and extra-rich party desserts. It will take a long time before you become accustomed to saying no to such alluring fare, but it really does become easier the longer you've lived with diabetes.

When you're invited out to dinner, one thing that helps is to eat something beforehand, not enough that you're stuffed but enough to make it easier to say no. Then if the hosts have food that you can eat, you can enjoy a little. If there's nothing you can eat, you won't be ravenous.

Another thing that helps is to remember that the main point of a social gathering is to socialize, not to stuff oneself with free food, although the evidence at some wingdings seems to contradict that theory. If you're not distracted trying to figure out how you can dump Mrs. Ennui and race to the dessert table for a second piece of chocolate cheesecake before it's all gone, you can enjoy the conversations a lot more.

When you join your friends at a potluck supper or a restaurant meal or just eat in the cafeteria at work, you not only have to find foods you can eat, but you also have to avoid insulting your friends and colleagues by refusing their offerings when you shouldn't eat them.

One challenge facing anyone on any kind of diet is the inconsiderate "friend" who keeps urging you to try some treat you know is not good for you: "Oh, come on. One bite won't hurt you." It helps if you decide ahead of time how you're going to respond to this.

What works for me is simply to say, "No, thank you." If they ask again, I say, "No, thank you" again. If several repetitions don't turn them off, I'll say, "I'm diabetic, and I can't eat that food." That usually stops the urging, but if I get the "one little bite" plea again, I'll say, "If I ate one bite, I'd eat the whole plate of cookies. And if I eat the whole plate of cookies, it would increase the chances that I would go blind someday." Anyone who persists after a refusal like that doesn't deserve to be dealt with.

Jennifer L. has another approach: "When it comes to diabetes, I discovered that I had to change *can't* to *don't* in my thinking and speaking. 'I *can't* eat pasta' means 'Poor me, someone or something is not allowing me to eat pasta.' I have no choice. It's beyond my control (which also means that sometimes if I do eat pasta, then it's a 'cheat' and there is the ensuing guilt and shame for being a bad diabetic).

"'I *don't* eat pasta' means that I have made a choice. I am in control (which also means that sometimes if I do eat pasta, I have just decided at that moment to make a different choice, no guilt; it's just my decision at that moment).

"A bonus to this way of thinking and talking is when you are out and about and someone offers you something you would rather not eat at the moment, *don't* works better than *can't* to get them to understand. If you tell them you can't have ice cream, they will tell you that you can, that just a little won't hurt. If you tell them you don't eat ice cream, what are they going to say? 'Yes you do'? And if they say, 'Well you used to,' you can always say 'I don't anymore.' "

Eating at work can be tricky

If you don't want your colleagues at work to know you're diabetic, you've got a special challenge. What can you do when Baxley, who loves to bake, brings in freshly baked coffee cake for morning break every day? Or how about those Danish pastries they pass around at staff meetings? Or the going-away parties that always feature home-baked treats?

As mentioned in Day 3, if you're overweight you can always announce that you've decided to stick to a strict weight-loss diet, which is usually true. If you're not, you can say you've learned you are allergic to wheat or you've decided to give up white sugar, or white flour, or your dentist told you to avoid sweets as much as possible.

Any of these strategies can backfire when thoughtful Baxley brings in gluten-free pastries or honey-sweetened Danish made with whole wheat. In that case, the only thing you can do is take one and break your diet or just eat a little bit, saying you're saving the rest for later and then give it to someone else.

Learning how to say no to those delicacies when you're so ravenous that even boiled cardboard would tempt you is more difficult. If possible, bring your own snack food so you can be absorbed in eating it when Baxley wheels out the coffee break array. One trick is to bring something that takes a long time to chew. Then you'll still be chomping away when everyone else has gobbled down their pastries, and you may not feel quite so deprived.

Bring something you can eat to potluck suppers

Eating at potluck suppers is always a challenge because most people bring foods that are high in starch and fat. I once went to a potluck supper at which the only dishes were sixteen different varieties of macaroni. If you bring something you can eat, make sure you're first in the dinner line. Otherwise, your dish may be all gone by the time you get to the table.

If you've eaten a little something ahead of time, it won't be a tragedy if there's only noodles swimming in grease by the time you get to the table. You can put a little on your plate and not eat any, and most people will be concentrating so hard on their own plates that they won't even notice.

Eating at restaurants lets you choose

Eating at restaurants has the advantage that you can usually choose what you order. If you need to have a lot of business meals, you'll, of course, face the same challenges as you do with the office coffee breaks. If your best client wants to eat at the House of Fat, where everything is served in a bowl of melted butter, or insists that everyone try the breaded Sweet and Sour Boar at the new Asian place where the cooks are all retired sumo wrestlers and the portion sizes are just as large, you may feel silly ordering grilled chicken with a salad instead. But "I'm watching my cholesterol" is always a good explanation if you don't want your clients to know about your diabetes.

Sometimes appetizers and side dishes have less carbohydrate and fat than the main entrées, and by ordering two or even three appetizers instead of one main course, you can avoid the worst offenders to your diet. Just explain to the others that you enjoy trying different things and ask the waiter to bring the appetizers when bringing the entrées to the other diners. Depending on their personalities, your business associates may be impressed with your independence and ability to break the "rules."

When you don't need to disguise your diabetes, eating out is a bit easier, but it's still very difficult at first. When everyone else is trying some delectable new ethnic treat that isn't on your diet, or when they're all pigging out at the pizza parlor, it's hard to sit there with your lean turkey on fiber bread and watch them eat as the delicious smells waft under your nose.

Take a taste. One thing that helps when you're with family or good friends (probably not recommended when eating with business clients for the first time) is taking a taste of what the others are eating. The first bite of anything tastes the best. Taking little bites of various dishes that other people have ordered, even the desserts, may make your BG levels go a little higher than they usually do after a meal, but it probably won't make them go through the roof.

At least taking a taste will be better than what would have happened if you had ordered a whole portion for yourself. Sometimes you'll discover that what they've ordered really isn't very good after all, and your "diet food" may taste the best. I once went to an Italian restaurant with friends who all ordered huge plates of pasta covered with red stuff. I ordered a salad with flame-broiled chicken strips on top. When my meal arrived, everyone stopped talking, looked at it, and asked what it was and how I'd managed to find it on the menu. They thought my meal looked better than theirs.

Some servers are helpful. When a restaurant isn't overly busy, some servers are good at letting you know which dishes have a lot of added sugar or starch or fat. When you explain that you have diabetes, some of them will even check with the cook to make sure. But others can't be bothered, especially when the place is crowded and diners are lining up to get in. You can usually sense which ones can be trusted. If you're not sure, you can stick with grilled foods and salads.

Take your own dressing. Unless I'm being taken to a fine place that I know will have good-quality olive oil and vinegar, I even bring my own salad dressing, because sauces and dressings are often full of added substances of all kinds. It's easy to put into your purse or pocket a small well-sealed plastic bottle of your kind of dressing, in a sealed plastic bag for insurance.

Take a doggie box. I also sometimes carry my own "doggie box" so I won't have to ask for one. I use one of those plastic containers with several compartments and a well-sealed cover, so I can save portions of all the parts of the meal and have a multicourse lunch the next day or give the portions I can't eat to someone else. For a person raised to belong to the Clean Plates Club, it also reduces temptation if you remove half of the meal to the doggie box before you even start to eat.

Check the diet drinks. One word of warning about "diet drinks" in restaurants. Studies have shown that ordering a diet soda in a restaurant doesn't guarantee that you will get one. Especially when they're busy, or if they've run out of diet drinks, some places will serve you a regular drink instead, figuring it won't make any difference. One solution to this problem is to carry with you the test strips designed to detect glucose in the urine. These strips change color in regular but not diet soda. (Although the strips detect glucose, not table sugar, they seem to work in commercial sodas. In the United States, regular sodas are usually sweetened with high-fructose corn syrup, which contains glucose. In other countries, table sugar may be used instead. If you can, check someone else's regular soda with the test strips before relying on them.) You can also use the strips to test for starch, but in this case you've got to put the food in your mouth for a minute or so to let the starch-digesting enzyme *amylase* break some of the carbohydrate down into glucose, which the test strip can detect.

What to order. I won't attempt to suggest what types of food you should order in restaurants. It depends on which type of diet you decide is best for you. You'll probably start out on some kind of American Diabetes Association exchange diet that limits fat, and it seems that every magazine or Sunday supplement or brochure you pick up wants to give you tips on cutting fat out of your diet. If there's anyone in America who hasn't been told at least 1,025 times to "select a lean turkey sandwich on whole grain bread for lunch instead of a cheeseburger and fries" or "choose a bran muffin with tub margarine for breakfast instead of bacon and eggs with home fries," that person must have been living in a cave in the Arctic for the past twenty-five years.

In case you *have* just returned from twenty-five years in the Arctic, ask your doctor or dietician for a pamphlet suggesting good restaurant choices for your particular diet.

Plan ahead if you eat on the run

Eating on the run, when you have no time to seek out a suitable restaurant, or maybe just need to grab a bite from a street vendor to keep you going, is even more difficult than eating in a restaurant because most fast food is both greasy (and so off-limits for a **low-fat diet**) and starchy (no good for a low-carbohydrate diet).

In this case, you just have to make the best of what's available. Be creative. If there's nothing in sight but a hot dog stand and you're on a low-carbohydrate diet, you could get the hot dog and throw away the bun. If you're on a low-fat diet, you could ask for a bun filled with sauerkraut and onions and tomato, or whatever kinds of garnishes they offer. If you're on an exchange diet, the hot dog would probably be OK with the bun as long as you don't load it up with extra calories.

Another solution when you know you'll have a busy day is to prepare ahead of time and bring snacks or stop in a suitable place in the morning and get enough to last throughout the day. If this happens a lot, you might consider preparing several daylong food packages and putting them in the freezer. Then if you had to leave in a hurry one morning in anticipation of a busy day, you could just grab a package from the freezer and head out the door.

Sometimes if you don't bring some food along, there may not be anything at all you can eat. In this case, you have to choose between going hungry and eating something like doughnuts that may cause food cravings for the rest of the day.

Learn to avoid psychological games

As I said earlier, learning to enjoy socializing in the presence of scrumptious food when everyone but you is guzzling down ambrosial treats is one of the most difficult burdens of having diabetes. Add to that the burden that some people take it as a personal insult if you refuse their offerings of food, even when they know you're diabetic.

Some people feel, consciously or unconsciously, that feeding you is a way of expressing their love or friendship. "You won't eat my food," a woman once said to me in a peeved tone, even though I'd told her I was diabetic and she never offered me anything but cheesecakes and tarts. She obviously felt that by rejecting her food, I was rejecting her—on purpose.

Some people with diabetes give in to these psychological games and eat foods that aren't good for them because they don't want to hurt their friends' feelings. Don't worry about your friends. Right now you have to think of yourself.

Sharing with others helps

It takes time to learn to deal with all these difficult situations, and I'm afraid there are no miracle solutions. But you should know that it usually gets easier the longer you've lived with diabetes.

Sharing your frustrations and angers and solutions to eating problems with others in the same boat—local friends or support groups or fellow travelers you meet through the Internet—will speed up the process of learning to cope with this most difficult aspect of managing your diabetes. As always, remember, you are not alone.

IN A SENTENCE:

■ *Maintaining your social connections without seriously breaking your diet is very difficult, but you can learn to do it.*

Stress and Blood Glucose Levels

Stress will increase your blood glucose (BG) levels. That's the condensed-book version of this chapter (very condensed). Maybe for now, that's all you want to know. If you're getting into the swing of things and want to understand how to fine-tune your BG level control, keep on reading.

There are many kinds of stress, and except possibly for some long-term emotional stress, they all increase BG levels, even in nondiabetic people. In order to understand how stress affects BG levels, you first have to understand how BG levels are controlled in nondiabetic people.

Normal control systems are like thermostats

In people without diabetes, BG levels are always fluctuating, going up a little and then down a little. But the body has a complex control system that, like the thermostat to your furnace, keeps the BG levels in a very narrow range, usually considered to be about 70 to 120 mg/dL (milligrams per deciliter) with normal meals. With a very large carbohydrate load, the BG levels might go up to 140 mg/dL, and a person still wouldn't be considered diabetic. After a huge slug of glucose (usually 75 grams) on an empty stomach—equivalent to the *glucose tolerance test*—the BG level could go up to 199 mg/dL and still be considered in the normal range if it came down again quickly. Because most people lose some control of their BG levels as they get older, children usually keep their BG levels in a narrower range than adults.

You could think of the normal control system as analogous to a furnace that keeps the temperature of your house high enough when it gets too cold and an air-conditioning system that keeps your house cold enough when it gets too hot. If you set the furnace to come on when it gets below 65 degrees and the air conditioner to come on when it gets above 70 degrees, you'll keep the temperature of your house in a narrow temperature range between 65 and 70 degrees.

When you have type 2 diabetes, it's as if you have the furnace, but the air conditioner is on the blink.

In the nondiabetic human body, when the BG level gets too high, the beta cells in the pancreas quickly secrete the hormone *insulin*, and the insulin brings the BG level down. When the BG level gets too low, the **alpha cells** in the pancreas quickly secrete the hormone *glucagon*, and the glucagon brings the BG level up. There are other controls, including nervous system signals, that fine-tune the system, but the glucagon/insulin ratio is the major player.

Glucagon is like the furnace in the analogy just described, and insulin is like the air conditioner. When your "air conditioners" are broken, signals that normally might produce small beneficial increases in BG levels may make your BG levels soar.

Different types of stress increase blood glucose levels

Stress includes physical stress such as infections, trauma, surgery, or intense heat or cold. In all these situations, insulin resistance (IR) increases and BG levels in nondiabetic people increase slightly. Another physical stressor is taking various drugs. Even pregnancy and adolescence normally increase IR.

Stress also includes emotional stress. For some people, chronic emotional stress seems to have relatively little physiological effect on BG levels. However, chronic emotional stress can affect how well you are able to maintain your diet and exercise programs. Depression might even make you stop taking your medications on time, or altogether. Thus chronic stress can have an *indirect* effect on BG levels.

Intense emotional stress that triggers the release of **adrenaline**, the **fight-or-flight response**, increases BG levels slightly in nondiabetic people and can make a diabetic person's BG levels soar.

Infections increase insulin resistance

Let's start with physical stress, such as infections. When your body is infected, it gears up to defend itself. One thing it does is to increase IR. This normally results in a small increase in the BG level, so the **white blood cells** that are sent out to fight the infection will have plenty of "food" (energy) to keep them going. As long as this increase is small, it's a good thing.

In nondiabetic people, when the increased IR makes the BG level go too high, the body just produces more insulin, and this brings the BG level down. When you have diabetes, you can't secrete this extra insulin when the BG level gets *too* high, so the BG level may skyrocket. And when the BG level gets too high, instead of helping the white blood cells fight infection, it seems to slow them down. This is why people with uncontrolled diabetes sometimes have sores that take a long, long time to heal.

When you have an infection of any kind, you should keep a careful eye on your BG levels. If they go too high, your doctor may want to give you some insulin on a temporary basis to bring the BG levels down enough that you can fight the infection. When the infection is gone, you'll usually stop taking the insulin. The better controlled your BG levels are normally, the less they will increase under conditions of stress, and not everyone with type 2 diabetes needs insulin when under stress.

Quite often, the increase in BG levels actually *precedes* the diagnosis of the infection. Your body is even smarter than your doctor; it can recognize an infection before there are any obvious signs, maybe one or two days before. So if you find that your BG levels have increased for no obvious reason, be on the alert for other signs of hidden infections, such as a bad tooth or a sore on a foot that you didn't notice, or even a cold that just hasn't shown its ugly face yet.

Trauma and other stresses also increase insulin resistance

Trauma and surgery affect people the same way that an infection does. Medical people call this *stress hyperglycemia*, and it's a normal response. IR increases and BG levels go up a little in nondiabetic people and a lot in those with diabetes. In these cases, the physicians dealing with the trauma or surgery should be informed that you are diabetic and should know what to do to keep your BG levels under control.

Other stressors such as adolescence, pregnancy, and even the fluctuations of the menstrual cycle can increase IR and affect your BG control. More and more young people are being diagnosed with type 2 diabetes and may have to deal with these additional stresses.

Drugs can make blood glucose levels go up or down

Steroids. Drugs can also raise BG levels. A major contributor to raising BG levels is **steroid** drugs, for example, **cortisone** and prednisone. In fact, these drugs can actually *cause* diabetes. There are obviously some conditions for which you really have to take such drugs, and in that case you should go ahead. You might have to take insulin on a temporary basis until the effects of the steroid wear off. The BG levels usually return to your normal levels when you stop taking the drugs. Long-term steroid therapy can cause enough damage that it can't be reversed.

Birth control pills and postmenopausal estrogens and progestins can also affect BG control. Reports on the effects of these hormones differ. Some say estrogens make BG levels go down and progestins make them go up, but others report just the opposite. It may depend on the specific estrogen or progestin preparation used, the dose, and the particular study group. The effect of combinations of the two hormones depends on what hormones are used and in what proportions. For example, in the past, birth control pills often made BG levels go up, but newer formulations often do not. In any case, if you are taking any of these drugs, you should keep careful watch on your BG levels to see if there are any significant changes.

Alcohol. Alcohol makes BG levels go down by reducing the amount of glucose made by the liver.

Glucosamine. Another popular drug, or dietary supplement, that may affect BG levels is glucosamine. This supplement is taken to treat arthritis, but there is evidence that it increases IR and makes BG levels go up in people with diabetes (YMMV, Your Mileage May Vary). Again, if you take this supplement, keep careful watch on your BG levels. It may take a month or even more before you see any change in either arthritic pain or BG levels, so don't conclude that it will have no effect on your diabetes control if you see no worsening after a few days or weeks.

Niacin and fish oils. Some people take niacin or fish oils to improve their lipid profiles. There have been contradictory reports on their effects on diabetes control. For some time, people were told that fish oil supplements (not the fish oils you get from eating fish) and niacin would increase BG levels in people with diabetes. More recent studies have reported that there is no significant effect on diabetes control.

Remember, YMMV. Formal studies are done on populations of patients. If 100 patients are studied and 25 get better, 25 get worse, and 50 stay the same, the study would seem to show no effect of a drug. But if you're in one of the groups that gets better or worse, the drug might help or hurt you. Some studies show effects, and others do not. So as always, if you try niacin or fish oils, monitor your BG levels closely to make sure they don't increase when you take them.

Some other drugs that may affect your BG control are listed in Table 3. Not everyone is affected by every drug on the list, and some people have reported effects from drugs not on the list. This list is far from exhaustive. Because new drugs come on the market all the time, you should ask your doctor or do an Internet search whenever you start a new medication to see if that drug could affect your BG levels and then monitor your BG levels to see if it does. Some drugs affect BG levels indirectly, by increasing the effectiveness of sulfonylureas.

TABLE 3
SOME DRUGS THAT MAY AFFECT BLOOD GLUCOSE LEVELS

INCREASE

Acetazolamide

Alpha agonists

Antipsychotics (some newer ones)

Beta blockers

Bumetanide

Caffeine (large doses)

Calcium-channel blockers

Cimetidine (Tagamet)

Counterregulatory hormones (e.g., glucagon, cortisol, adrenaline)

Cyclophosphamide

Cyclosporine

Diazoxide

Epinephrine-like drugs (decongestants and diet pills)

Fish oils

Furosemide

Glucosamine

Indapamide

L-Asparaginase

Lithium

Minoxidil

Niacin (nicotinic acid)

Nicotine (large doses)

Nonsteroidal anti-inflammatory drugs

Older contraceptive formulations

Pentamidine isethionate

Phenobarbital sodium

Phenytoin (Dilantin)

Steroids (cortisone, prednisone, progestins)

Thiazide diuretics

Thyroid preparations

DECREASE

ACE (angiotensin-converting enzyme) inhibitors

Alcohol

Alpha blockers

Fibric acid derivatives (Clofibrate)

Salicylates and acetaminophen (large doses)

Warfarin

Short-term stress can trigger adrenaline release

Long-term emotional stress, even major stress such as grieving for a departed spouse, parent, or child, probably won't affect your diabetic control unless the natural depression that follows such events makes you careless about your treatment program. However, short-term stress that triggers the release of adrenaline can have a major effect on BG levels.

For example, I depend on my computer for my income, and I once had to replace a fan on my computer's Pentium processor. The technician talking me through the procedure didn't seem very sure of what he was telling me, so I was very nervous, so nervous I dropped the Pentium processor on the floor. By the time I hung up the phone, I was literally shaking. Out of curiosity I tested my BG level. It was up to 200 mg/dL. So I decided to take a walk to calm down, and after thirty minutes of walking, it was back down to about 85.

Adrenaline causes insulin resistance

During a stressful fight-or-flight response such as the one I've just described (I wanted to flee, but I didn't know where; I wanted to belt the technician, but he was in Idaho), the body secretes a lot of adrenaline. Like glucagon, adrenaline makes the BG level go up by stimulating the liver to produce more glucose and export it into the bloodstream to send to the muscles. It does this because whether you decide to flee or fight, your muscles will need more than the usual amount of energy.

Another reason to increase the BG level is that some kinds of stress reduce the blood flow to the brain. Because it won't help to have strong muscles if your brain decides to take a nap, the higher BG level also provides enough glucose to the brain to keep it working even when its blood flow is slowed.

The adrenaline also keeps the liver from breaking down glucose for its own energy needs. Instead, it ships the glucose out to the muscles, which are more important in a fight-or-flight situation. (The liver is "mother-like" and does a lot of metabolic chores like this for other parts of the body.) At the same time, adrenaline speeds up the metabolism of glucose in the muscles so the muscles can extract as much energy as possible out of the glucose that was kindly sent to it by the altruistic liver.

Problems happen, however, when instead of using up that extra glucose for fleeing or fighting, you just sit quaking behind a podium before giving a speech, or in the wings before going on stage for a play or a concert, or in a waiting room for a job interview. All that glucose just hangs around in the blood, and your BG levels go high, as mine did when I dropped the Pentium processor.

In a nondiabetic person under the same conditions, when the BG level increased just slightly, the pancreas would shoot out some extra insulin and bring it down. When you have diabetes, your pancreas can't do that. So your BG level goes sky-high.

Low blood sugar also triggers the release of adrenaline, and this causes some of the same symptoms as short-term stress, including shaking, nervousness, sweating, and hunger (see Month 2). Interestingly, caffeine also triggers the release of adrenaline, and some people report that a "caffeine high" feels a lot like a "BG low."

Some people also find that black coffee increases their BG levels. Others do not. Studies have shown that caffeine increases BG levels, but these studies usually used large amounts. One or two cups probably won't matter. If in doubt, test your BG levels after consuming nothing but coffee and find how it affects you.

Some other hormones also increase insulin resistance

Adrenaline isn't the only **stress hormone**. Under stressful conditions, other hormones called *counterregulatory hormones* are also produced. These include *growth hormone* and *cortisol*. These hormones counteract the effects of insulin. In other words, they cause increased IR.

In fact, in certain disease states, levels of these counterregulatory hormones can be increased enough that the resulting IR actually *causes* a diabetic condition. Too much growth hormone in adults produces acromegaly, and too much cortisol produces Cushing's disease; both these diseases are associated with diabetes.

You don't need to remember the details at first, but you should understand that the orchestration of BG levels during stress, and even during nonstressful times, is very complex. Most of the hormones, such as insulin, glucagon, adrenaline, cortisol, and growth hormone, have multiple effects, and I've mentioned only the primary ones.

Like a complicated engineering system with checks and balances and counterchecks and counterbalances, the body has many different controls that interact to produce reactions to the stimuli of everyday life. When one of the control systems in the body is defective, sometimes another one can step in and take over. This is one reason we see YMMV in diabetic control. Some of you may have controls that are "rusted" at one point of this complex system, and others may have defects at some other point.

In general, stress will make your BG levels go up. It's important, especially at first, to test under different conditions of stress to see how stresses of various kinds affect *your* BG control. Then with experience, you can anticipate these changes, or when you encounter unanticipated stress—for instance, if you encounter a saber-toothed tiger in your backyard or your dentist tells you that you need a root canal job—you will know what action to take to prevent your BG levels from going too high.

IN A SENTENCE:

■ *Stresses of many kinds will make your blood glucose levels increase.*

First-Week MILESTONE

By the end of your first week, you've come a long way in understanding and accepting your diabetes:

- You know that your diabetes is not your fault—you just have genes that are unsuited to a modern lifestyle.

- You've learned what diabetes is and how different foods, exercise, and stress can make your blood glucose levels go up or down.

- You've been introduced to different dietary philosophies.

- You know how to test your own blood glucose levels, and the importance of keeping those levels close to normal.

- You understand that sharing your experiences with others can help you accept and deal with your diabetes.

living

You're Chairman of the Board

After a week with this blasted disease, I hope you're beginning to realize that you're going to have to mobilize your emotional resources and take charge of managing your diabetes at some point.

That doesn't mean you should fire all your health-care providers, enroll in medical school, and get a PhD in pharmacology on the side. You need the knowledge and experience of a whole mess of people to help you get a grip on this thing. But a large part of the treatment of diabetes involves daily choices of foods and exercises, so in the long run, like the chairman of the board, you are the one who is going to make a lot of the decisions.

Right now, it's up to you to make sure you are getting all the medical appointments and tests you should have.

Some have a health-care team

When you read diabetes magazines and books written by diabetes groups such as the American Diabetes Association (ADA), they always talk about your *health-care team*. This conjures up images of five or ten medical professionals sitting around a table discussing your case and deciding on the optimal, coordinated treatment for you. Or maybe they're gussied up in colorful costumes standing outside your house chanting, "Rah, rah, rah. Sis, boom, bit. Diet and exercise. You can do it!"

These publications suggest that your health-care team may include a **primary care provider (PCP)**, often an internist or family physician; an **endocrinologist** (often called just an *endo*), a doctor who specializes in endocrine diseases including diabetes, or even a **diabetologist**, usually an endocrinologist who has decided to specialize even more; a *diabetes nurse educator*, who may also be a *certified diabetes educator (CDE)* to train you in things like using your blood glucose (BG) meter; an **ophthalmologist**, an eye doctor with an MD who specializes in eye diseases rather than in prescribing lenses, or even the more specialized *retinologist*, to check your eyes for retinopathy; a *podiatrist*, a foot doctor to check your feet; a *registered dietician (RD)* to work out a diet for you; a *pharmacist* to explain the effects of drugs to you; an *exercise physiologist* or a *physical therapist* to work out an ideal exercise program for you; a *social worker* to make sure you have no situations at home that would interfere with your diabetes management; and even a *mental health professional* to help you cope with the psychological stresses of this disease. The theory is that even if they don't sit around the table all day discussing your fascinating case, these specialists at least all communicate with each other and coordinate their efforts to offer you the best care possible.

If you have excellent insurance, you may have such a team working on your case. In reality, though, even if you have consulted all these medical specialists, you will probably find that they don't communicate very well with each other, if they communicate at all. You may have to tell your family physician what the ophthalmologist found, for example. Or an endocrinologist may tell you to do something that is different from what the internist said, which is different from the advice you got from the CDE.

You may not even have a team working on your case. This may be your choice. You may not have the time, financial ability, or inclination to consult so many people. Or this may be your insurance company's decision. Some health maintenance organizations (HMOs) may have rules about how many specialists a person with diabetes can see. And some family physicians may believe that they can manage diabetic patients by themselves without help from specialists, as was usually done in the past.

Thus you may have to orchestrate your visits to any specialists yourself. If your health insurance will pay for office visits to anyone, or if you're trying to figure out some way to spend a lot of extra cash, you're in luck. You can see them all. Otherwise, you'll have to decide which ones are most important for your care and then either persuade your PCP to refer you to them or to pay for the visits yourself.

Visiting an eye doctor is essential

One *essential* appointment is a visit with an *ophthalmologist*, who will check your eyes for signs of retinopathy. You may have had elevated BG levels, especially after meals, for five or ten years, or even more, before being diagnosed. If the BG levels have been elevated a lot, especially if they've been high all day, not just after meals, you could already have some damage to the retinas of your eyes.

Make sure the eye doctor does what is called a *dilated examination*, which means you have drops in your eyes that dilate the pupils so the doctor can see to the edges of the retina. This is important. Diabetic retinopathy usually starts at the edges, which are difficult to see without dilating the pupils. Otherwise it's like looking through a keyhole and trying to see the edges of a room.

Retinologists are even more adept at detecting very early signs of retinopathy than ophthalmologists. Some people say their ophthalmologists told them their eyes were fine but a retinologist said there were subtle signs of problems. Sometimes the retinologist injects a dye into your bloodstream and then takes lot of photographs of your retinas, which not only allows careful scrutiny of the photographs at leisure but also provides a record of your retinas to compare with future studies, to see if there have been any changes. It would be nice if everyone could see a retinologist on diagnosis, but some insurance plans don't want to pay for the visits without a referral.

If you do have signs of retinopathy, it doesn't mean you'll go blind. These days, laser treatments to the eyes can stop the progression of this complication pretty well. And bringing your BG levels down close to normal should keep new lesions from occurring.

If your ophthalmologist looks at your eyes and finds no signs of damage, this will be a big weight off your back, but don't feel you're out of the woods and never go back for an appointment. You should have your eyes examined for this complication at least once a year, maybe even every six months, just to make sure that if retinopathy does occur, you can stop it in the very earliest stages.

You may want other specialists

Whether or not you need to see the other specialists really depends on your own personal needs. If you've always wanted an excuse to take up mountain climbing and are able to buy proper equipment and join a mountain-climbing class and get your exercise by yourself, you don't need to see an exercise specialist for help in that area. But if you've got severe arthritis and a little bit of heart failure and any kind of movement is difficult for you, then a visit with a *physical therapist* should help you to design an exercise program that would be appropriate for you.

If you love reading books about food and nutrition and are good at working with numbers, you can probably design your own diet plan that will work with your food preferences as well as the dietary philosophy you think is best for you (see Day 4). If that seems like too much trouble, then a visit with a *dietician* may be a great help. Like physicians, dieticians vary greatly in their ability to communicate with their clients. Some of them have great gifts in listening to your food preferences, lifestyle, and budgetary constraints and coming up with a diet that will be wonderful for you. Others, alas, tend to give all their diabetic patients pretty much the same diet, which may not work for you.

In my case, which I'm afraid may be all too common, a nurse handed me an ADA exchange diet (see Day 4) pamphlet for a 1,500-calorie diet and told me to follow it. That was the nutritional component of my healthcare team. If I'd followed that diet, I would have gained weight (I'm small) and would have had to eat less broccoli and spinach than I was accustomed to and more small dinner rolls. That didn't seem very sensible to me. So I pared down the total calories by eliminating some starch exchanges and substituted three vegetable exchanges for most of the other starch exchanges (three vegetable exchanges have about the same number of carbohydrate as one starch exchange) so I didn't have to rush out to the store for a six-month supply of small dinner rolls. I was hungry all the time, but I lost thirty pounds.

It's important to find the right doctor

Whether or not you need to see an endocrinologist or a diabetologist depends on both the complexity of your disease and the personalities and expertise of the various physicians involved. The diabetologist should know a lot more about diabetes and the latest therapies than the average PCP, who must keep up to date with not only diabetes but also hundreds of other diseases, both minor and serious.

On the other hand, sometimes the ability to listen to the patient is more important than expertise. When Fern H. asked her family doctor about getting a C-peptide test, he said he'd never heard of it, so she decided to see an endocrinologist instead. When she questioned the endocrinologist's recommendation to take an expensive drug, he yelled at her, "You'll take what I tell you to take," so she tried another doctor. She wasn't too thrilled with him either.

"Had my endo appointment Friday and just fired another one. I'm better off with my family doctor. At least he listens! The endo told me my numbers were great: 104 to 183 is great? He said a C-peptide was a waste of time and money. He wasn't even going to do a blood lipid, but I insisted. All he cares about is the A1c. I'm going to stick to my sincere, helpful family doc. I'd rather discuss options with my GP, and we can make decisions together. I won't relinquish my control to any MD." She then returned to her family doctor, who in the meantime had learned about the C-peptide test, and he said, "We can learn together." This still works for her.

All endocrinologists are obviously not this controlling, and all family physicians are not such patient listeners, but choosing the best medical people for your own particular situation will depend on their personalities and yours, as well as their expertise. Fern is very independent. If you're not quite so independent, you may want your physician to tell you what to do, especially at first.

You have to take charge

The most important thing, however, is to not sit back passively and stick with a particular health-care person you don't feel is right for your diabetes control. For example, if you've been having A1c's of 9 and 10 and your PCP doesn't suggest making some major changes in your treatment, find another one. Having diabetes means spending a lot of time with health-care providers, and you might as well get the best you can find.

If your PCP doesn't suggest that you consult a dietician and you think you need one, ask for the referral. If the PCP refuses, see if you can make an appointment on your own. Even if you have to pay the bill yourself, it may be worth it in the long run. One office visit bill is a lot cheaper than years living with complications from failing to find a diet that you are able to follow.

Even if you have a wonderful PCP who listens and seems to be knowledgeable about diabetes treatment, you may eventually end up knowing more about diabetes than your doctor does. The doctor goes home at night and thinks about other things. You live with your diabetes twenty-four hours a day, 365 days a year. So you might as well start now and learn about things that should be asked and done when you see your doctor.

If the doctor omits something you think is important, don't feel too shy to ask about it. For example, some people feel that every visit to a doctor should include a careful examination of your feet, because people with uncontrolled diabetes are prone to foot infections that are hard to heal. Some people take off their shoes at every visit to remind the doctor to do the foot inspection. However, if your diabetes was discovered in the very early stages and you're still under excellent control, with no signs of neuropathy, you might get more from the doctor's limited time by discussing something else.

Your physical exam may include special tests

You may have had a thorough physical exam when you were diagnosed. You were probably still in shock and not paying much attention. If you were diagnosed after a routine blood test, you may be seeing your doctor for the first time after your diagnosis. By now, your shock should have abated a bit, and you may be able to pay more attention to what is involved in your examination.

A physical exam for a person with type 2 diabetes usually involves the same routine steps as any other physical exams. Because people with diabetes are more prone to heart problems than others of the same age, your doctor may also pay special attention to your cardiac health, including an electrocardiogram.

Hemochromatosis. Ask your doctor about the possibility of *hemochromatosis*, which can cause diabetes, especially if anyone in your family has had this hereditary disease. This is described in Month 2.

Pedal pulses. Make sure your doctor checks your *pedal pulses*, the pulses in your feet, and tells you if they are normal or not. This is because people with diabetes are more susceptible to **arteriosclerosis**, or hardening of the **arteries**, which can reduce circulation to the feet and eventually make you prone to slow-healing foot infections.

Tuning fork. Another test that should be done is the tuning-fork test. In this simple test, the doctor puts a tuning fork on an anklebone and asks you to say when you no longer feel the vibration. This is testing for signs of neuropathy. A person with no neuropathy should be able to feel the tuning fork until the tester no longer sees it vibrate. Loss of this sense of vibration is one of the first signs of neuropathy, so if you have no loss in this area, there's a good chance you don't have other nerve damage.

Filament test. Another way to test for neuropathy is to touch your feet with a thin filament. If you can feel it, your nerves are OK. However, studies have shown that the tuning fork detects nerve damage at an earlier stage.

If there's any sign of nerve damage or of poor circulation, make sure your doctor checks your feet at every visit because small cuts or sores could turn into major problems.

Heart rate variability. When sensory nerves are damaged by high BG levels, you may feel tingling or pain. But when internal, **autonomic nerves** (see Month 10) such as the *vagus nerve* are affected, there are no clear symptoms. Such damage may lead to digestive problems or "silent" heart attacks that lack the usual symptoms of pain or pressure. The latter can be deadly because you won't know to seek help.

There is a noninvasive test for **autonomic neuropathy** called the *R-R interval* or *heart rate variability (HRV) test*. Some doctors say there's no point in testing for this because there's nothing they can do about it.

Nevertheless, there is something you can do about it. Knowing you were at risk for a silent heart attack might make you more vigilant and careful with your lifestyle modifications. So if your doctor isn't aware of this test, ask about it. There are now gizmos and software that are supposed to let you measure your own HRV. These may be fine for healthy athletes wondering about their fitness, but properly interpreting the implications of an HRV test for autonomic neuropathy requires an understanding of cardiac physiology and is best done by a physician.

Lab tests. Your doctor may order a lot of lab tests, including the hemoglobin A1c test and tests for kidney function. See Day 5 for an explanation of the most common tests.

Reducing worry. Not all physicians perform all these tests when you're diagnosed, because it usually takes ten or more years for diabetic complications to show up. However, you may have had high BG levels for a long time before you were diagnosed. In fact, sometimes it might have been early signs of complications that prodded you into seeing a doctor in the first place. Being checked for all the major diabetic complications soon after your diagnosis means that you know right away whether you have any early signs of them. Otherwise, you may worry about the unknown. Worrying is stressful, and stress makes your blood pressure and BG levels go up.

Take charge and stay well

If you have no signs of protein in your urine, no loss of sensation on the tuning-fork test, no loss of your pedal pulses, and no signs of retinopathy in your eye examination, you are very lucky. You probably have no diabetic complications. Now your job is to make sure your BG levels stay as close as possible to normal so you will never develop any such complications.

Insist on getting copies of all your lab tests, even if you're not ready to try to understand them all. For one thing, if you decide to change doctors, you'll have your own record of what your lab tests were in the past. In addition, knowing your lab test results helps you understand where you are in your diabetes control.

One doctor told me my A1c results were "normal," but I asked for a copy of the report. When I got it, I found my A1c results were above normal, in the "well-controlled diabetic" range. I asked the doctor about it and he said, "Well, that's normal for a diabetic."

In order to control your diabetes, you need to have the correct facts. Unfortunately, you must sometimes insist and persist and demand. It's not always easy being chairman of the board, but it's worth the effort. It's your best chance at ensuring that you stay complication-free for many a year.

IN A SENTENCE:

▪ *Taking charge of your diabetes is an important part of controlling the disease.*

Guarding Your Beta Cells

The cells in the pancreas that produce insulin are called *beta cells*, and to control your diabetes, you want to keep your beta cells as healthy as possible. High blood glucose (BG) levels are toxic to beta cells. This is called **glucotoxicity**, and the good news is that it's partially reversible if you can get your BG levels close to normal. The longer your beta cells are exposed to high BG levels, the more apt they are to suffer permanent damage.

There are vicious and virtuous circles

Although no one yet understands exactly how glucotoxicity works, high BG levels seem to increase insulin resistance (IR) or decrease the ability of the beta cells to produce insulin, or both. More IR and less insulin production make the BG levels go higher, and that causes more glucotoxicity, which further impairs the beta cells and increases IR. You get the picture. You're caught in a vicious circle.

On the other hand, if you can get your BG levels close to normal, by whatever means it takes, the vicious circle reverses. Your beta cells become more responsive and your IR lessens. This causes lower BG levels, which causes even less glucotoxicity, which makes your beta cells work even better. Now you're in a positive circle, a sort of virtuous circle.

Does this mean that bringing your BG levels back to normal will cure your diabetes? Unfortunately, no. While caught in the vicious circle of glucotoxicity, some of the beta cells may have stopped working, and scientists don't yet know how to revive them. This is why it's important to bring your BG levels back to normal as soon as you can before too much damage has been done—and to keep them there.

Look out for a trap

This reversal of glucotoxicity sometimes can be a trap. Carmen W. was able to bring her BG levels back to normal just with diet and exercise. The glucotoxicity abated, and she found she could even eat a few desserts without having her BG levels levels go above normal. "I was thrilled. I thought I was cured. I'd planned to stick to my diet anyway, but I got into the habit of eating a nice dessert once a week as a treat. Then it was once a day. Then it was lots of bread, as well as dessert, at almost every meal. I sort of forgot about my diet (I was cured, right?) and went back to eating the big, high-fat, starchy meals the rest of the family enjoyed. I never tested anymore because I figured I was cured, and I hated to prick my fingers."

Then after some months, Carmen noticed she was thirsty a lot, and she seemed to have to get up a lot at night. One day she tested and was aghast to see that her BG level had reached 400 mg/dL. Carmen knew what to do. She went back to her diet and started exercising again. Unfortunately, this time, the diet and exercise didn't do the trick. Months of high BG levels had knocked off a few more of her beta cells, just enough to make controlling her diabetes difficult, and she had to start taking oral drugs.

The same trap can occur in people with a lot of weight-associated IR. If the diabetes is diagnosed at an early stage, and if you are able to lose a lot of weight, sometimes there are still enough beta cells left to cope with the smaller demand for insulin, and the BG levels return to normal without drugs. But you still have the diabetes genes, and if you regain the weight, the BG problems will return.

This achievement of normal BG levels with weight loss occurs more often in younger people who are diagnosed very early in the process, before many beta cells have conked out. There's no guarantee it will work. If you're overweight, some health-care people may tell you that if you'd just lose a few pounds, your diabetes would "go away." Yes, your IR will go down, and you'll find it a lot easier to control your diabetes. But having type 2 diabetes genes itself also causes IR, maybe about half the total IR found in someone who is very overweight. As with other things, YMMV

(Your Mileage May Vary). It's definitely worth a lot of effort to try to dump the weight, but don't expect miracles. Even if you become sylph-like, you may still have some problems with your BG levels.

First you produce more insulin than normal

People have studied the way insulin-resistant people lose beta cells. You presumably start off like everyone else, producing just the right amount of insulin to keep your BG levels normal. Then, as your IR develops, you start producing even more insulin than other people. By doing this, you are able to keep your BG levels in the normal range.

Then when the beta cells become exhausted and start to fail, your insulin production falls, until it reaches the "normal" level again. But remember, this would be the normal level if you had no IR. When you have IR, the "normal level" is insufficient to let the muscle cells take up the glucose in the blood, and your BG levels will be high. Eventually your insulin levels may drop even below normal.

Figure 2 illustrates this process. It shows the amount of insulin people produce during a glucose tolerance test compared with the fasting BG level. Increased fasting levels suggest increased IR.

You can see that people with normal fasting levels (no IR) produce a certain amount of insulin. As the fasting levels increase, people produce *more* insulin than normal. In other words, they need more insulin to take care of the same amount of glucose. They are developing IR.

Studies have suggested that at a fasting BG level of about 120 mg/dL (milligrams per deciliter), the beta cells are working as hard as they can to keep the BG levels in the normal range after meals, when the demand is the greatest. This represents the peak of the curve. When the fasting levels get higher than that, some beta cells begin to become "exhausted" and expire. Now the insulin levels after meals begin to fall.

When the fasting BG level reaches about 140 mg/dL, the beta cells are working as hard as they can just to keep the *fasting* BG levels from increasing any more. When the fasting BG gets even higher than that, some beta cells give up the ghost even when you're not eating anything at all, and the fasting insulin levels begin to fall. By the time the fasting BG levels have reached about 200, the insulin levels are far *below* normal after a meal.

The sooner you are diagnosed, the better

What this all means is that **the sooner you are diagnosed and work to keep the BG levels low, the more beta cell function will remain, and the easier it will be to control the diabetes**. Not taking your

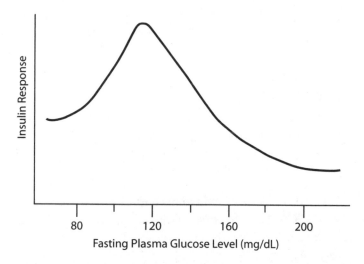

FIGURE 2. Variations in insulin secretion as the beta cells become "exhausted." The vertical axis shows how much insulin is produced during a glucose tolerance test (GTT). The horizontal axis shows the fasting blood glucose (BG) levels, which increase as the diabetes gets progressively worse. Notice that at first the amount of insulin produced in the GTT increases. This is a sign that insulin resistance is increasing, so the beta cells have to produce more insulin to deal with the glucose in the test. Then, at a fasting BG level of approximately 120 mg/dL, the beta cells begin to deteriorate. At a fasting BG level of about 150 mg/dL, they produce "normal" amounts of insulin in the test, that is, amounts that would be normal with no insulin resistance but are subnormal under conditions of insulin resistance. Eventually, they aren't able to produce even normal amounts of insulin during the test. They are "exhausted."

diabetes seriously because you were told you have "borderline diabetes" just means you are creating more problems for yourself in the future. Physicians aren't apt to tell their patients, "You have a borderline brain tumor. Watch your carcinogens." The best time to treat a cancer is when it's small. Diabetes should be treated the same way, when the damage is small.

Unfortunately, current diagnostic criteria say that you don't diagnose anyone with diabetes until the fasting BG levels reach 126 mg/dL. This means that thousands of people have fasting BG levels high enough to cause some beta cell exhaustion, but they're not being told that they have a problem. By the time they're diagnosed, it may be too late. They have enough beta cell damage that they won't be able to restore normal BG levels even if they reduce their IR by losing a lot of weight. Doctors didn't use to diagnose you as diabetic until the fasting levels were above 140, which meant even more beta cell damage had probably occurred.

Lipids are also toxic

High levels of fats in the blood seem to have an effect on the beta cells that is similar to glucotoxicity and is called **lipotoxicity**. Some say both effects work the same way and call it *glucolipotoxicity*. So controlling your BG levels but allowing your blood fat levels to skyrocket is not a good idea for the sake of your beta cells as well as for your cardiovascular health.

People who are overweight tend to have more fatty acids (see Day 3) in their blood whether they consume a lot of fat or not. Thus losing weight may help reduce lipotoxicity as well as reduce IR and glucotoxicity and is therefore a good thing to do.

In Week 3 I'll discuss how all this affects decisions about what kind of treatment you should get for your diabetes. Now you know that by keeping your BG levels down, you can turn a vicious circle into a virtuous circle. **High BG levels promote high BG levels, but low BG levels promote low BG levels.**

If only chocolate cheesecake would promote low BG levels, most of us would have it made. Sticking to a strict diet and exercising a lot takes work, but it's worth it. Be good to your beta cells. Without glucotoxicity, they will be nicer to you.

IN A SENTENCE:

▪ *High blood glucose levels are toxic to beta cells, and the sooner you can get them close to normal, the easier it will be to control your diabetes.*

Paying
the Bills

Diabetes is an expensive disease. Testing four times a day with test strips that cost about a dollar a strip, list price, today and undoubtedly more in the future, means almost $1,500 a year in test strips alone (so you can see why the meter companies are happy to give away meters to get you to buy their strips; you can find strips discounted, and although some meters use cheaper strips, meters vary in accuracy, so you have to balance accuracy with cost). Prescription medications add to the cost.

Proper care of diabetes includes not only drugs and supplies for blood glucose (BG) testing but also regular visits to a myriad of health-care specialists as well as regular laboratory tests such as the hemoglobin A1c. Because there is not yet a cure for diabetes, this diabetes care will probably continue for a long time. Insurance companies are all too aware of this fact, which is why if you already have diabetes, they are not keen on enrolling you in their insurance plan. However, the Affordable Care Act of 2010 mandates that insurers can no longer deny coverage if you have a preexisting condition. One exception is "grandfathered" individual plans created before March 23, 2010. If you have one of these plans, see if you can switch to another plan that covers preexisting conditions. Obesity counseling is now covered in Affordable Care plans.

However, no matter how expensive all this preventive care is, it's a droplet in the bucket compared with the cost of treating diabetic complications such as kidney failure requiring **dialysis** or a kidney transplant, or foot ulcers that cause gangrene and amputation. For example, a 1993 study showed that the cost of diabetes care for a sixty-four-year-old man without complications was just over $2,000 per year. The cost of treating end-stage kidney disease was $15,675 a year, almost eight times as much. That's from just one complication alone. Thus your insurance company should be more than willing to help you keep your BG levels close to normal. The important words here are *should be*. They may be reluctant. This is because many patients change insurance providers frequently. So one company may not want to pay for a lot of preventive care that will save money for another company.

Insurance usually pays for supplies

Most states now have laws requiring insurance companies to cover treatment for type 2 as well as type 1 patients, although the breadth of treatment can vary. In 2015, these laws were in place in forty-six states. Idaho, North Dakota, Ohio, and Alabama have no state mandates. Medicare now also covers 80 percent of the costs of testing supplies for type 2 patients. This is actually a cost-effective move for them. The lower your BG levels are, the lower their expenses will be in the long run.

If you're ordering supplies by mail, be cautious about companies that promise to bill your insurance company directly, with no or little expense to you. Some of these companies bill your insurance company at inflated rates. Some people have found that their entire insurance allowance for supplies was exhausted in a few months, leaving them responsible for the bills for the rest of the year.

Laws can't force you to use the testing supplies your insurance pays for. That's up to you. By now you should have a BG-testing meter, and you should be comfortable using it. Your BG levels should have dropped as a result of either diet and exercise or some kind of drug treatment, or maybe even dieting most of the time and making a lot of plans for exercising tomorrow. No one is perfect. But every bit helps.

You'll have other expenses

Following a good diet for your diabetes can also be expensive, and alas, no matter how good your insurance is, the insurance company is not going to pay the grocery bills. Low-carbohydrate diets especially, with their emphasis on meat and nonstarchy vegetables, can be an added expense. Low-fat diets are usually cheaper.

However, even if fish, lean meats, and fresh, out-of-season vegetables and fruits seem expensive—and they are more expensive than white bread and jam or casseroles that consist mostly of noodles or white rice—they're usually a much better buy than the fast food or prepared foods you may have been eating before. Whatever the cost, it's cheaper in the long run to eat good food than to pay a doctor's bill because you let your BG levels get too high.

Other expenses related to your diabetes care, such as vitamin pills or exercise equipment, or time lost from income-producing work because you are exercising instead, also add to the financial burden.

Medical insurance is important

What all this means is that when you are diagnosed with diabetes, some of the spontaneity may have to go out of your life. Good medical care today is out of reach of the average person who lacks insurance. Thus you can no longer afford to simply quit a job you don't like and start looking for something else. First you need to do some research to find out what effect this move will have on your health insurance. Research first and quit later.

When you have insurance. If you already have a good insurance plan when you're diagnosed, you're in luck. You can't be dropped just because you have diabetes. Your job is to find out how much care your plan will cover. Many plans will pay for diabetes education as well as visits with a dietician, exercise specialist, and endocrinologist. Others may be more limited. Many plans will pay for certain coverage only if your doctor prescribes it, so don't be too shy to ask.

If your plan says it won't pay for something you think would help you with your control, don't give up. Try to persuade the insurer (preferably with the endorsement of your doctor) that you are doing your best to take an active part in controlling your diabetes, and point out that anything they can do to help you with this goal will reduce their costs in the long run. For example, if your plan routinely covers the cost of one hundred test strips every three months for people with type 2 diabetes, enough to test about once a day, and you think you could get better control if you tested more often, ask for a prescription for more. If it won't go through, ask your doctor to write a letter explaining that you're working hard to control your diabetes and more strips would help a lot, especially in your first year.

Better control should reduce your medical costs not just in the future but now. For example, one study calculated that costs for patients with "improved" A1c values were almost $1,000 a year lower than those of less well controlled patients. Talking about the bottom line is speaking a language insurance companies understand.

If your insurer still won't budge, consider paying for whatever it is yourself if you can possibly afford it. In the long run, the cost of one visit to a specialist or one piece of equipment will be tiny compared with the personal cost of complications that might result from poor control.

Unfortunately, many employers have to bid out for the cheapest medical coverage available, and if they change insurance providers, you may have to find a whole new health-care team after you've become comfortable with one group of people.

If you work for a large company with a large pool of mostly healthy people, the fact that you are diagnosed with diabetes probably won't make much difference in the employer's choice of insurance plans. But even though rising insurance costs are the result of many factors, if your company is small, your employer may make you the scapegoat and blame you for escalating insurance costs. Although the employer is not legally allowed to discriminate, you may find subtle discrimination that is difficult to prove. Another problem with small companies is that they, like churches and federal agencies, are often exempt from federal regulations concerning health-care benefits.

As with the rest of your care, you will have to be "chairman of the board" when it comes to dealing with your health insurance. Insurance plans keep changing their rules, and state insurance laws keep changing. It's up to you to find out exactly what your insurance will and will not cover. If in doubt about the rules in your state, consult the state insurance commissioner.

Leaving your job. If you leave or lose your job, or if you are widowed, you will be eligible for COBRA (Consolidated Omnibus Budget Reconciliation Act) insurance, which means that for eighteen months (twenty-nine months if you're disabled) you can continue to receive the benefits you had when you or your spouse was an employee, but you have to pay the insurance premiums yourself. This may seem expensive, and you may have to pay slightly more than the employer paid, but it's probably a lot cheaper than paying for your diabetes care by yourself.

Changing jobs. If you're considering changing jobs, find out what kind of insurance you'll get at the new job and see if your new salary will make the move worthwhile. But don't be a slave to insurance. Some people spend their lives in dead-end jobs just because they come with good benefits. It doesn't make sense to turn down a $10,000 raise and a job that offers the possibilities of advancement just because you'd lose $5,000 worth of health insurance. If the new job does include health insurance, make sure your diabetes care won't be excluded for twelve months because it's a preexisting condition. Do some calculations, and figure out what will be in your best interests in the long run.

Federal insurance. If you have federal health insurance coverage through Medicare (800-633-4227), Medicaid (see your local social services office), or the Department of Veterans Affairs (800-827-1000), your diabetes care will be covered, although they may not allow as many extra visits to specialists as a top-notch private insurance plan.

When you're not insured. With the Affordable Care Act, you should be able to enroll in a health-care plan if you can afford one of the plans available in your state. They can't refuse you because of your diabetes.

If you won't be getting insurance through your employer, see if any of the associations you belong to offer group health insurance rates, which are lower than individual rates. If you don't belong to any associations, consider joining one if the savings in health insurance would be more than the cost of membership.

Research before you buy. Before you sign up for a plan, it's up to you to find out exactly what it covers. The old *fee-for-service* plans, in which you could choose your doctors and the insurance company would pay, are less common these days. Most plans involve some kind of *managed care* in which a "gatekeeper," a sort of medical St. Peter who decides who gets expensive treatment and who goes to another place, decides whether or not you are allowed to see certain specialists. Sometimes the gatekeeper is your primary physician and sometimes the insurance company, often a clerk who simply follows rules without really understanding the ins and outs of diabetes care. Even within the managed care plans, there are different types. In some you are limited to specific doctors in the plan; in others you can see doctors outside the plan but you have to pay a greater percentage of the cost. Find out what you're buying before you buy it.

If your income is limited and you have to buy your own insurance, do some pencil pushing and think about a large-deductible policy, which will be much cheaper. With the large-deductible policy, you have to pay for most of your lab tests yourself. Paying an extra $1,000 per year so the insurance will cover $400 worth of lab tests doesn't make sense. However, with a large-deductible policy you are taking a risk. If you have serious medical problems, you'll have to pay a lot more.

For example, in one case, a $10,000-deductible policy cost about $1,200 per year less than a $250-deductible policy. Both offered office visits with a small copay. If you're relatively young and, except for the diabetes, you're relatively healthy and very lucky, in ten years you could save $12,000 with the cheaper policy.

But if you had any expensive illnesses, you could have up to $17,000 in out-of-pocket expenses per year with the cheaper policy, which pays only 80 percent once you've reached your deductible amount, until the ceiling of $17,000 is reached. This is compared to only $2,250 with the more expensive policy. If you're older and at greater risk of serious illness, the more expensive policy might make more sense for you.

One advantage of paying for your own lab tests is that you can decide which tests you really want to have and how often you want to have them. If you want a hemoglobin A1c test every three months and the insurance company will only pay for it twice a year, most people would have the test only twice a year. If you're paying for it yourself, you can have it done every three months if you like.

The problem with this approach is that it's human nature to scrimp on expenses when you're paying the bill. Let's say you've calculated that unless you have a major medical crisis, you can save $500 a year by having a $2,000-deductible policy and paying for your A1c test four times a year, as well as other expected medical costs you'll incur yourself. But the test costs about $50, and when the time comes, it might be very tempting to put it off and spend the $50 on something else. If you are likely to do this, you might be better off paying more for the lower deductible.

Free drug programs exist

If you really can't afford your diabetes medications, most drug companies have special programs that offer free drugs to people in need. In general, your doctor has to apply for the programs, and a lot of paperwork is involved. Then you get free drugs for about three months, after which you have to apply again. Not all drugs are available this way, but it never hurts to try. Your doctor can call the Partnership for Prescription Assistance (800–762–4636 or go to www.pparx.org), or you can find out which company makes the drug you need and ask it how to apply.

Numerous groups offer help in researching where to get free drugs. They charge five dollars per drug. This might be worthwhile if you can't get the information from the partnership (which does not charge a fee). But be careful. There have been complaints about a few of these groups.

Don't forget to ask your doctors about free samples. They'll often have enough to tide you over until you've found a permanent source.

There are programs for the uninsured

Lions Clubs often offer free or low-cost programs for eye-care problems. Many hospitals offer free or reduced-price programs under the

Hill-Burton Program (800–638–0742). Many cities have walk-in clinics for people without insurance. And the federal Bureau of Primary Health Care (888–275–4772) sponsors health-care centers that provide care regardless of insurance status.

If you don't have good insurance and you feel you're not getting very good diabetes care, one way to get at least some good care is to enroll in research studies at major hospitals and universities, if you live within a reasonable distance of such sites.

Clinical trials. There are different kinds of studies. Some of them are *clinical trials* of new drugs, or new ways of using old drugs, usually sponsored by drug companies, which are required to test the effects of new drugs on a certain number of people before they go into the marketing phase.

The advantages of taking part in such trials are free physical exams, lab work, and drugs. But find out something about the people involved in the trial and exactly what the drug is and what its possible side effects are before you enroll.

Sometimes drug companies pay private physicians huge sums to enroll patients in such trials. If this is the case, the physician who suggests that you enroll may not have your best interests at heart and might push you to sign up so he or she can get the bonus payment from the drug company. One headline in *Practice Trends*, a journal for physicians, said, "Research Projects Can Add to Your Bottom Line" and began, "If the prospect of participating in scientific studies while adding thousands of dollars to your annual income sounds intriguing, consider incorporating research projects into your practice." The article said some drug companies pay physicians $350 per patient on enrollment and another $350 if they complete the project, and the physician is not required to inform the patient that he or she is making money from the research.

Nevertheless, some trials may benefit you, and some physicians may learn more about diabetes by participating in a diabetes drug trial, which would benefit you as well. But be cautious. Don't sign up for any trial that you think is not in your best interest.

Research studies. Another type of study is the research study, done only at major research hospitals. These studies are usually funded by government grants, not by drug companies, and are conducted by research scientists trying to understand how diabetes works.

The advantage of this type of trial is that you not only get free medical exams and tests, but you also have contact with some of the best diabetes doctors there are. Furthermore, because this is their own research, not just a routine test for a drug company, they are usually greatly interested in the results and in how you react to whatever it is they are studying.

In both the clinical trials and the research studies, you will first be screened to see if you qualify for the study. This means a free physical exam, often with extras like an electrocardiogram, as well as a lot of lab tests. You may be rejected from the study on the basis of the results; for example, if your A1c was too low or too high, or if they found something else that would suggest that the study drug wouldn't be a good idea for you. But even if you're rejected, you've had some medical care at no cost to you.

Even with the research studies, don't rush into something that doesn't feel right for you. Ask questions before you sign on the dotted line. What are the potential side effects of this drug or this treatment? Can you drop out if you think the treatment is hurting you? Will you actually get the drug or treatment in the study, or is there a chance that you will get a placebo instead? Does that matter to you? That is, are you participating because you want to take the drug or because you want the free medical tests?

Good medical care is expensive, and finding ways to pay for it can consume a lot of time. But like the rest of diabetes control, it's worth the effort. You deserve the best.

IN A SENTENCE:

■ *Diabetes is expensive, so make sure you have the best insurance you can afford.*

Diabetes Drugs

Sulfonylureas stimulate insulin secretion

Today there is a whole range of drugs available for treating type 2 diabetes. *Sulfonylureas* were the first drugs developed for diabetes, starting shortly after World War II, when it was noticed that sulfa drugs used to fight infection often brought blood glucose (BG) levels down. They are still used, but there are now second-generation sulfonylureas that are more effective than the early drugs. Some examples are glimepiride (Amaryl), glyburide (DiaBeta, Glynase, Micronase), and glipizide (Glucotrol).

These drugs work primarily by whipping your sluggish *beta cells* into producing insulin whether or not you eat. The sulfonylureas make the beta cells produce insulin all day, so if you miss a meal or don't eat enough carbohydrate with a meal, the insulin can make your BG level go too low. Thus if you take a sulfonylurea, it is essential to maintain a regular meal schedule with a certain amount of carbohydrate with each meal or snack, whether or not you are hungry. Some people gain weight when they use sulfonylureas. If being overweight has contributed to your insulin resistance (IR), a sulfonylurea may not be the best drug for you.

119

Some people say that constantly flogging your pancreas to produce more insulin will make it even more "exhausted" and wear it out faster. If simply producing a lot of insulin is what exhausts beta cells, this idea makes sense. However, there is little real evidence for this theory. Note that a lack of evidence doesn't mean that something isn't true; it may just mean that no one has done the right experiments yet. In the British UK-PDS study I mentioned in Day 6, beta cell function in people treated with sulfonylureas didn't deteriorate any faster than in those on insulin, metformin (discussed later), or diet and exercise. Some people have concluded from this study that beta cell deterioration is inevitable, no matter what you do. However, people in all four groups studied kept their BG levels higher than normal, in some cases quite a bit higher.

In 1970, a study called the University Group Diabetes Program (referred to as the *UGDP study*) found that people taking sulfonylureas had higher rates of heart attacks than those who did not. Many physicians now feel that this study was flawed and should be ignored, but because of the study, the package inserts for the sulfonylureas warn people of this possibility. Sulfonylureas work by closing certain potassium channels in the beta cell. Heart cells also contain potassium channels, and some of the sulfonylureas do act on the heart-cell potassium channels.

A study reported in 2006 suggested that the older sulfonylureas are associated with higher rates of cardiac deaths, and it recommended using the newer sulfonylureas and then only as third-line drugs after a biguanide or thiazolidinedione (see later in this chapter) had been tried. In 2014, another study showed higher rates of cardiovascular disease in women with long-term use of sulfonylureas than in those using metformin. A meta-analysis reported in 2015 showed no increase in mortality with sulfonylurea use. However, the issue is still controversial, as other meta-analyses have shown increased cardiovascular risk.

Some new drugs work faster

Since 1997, a new type of drug has been available. Like the sulfonylureas, these drugs work by stimulating your pancreas into producing more insulin. However, unlike the sulfonylureas, these agents work for only a short period of time. You take them right before meals, and they do their work and then quit. As a result, the risk of getting low blood sugar (**hypoglycemia**) is much smaller. If you don't want to eat, you don't take the drug, which means you don't need to eat when you're not hungry. This may help prevent weight gain, although weight gain is listed as a possible side effect.

Repaglinide (Prandin) and nateglinide (Starlix) are the two drugs of this type currently available. Repaglinide is considered in the *meglitinide* class. Nateglinide is classified as a *phenylalanine derivative* and is said to work faster. There is some confusion about the classification of these two drugs, and you may see nateglinide called a *meglitinide*. For our purposes, it doesn't matter what you call them. What matters is whether or not they work.

There is some evidence that when you use these drugs, the beta cells produce more insulin if you eat a lot of carbohydrate and less insulin if you eat less, which better matches the insulin output with the need and again reduces the probability of hypoglycemia, although it still exists.

Repaglinide is excreted in the feces, rather than the urine as many drugs are, and this would be beneficial if your kidney function is not good.

Biguanides work mainly on the liver

Another type of drug is the *biguanides*. The only such drug available in the United States today is metformin (Glucophage). This drug seems to have many different effects, but its main action seems to be to keep the liver from producing too much glucose when you don't need it. There is some evidence that it also improves *endothelial* (blood vessel lining) function.

You may remember the discussion of insulin and glucagon in Day 7. Insulin makes the BG level go down, glucagon makes it go up, and it's the ratio of the two that is important. When you have type 2 diabetes, you don't have enough effective insulin; you may have a lot of insulin, but it doesn't work very well. In addition, people with type 2 diabetes usually have more glucagon than normal, a sort of double whammy.

Glucagon is one of the hormones that tells the liver that the BG level is too low, so it should snap into action and crank out some glucose to bring the BG level back up again. That's fine when the BG level really is low; it's what keeps you from passing out from hypoglycemia. But when you have type 2 diabetes, the extra glucagon often tells the liver to keep spewing out glucose even when the glucose level is already high.

Insulin is glucagon's opposite. Insulin tells the liver to stop spitting out glucose. But when you have IR in your muscle cells, you usually have IR in your liver as well. So the extra glucagon is telling the liver to crank out extra glucose, and because of IR in the liver, the insulin is unable to turn it off. You can think of glucagon as the accelerator for glucose production by the liver and insulin as the brakes. When you have diabetes, not only are your brakes rusty, but your accelerator is stuck on high. The net result is the production of a lot of glucose by the liver even when your BG level is already high enough.

Metformin is supposed to stop this process. It also seems to help some people lose weight by reducing their appetite. It is thus often the drug of choice for overweight people with type 2 diabetes. Some physicians even prescribe it for weight loss in nondiabetic patients.

Metformin sometimes has side effects of nausea, gas, and bad diarrhea. Many people can control these side effects by taking the drug with meals and by starting with small doses and increasing the doses slowly. Some find that yogurt helps. Others are never able to tolerate it.

Metformin can also have a very serious side effect called *lactic acidosis*, which can be fatal. An earlier-generation biguanide, phenformin, was removed from the market because of this side effect. Because poor kidney or liver function can contribute to lactic acidosis, anyone with evidence of either should not take metformin. Fortunately, lactic acidosis is very rare, but if you take this drug you should insist on getting the package insert that comes with the drug. Carefully read the symptoms of this rare occurrence, and stop taking the drug immediately and consult a physician if you have any symptoms of lactic acidosis. Metformin should also not be used if you drink a lot of alcohol or have congestive heart failure.

Alpha-glucosidase inhibitors slow down starch digestion

Another class of drugs called *alpha-glucosidase inhibitors* keeps carbohydrates from breaking down into sugars in the intestines. Acarbose (Precose) and miglitol (Glyset) are such drugs.

You may remember that carbohydrates are composed of sugars. The long chains are called *polysaccharides* (many sugars). The intestines can't absorb polysaccharides, even when they are broken down into *disaccharides* (two-sugar units). They expect enzymes to break the polysaccharides down into *monosaccharides* (single sugars) like *glucose, fructose,* or *galactose,* which can be taken up by the cells of the intestinal wall.

Drugs like acarbose keep the enzymes (called *alpha-glucosidases*) from doing their job, so much of the carbohydrate you eat just passes right through your intestine. The glucose it contains never reaches your bloodstream, and your BG level doesn't go up as much after a meal. Because they work on the enzymes that break down polysaccharides, however, they have no effect if you eat a monosaccharide like glucose or fructose. They are also less effective with milk sugar, or lactose (only 10 percent inhibition, compared with 90 percent for starch). Furthermore, because they work on the carbohydrates that you eat, they must be taken with the first bite of any meal.

These drugs don't need to get into your bloodstream to be effective; they do their work in the digestive tract. For this reason they are thought to have fewer potential side effects on other organs, although they can cause reversible liver damage if used at high doses.

The glucosidase inhibitors do have one unfortunate side effect. Even though your own digestive enzymes can't break down the polysaccharides when you eat them, the intestinal bacteria can. They munch happily away on the carbohydrate you didn't get to use and produce gas. Some people can tolerate the results, but some can't.

Thiazolidinediones reduce insulin resistance

Another class of drugs is the *thiazolidinediones (TZDs)*, often called the *glitazones* by people like me who can't pronounce their formal name. These include pioglitazone (Actos) and rosiglitazone (Avandia). Another glitazone, troglitazone (Rezulin), was withdrawn from the market after more than sixty people using the drug suffered fatal liver damage, and Avandia now comes with a "black box" warning that it may cause cardiac problems and should not be used in people with congestive heart failure.

These drugs seem to work primarily on the underlying problem in most people with type 2 diabetes: insulin resistance. Many people who use insulin (see Week 4 and Month 5) find that their insulin needs are greatly reduced when they also take one of the glitazone drugs.

Unlike the other diabetes drugs, the glitazones somehow change the expression of certain genes and stimulate the formation of new fat cells. More fat cells? You might think that this is the last thing you want. But these new "baby fat cells" are more sensitive to insulin than the older fat-stuffed cells, and this helps keep your BG levels down. This process takes time, and it may take several weeks before you see any results from using these drugs and even more before they have their maximal effect.

Because of the fatal liver damage from the first-generation glitazone, if you have any kind of preexisting liver problems, these drugs should not be used. Even though the newer drugs are supposed to be kinder to the liver, it's essential to make sure your liver function is tested regularly when you use them. Some people find that when they take these drugs they retain fluid and thus gain weight. The weight gain usually reverses if you stop taking them.

Since the glitazones can potentially cause fluid retention, they should not be used if you have any signs of heart failure, especially if you're also using insulin. In a small number of people, especially those who see fluid retention in the extremities, the glitazones can cause macular edema, an eye condition (see Month 10).

The glitazones also seem to have beneficial effects. They reduce **inflammation** (thought to be important in causing diabetes; see Month 6), improve endothelial function, and increase levels of a beneficial hormone called **adiponectin** (see Month 7). In one study of people with prediabetes, treatment with a glitazone reduced the incidence of type 2 diabetes even several years after the drug was no longer being used. Some studies suggest that the glitazones help preserve beta cell function.

Most drugs have several effects

I've focused so far on what are considered to be the primary effects of some of the types of oral diabetes drugs. Most of them are reported to have other effects as well, and there is some overlap in their effects. For example, metformin and the sulfonylurea glimepiride may decrease IR, like the glitazones. The sulfonylurea glipizide may help with insulin secretion after eating, like the fast-acting insulin-releasing agents. The sulfonylurea glyburide appears to do both, although to a lesser degree. Metformin may inhibit the uptake of carbohydrate from the intestine, like the alpha-glucosidase inhibitors. The glitazones and metformin may also have a beneficial effect on lipid profiles.

Thus when choosing a drug for you, your doctor should take into account your need to lose weight, the amount of IR you have, your lipid profiles, your diet plan, your lifestyle, and the health of your liver and kidneys.

The incretins are hormones

It has been known for many years that when glucose is injected into a vein, less insulin is produced than if you eat the same amount of glucose. This suggested that something in the digestive tract stimulates the release of insulin.

And, indeed, it was found that when you eat, the gut produces several hormones that stimulate the beta cells to release insulin. These are called **incretins**. Two of them are *glucagonlike peptide-1* (**GLP-1**) and *glucose-dependent insulinotropic peptide* (**GIP**), formerly known as *gastric inhibitory peptide*. Other gut hormones such as **grehlin, obestatin** (which have opposite effects on appetite), and *oxyntomodulin* (which reduces appetite) have effects on appetite, and even more gut hormones will undoubtedly be discovered in the future.

If you have type 2 diabetes, you produce less GLP-1 than normal. You produce normal amounts of GIP but are most likely resistant to its action. In other words, you're GIP-resistant, just as you are insulin-resistant.

Hence, a lot of the research has focused on GLP-1, as you are most likely sensitive to its actions if you can increase its levels.

Both GIP and GLP-1 are made up of chains of *amino acids*, which are the building blocks that make up proteins. Short chains of amino acids are called *peptides*; longer chains are called *polypeptides*, or *proteins*.

Most peptides and proteins can't survive the acid environment and digestive enzymes in the stomach, so like the protein insulin, GLP-1 and GIP can't be taken in pill form; they must be injected.

When GLP-1 is injected, it has several beneficial actions. First, it inhibits the secretion of the hormone *glucagon* (see Days 6 and 7). People with type 2 diabetes have not only too little insulin for their needs but too much glucagon, so reducing the amount of glucagon produced after meals is a good thing for us.

You recall that glucagon opposes the action of insulin. Among other actions, it stimulates the liver to produce and release glucose to keep the BG level from falling too low between meals. The problem is, when you have type 2 diabetes, it keeps on stimulating the liver even after you've eaten and contributes to your high postmeal BG levels.

Like fat, GLP-1 also delays gastric emptying, which is often accelerated in people in the early stages of diabetes (*delayed* gastric emptying, or **gastroparesis** [see Month 10], is a late complication). This delaying caused by GLP-1 means that if your beta cells still produce some insulin but just not enough to cover large glucose loads, the delay in gastric emptying may mean your beta cells can cope better with the mealtime influx of carbohydrate.

GLP-1 also acts on the brain to increase satiety, which is a good thing if you tend to eat too much, and feeling full after eating just a little food should result in weight loss. GLP-1 stimulates the beta cells to produce and secrete more insulin. There are some indications that it actually restores the phase-one insulin response (see Month 7) and increases the proliferation of beta cells.

One nice thing about GLP-1 is that its effects on insulin stimulation and glucagon suppression are glucose dependent. It won't have these effects unless your BG levels are greater than about 90 mg/dL, and this reduces the risk of hypoglycemia.

All this sounds wonderful. There's just one catch. GLP-1 doesn't last very long in the body; it's quickly destroyed by an enzyme called *DPP-4* (*dipeptidyl peptidase 4*). In order to see results from GLP-1, you'd have to receive a constant infusion of the hormone.

Exenatide 1 (Byetta) mimics the actions of GLP-1. Because GLP-1 is so quickly destroyed in the body, researchers sought compounds similar to GLP-1 that would have the beneficial actions of the natural hormone (called *GLP-1* **mimetics**, or drugs that mimic the action of GLP-1) but would last longer in the body. They discovered one in an odd place: the saliva of the Gila monster. It is called *exendin-4*. A synthetic version of exendin-4 is called *exenatide 1 (Byetta)*.

Byetta was approved by the Food and Drug Administration (FDA) in 2005. It is injected before meals, and a common side effect is nausea, which usually improves with time. Results so far have varied. Some patients say it's a miracle drug. They've lost significant amounts of weight, and their BG levels have improved. Others find it doesn't work for them.

Some patients are reporting on the Internet that they get cold extremities, constipation, pains in their teeth, and hair loss when they take the drug. However, these claims have not been analyzed statistically. Another side effect is the production of antibodies against exenatide. If you inject insulin, you also produce antibodies against insulin, but in most people this doesn't cause a lot of problems. No one knows the long-term effect of antibodies against exenatide, or, for that matter, the long-term effects of taking any new drug.

Because exenatide (Byetta) delays gastric emptying, it should not be used if you have any signs of gastroparesis. For the same reason, drugs that require rapid absorption should be taken an hour or so before or after injecting Byetta.

Long-acting incretins are now available. Byetta has to be injected twice a day, which some people find inconvenient. There are now four FDA-approved longer-acting incretins: *liraglutide (Victoza)*, which is injected once a day, and three versions that are injected once a week, namely, exenatide extended-release (Bydureon), albiglutide (Tanzeum), and dulaglutide (Trulicity). Liraglutide has also been FDA approved for weight loss. Other incretins are in development.

If postmarketing studies show unacceptable side effects from any of these products, they will be removed from the market. Some studies show increased rates of pancreatitis and thyroid cancers with some incretins, but a recent study showed no increase in acute pancreatitis from some incretins. The risk/benefit ratio is debated among clinicians.

DPP-4 inhibitors keep GLP-1 active. Recall that one reason we can't simply inject the natural hormone GLP-1 is that it's quickly destroyed by the enzyme DPP-4. So another approach to goosing up your incretin levels is to inhibit the enzyme that breaks your natural GLP-1 down. As a group, these drugs are called *gliptins*, or *DPP-4 inhibitors*. Unlike exenatide, they don't cause nausea. However, they also do not usually result in weight loss.

FDA-approved DPP-4 inhibitors include sitagliptin (Januvia), alogliptin (Nesina), saxagliptin (Onglyza), and linagliptin (Tradjenta). Still more of these drugs are being developed, and some of them have been approved in

Europe or Japan. They are also available in combinations with other drugs like metformin and pioglitazone. Other DPP-4 inhibitors were removed from the market because of unacceptable side effects.

These drugs should be used with caution in people with prior history of congestive heart failure, and in spring 2015 an FDA advisory committee recommended that the labels of two of them, saxagliptin and alogliptin, warn about this increased risk. Some members of the committee thought that this warning might apply to other drugs in this category; a subsequent trial of sitagliptin showed no increased risk. Note that this is an advisory committee, and the FDA is not required to act on its recommendation. A majority of the committee did not consider the risk high enough to remove the drugs from the market.

However, on the positive side, a recent study suggested that these drugs may reduce the risk of autoimmune diseases.

Although they do work to increase GLP-1 levels, the DPP-4 inhibitors also act on other peptides in the body, and the long-term effect of their use is unknown. Their effects on cancer rates are controversial. Some people report slow wound healing while taking the drugs, but some studies show improved healing of wounds in mice and humans.

SGLT-2 inhibitors make you excrete more glucose

The kidney is an amazing organ. It not only filters waste products and toxins from the blood, but like the liver, it also produces glucose when BG levels are low. The kidney is constantly working to keep the levels of various substances in the blood at healthy levels.

The section on nephropathy in Month 10, Living, gives some information on how the kidney works. Essentially, all the molecules in plasma, except proteins, are absorbed into the kidney. But later the useful ones are reabsorbed back into the blood. When BG levels are normal, almost 100 percent of the glucose is reabsorbed back into the blood.

This means you don't lose glucose calories in your urine, which would be beneficial in an environment in which food was scarce, which was true for most of human evolution.

In order to reabsorb the glucose into the blood, the kidney uses glucose transporters called *sodium-glucose transporters,* abbreviated **SGLT**. If these transporters are blocked, the glucose can't get back into the blood and is excreted in the urine. SGLT-2 inhibitors currently FDA approved in the United States include canagliflozin (Invokana), dapagliflozin (Farxiga), and empagliflozin (Jardiance). More are under development.

Glucose also gets into the urine when BG levels are higher than about 200 mg/dL, which is why having glucose in the urine is a sign of high BG.

Different people may have slightly different thresholds for "spilling" glucose into the urine. Kidney damage can also cause spilling of glucose.

The transporter that is responsible for reabsorbing 90 percent of the glucose into the blood is called *SGLT-2*, and it's this one that is blocked by the new SGLT-2 inhibitors. There's also a similar transporter called SGLT-1, which absorbs 10 percent of the glucose in the kidney and is also responsible for absorbing glucose from the gut. If this transporter is blocked, you can't absorb dietary glucose, and this can result in diarrhea. So researchers have developed drugs that work only on SGLT-2.

Blocking reabsorption of glucose in the kidney reduces the BG concentration. It can also cause slight weight loss, as you're losing calories (up to about three hundred calories a day) in the urine. Some people also find that their blood pressure goes down on these drugs. One advantage is that they rarely cause hypoglycemia.

However, high levels of glucose in the urine can cause genital infections. And the drugs don't work well in people with impaired kidney function. In spring 2015, the FDA reported that SGLT-2 inhibitors can cause **diabetic ketoacidosis**, or **DKA** (see Month 2), in people with type 2 diabetes. DKA is usually found in people with type 1 diabetes who have very high BG levels, but the DKA found with SGLT-2 inhibitors occurs with normal BG levels. Signs of DKA include difficulty breathing, nausea, vomiting, abdominal pain, confusion, and unusual fatigue or sleepiness. DKA is serious and can be fatal if not treated, so although this side effect is not common, if you have these symptoms while taking an SGLT-2 inhibitor, don't wait to seek medical treatment.

Bile acid sequestrants lower both glucose and LDL

Bile acid sequestrants have been used for decades to lower **LDL** (*low-density lipoprotein*) cholesterol, and it has recently been discovered that they also lower BG levels, thus having two effects that should be beneficial in people with type 2 diabetes. The only sequestrant approved by the FDA for lowering BG levels in type 2 diabetes is colesevelam (Welchol).

The sequestrants lower cholesterol by binding to the bile in such a way that it can't be absorbed from the intestine. Normally, bile cycles from the liver through the bile duct to the intestine, where it helps to emulsify cholesterol. When its job is done, it's taken out of the intestine and sent to the liver, where it's recycled.

When the bile is bound to the bile acid sequestrant, it just passes through the intestine and out with the feces. Then the liver has to make more, and because bile is made from cholesterol and the liver's cholesterol supplies are lowered, the body makes more LDL receptors on liver cells and removes more cholesterol from the blood.

The mechanism for lowering BG levels is not yet understood, however. It is now thought that bile acid sequestrants are signaling molecules and may increase levels of GLP-1 and affect beta cells as well as hepatic glucose metabolism.

Because the drugs have been used for years to lower cholesterol, their side effects are known. One advantage of the drugs is that they don't cause weight gain or hypoglycemia, but they can increase triglycerides, and constipation is a common side effect.

Bromocriptine works in the brain

Bromocriptine is a *dopamine agonist*, meaning a drug that works on dopamine receptors (specifically, D2 receptors) in the brain to produce the same effects as dopamine would produce. It's been used in dopamine-deficiency diseases like Parkinson's for some time. So you may wonder what it has to do with diabetes.

There is evidence that insulin resistance and obesity are regulated in part by the brain. It seems that people with type 2 diabetes lack the normal early-morning surge of dopamine that is seen in healthy people, and fast-acting bromocriptine restores this morning surge. Although no one yet knows exactly how bromocriptine works for diabetes control, it does increase insulin sensitivity, reduce postmeal BG levels by suppressing hepatic glucose production, reduce hemoglobin A1c (although not by a lot), reduce fasting and postmeal lipid levels, and reduce cardiovascular events.

The drug that has been tested in humans is a fast-acting formulation of bromocriptine mesylate (Cycloset), which produces a surge of dopamine that doesn't last long. In 2009, Cycloset received FDA approval for treating type 2 diabetes. Other formulations of bromocriptine had previously been approved for other indications, but they produced longer increases in dopamine levels. This previous use means physicians had some experience using the drug.

To try to understand how hormone surges in the brain could help with diabetes, think of hibernating animals. They put on weight in the fall, even when they don't eat any more than they ate in the summer, and one reason is that decreasing day lengths trigger hormone surges that tell the body to store fat. These hormones change their insulin sensitivity.

If, for some reason that no one yet understands, some people have hormone levels that would be suitable if they wanted to store fat, but they have these hormone levels all year round, then fixing the hormone levels with a drug should help them to lose weight as well as increasing insulin sensitivity. And increased insulin sensitivity can have many healthy results.

Bromocriptine is an ergot derivative, and the drugs do have side effects. Nausea, fatigue, vomiting, and headache are the primary ones, but some report dizziness and other central nervous system effects. At higher doses of bromocriptine, some people report hallucinations, but the doses of Cycloset approved for diabetes treatment are much lower.

Pramlintide (Symlin) is for insulin users

When the beta cells secrete insulin, they also secrete another protein called *amylin*. Hence people who are producing almost no insulin are also producing almost no amylin.

Amylin does almost all the same things that GLP-1 does: it reduces glucagon levels, slows down gastric emptying, and increases satiety, thus resulting in weight loss. However, it does not stimulate the production of insulin.

Like the GLP-1 **analogs**, an amylin analog has been produced. It is called *pramlintide* (*Symlin*). Like exenatide, amylin is injected at mealtimes. And like exenatide, amylin tends to cause nausea, especially at first.

Because exenatide stimulates some insulin release, if you have some beta cells left, it would make sense to use exenatide. If you don't have many beta cells left, amylin should work about the same. It has been approved for use by insulin users, but because it delays gastric emptying, it's important to adjust mealtime insulin doses (see Month 5) when using the drug, to avoid hypoglycemia.

Exenatide and amylin seem to increase the feeling of fullness, so they might be worth investigating if you think you are overweight because your appetite is unusually large.

Combination drugs may be easier to take

When new drugs are approved by the FDA, drug companies usually market them as single drugs, with high prices. If the drug is successful, when the company's patent expires, other companies will produce generic copies of the drug, resulting in competition and usually forcing the drug companies to reduce their prices for the brand-name drugs.

One way the companies try to protect their patents is to get FDA approval of the brand-name drug for special patient populations, for example, for children. Another way is to produce brand-name combination drugs, combining two different drugs in one pill, and get FDA approval for the combination.

With so many oral drugs now on the market, there are many possible combinations. These include metformin and a glitazone (Actoplus Met, Avandamet); metformin and a sulfonylurea (Metaglip, Glucovance); metformin and a gliptin (DPP-4 inhibitor) (Janumet, Kombiglyze, Jentadueto, Kazano); metformin and an SGLT-2 inhibitor (Invokamet, Xigduo); metformin and repaglinide (Prandimet); a gliptin and an SGLT-2 inhibitor (Glyxambi); a gliptin and a glitazone (Oseni); a sulfonylurea and a glitazone (Avandaryl); and a glitazone and a sulfonylurea (Duetract).

It may be easier to take one instead of two pills, and sometimes it's cheaper. The problem with combinations is that you're locked into one or a few combinations of dosages; it's difficult to change the dosage of one of the drugs without changing the dosage of the other one.

Insulin also works

Insulin is, of course, another option, and not necessarily a last resort, especially if your main problem is low beta cell output instead of a lot of IR. Because it is such an important option, I discuss it in more detail in Week 4 and Month 5.

New drugs are being developed

Because type 2 diabetes is becoming epidemic in this country, selling new diabetic drugs is very lucrative. You can get a starting dose of metformin for less than $8 a month, sometimes free with Medicare Plan D, or $4 per prescription at some stores. Newer brand-name drugs can cost more than $500 a month, and the prices will undoubtedly continue to rise. Drug companies are working overtime to develop new drugs to treat this disease, and you can expect to see many new drugs announced in the years ahead. Research is also going on, exploring drugs that reduce the complications caused by high BG levels (see Month 10).

Not long ago, the only choice doctors had was either insulin or a first-generation sulfonylurea to treat patients with type 2 diabetes who couldn't control it with diet and exercise alone. Now there are eight or nine different classes of drugs, with several drugs in most of the classes. At the rate things are going, there will soon be a vast variety of drugs, each attacking type 2 diabetes at a different site.

New oral drugs are being approved all the time, so if your drug isn't mentioned here, it's probably a new one.

Check postmarketing studies

Drugs can be approved before large numbers of people have taken them, and side effects may show up when more people take the drugs. So if you're taking a new drug that hasn't been on the market long, be alert for reports of new side effects, or ask your doctor about them. Sometimes a drug that appeared to be safe initially turns out to increase rates of heart disease or cancer. So older drugs are usually safer as well as cheaper.

IN A SENTENCE:

▪ *There are many different types of diabetes drugs, and they work at different places in the body.*

Depression

Having diabetes can be depressing. In fact, there is a statistical association between diabetes and depression. More people with diabetes are diagnosed with depression than other members of the population.

Some people think this means that some kind of hormonal changes associated with diabetes cause depression. I think that anyone who *doesn't* get depressed when they are told they'll have to be on a strict, calorie-limited diet for the rest of their lives, not to mention spending a lot of their precious leisure time on an exercise bicycle, is probably a bit loony.

Of course, there's a difference between just feeling sad, which is a natural reaction to learning that you have any kind of chronic, incurable disease, and clinical depression, which includes feelings of hopelessness that last for weeks or months. The latter condition is serious and requires some kind of outside help. Clinical depression is nothing to be ashamed of. Like diabetes, it is a medical condition that requires medical treatment. The sooner you are able to get help, the less you will suffer. Don't wait.

Just feeling blue is common

The other kind of depression, just feeling blue and tired and not interested in doing anything for a while, is more common with diabetes. This depression often occurs after diagnosis. One day you're just like everyone else, and suddenly you're different. You can't do the ordinary things that everyone else can do. A friend bakes bread and serves it slathered with fresh butter and homemade raspberry jam, but you can't have any. So you sit there and smell the freshly baked bread and watch the others eating as they comment on how delicious it is. Then they start discussing their favorite kinds of sweet rolls, and their favorite bakery, and their favorite kinds of pie. And you know you can't have any, maybe forever. You're not like everyone else anymore; you're an outsider. Is it any wonder you might get a little blue?

Professionals want to cheer you up

Many of the authors of pamphlets and magazines written for people with diabetes realize that it's a bit depressing to get a diagnosis of diabetes, so they want to cheer you up and remind you of all the good things you can still do. One brochure for a diabetes drug is illustrated with photographs of people smiling happily as they take vigorous walks, grinning from ear to ear as they prepare salads with low-fat dressings, smiling adoringly at spouses as they stick needles into their fingers to draw blood for blood glucose tests, and looking rapturous as dieticians point out the tiny serving sizes that will be allotted to them for the rest of their lives. I once went through a copy of *Diabetes Forecast*, the magazine of the American Diabetes Association, and couldn't find a single picture of anyone who wasn't smiling.

This outlook is understandable. If people published magazines showing people sobbing uncontrollably, or shrieking with pain when jabbing their fingers, or sitting in the corner while everyone else ate cake and ice cream, no one would want to read them. A cheerful attitude and stories of people with diabetes who overcame their handicap and lead happy, fulfilling lives can sometimes be inspiring. It's especially important for children to see successful role models.

But sometimes the feeling that no one understands what you're going through can be more depressing than the disease itself. "Don't think you'll never be able to eat delicious food again," wrote one author in an article for the newly diagnosed. "Diabetes diets can be both delicious and varied." Yeah, right. Especially if you want to eat lettuce, low-fat dressing, and lean turkey breast day after day while everyone else is chowing down on pizza and cornstarch-thickened Chinese sauces. Of course the foods you eat *can* be varied and delicious. If everyone were on the same diet, there wouldn't actually be much of a problem. People in some parts of the world eat rice and beans three times a day and don't get depressed because everyone else is eating rice and beans too. It's having to watch other people eat even more delicious foods three times a day, 365 days a year, that can get depressing.

Putting food in front of starving people and not letting them eat it is considered a form of torture. Yet people with type 2 diabetes, who are often hungry all the time because they are on low-calorie weight-loss diets, are expected to smile happily as they endure this day after day, year after year.

"I spent the holidays watching my family eat delicious foods," said Virginia P. "I felt like Tantalus." Tantalus was the son of Zeus who was punished in Hades by constant hunger, surrounded by food. Whenever he reached for fruit from a heavily laden tree, it flew just out of his reach. The word *tantalize* comes from his ordeal.

Some professionals aren't sympathetic

Most medical people don't really understand what a person newly diagnosed with diabetes is going through. Some can be quite unsympathetic. "I went into my doctor, literally breaking down into tears, saying how depressed I was and how unfair it was I developed diabetes," said Dawn A. "She just about yelled at me. Just what I needed! But she told me that I should be thankful that all I was in there seeing her for was diabetes. She told me I was lucky that I wasn't being treated by her for cancer or some other incurable disease. I was *lucky* to have diabetes, because in the grand scheme of things, diabetes was controllable."

Of course the doctor was correct. But that's like telling someone he has six months to live but he should leap with joy because someone else has only three weeks. We all expect to be the lucky ones, the healthy ones. Finding out we're not is depressing.

Family members may not understand either. "When I phoned my sister-in-law," said Annie Mae G., "and told her the reason I was declining her dinner invitations was because she never served anything I could eat, she said, 'Well, you can't expect us to keep up with the ins and outs of your latest diet,' as if my diabetic diet was some kind of self-imposed fad thing I changed from week to week. It's not. It's going to be medically necessary for the rest of my life."

Being different and not being understood is often harder than the medical management of the disease. Think about it. Imagine that everyone else didn't have to worry about elimination, that their wastes just somehow evaporated from their skin, but you had a disease that required you to go to the bathroom instead. You would probably feel like a pariah. No one else would have to leave the classroom or stop during a trip or get up at night to do this disgusting thing that you had to do. "Why me?" you might ask.

But when everyone in the world has to go to the bathroom, it never seems like a particularly odious chore. It takes a few minutes a day, but mostly we don't think about it.

Diabetes management can be the same. It means extra effort, extra work, extra planning, and extra willpower. But it's doable, in most cases. Once you accept the reality of this disease and work its management into your normal lifestyle, the depression will tend to lift.

So you're different. So what. Lots of people are different; why should you be exempt? So you can't eat a lot of cake and pie. So what. Lots of people in the world go to bed hungry every night. Is giving up a little pie and cake really that bad?

There's also a positive side

I enjoy my food a lot more than I used to, when I often ate more than I needed because the food looked so good and I was raised to clean my plate. After dinner I sometimes felt so stuffed I was uncomfortable. Now I concentrate on taste more than quantity. The first bite of everything usually tastes the best. By limiting the number of bites, I get a larger percentage of the best part of the food. I no longer eat something I don't like just because it's on the plate. With time, most people also come to realize that lifestyle changes like eating less and moving more make them feel better, that in general their life has improved.

For about thirty years, before my diabetes diagnosis, I had been trying to lose a little weight, starting when I thought 115 pounds was too much. But in all those years, instead of losing weight, I managed to gain forty pounds. I'm sure you've been through it all, repeatedly telling yourself, "*Tomorrow* I'll be really good."

But when I got the diabetes diagnosis, I knew this was different. This was serious. I was hungry pretty much twenty-four hours a day, but I still managed to lose about thirty pounds. I slowly switched to a low-carbohydrate diet and stopped being hungry all the time. So far, I've managed to keep most of the lost weight off.

Having diabetes has had other benefits in my life. I've made a lot of friends all over the world by way of the Internet. The disease has rekindled my earlier interest in biochemistry, which I studied in graduate school. Rather than seeing it as a handicap, I see diabetes as a fascinating, incredibly complex puzzle to be solved. Answers, no matter how trivial, have more potential benefits to other people than solving a crossword puzzle.

I've always enjoyed testing things. So of all the diseases I might have gotten, I'm lucky to have gotten one that gives me an excuse to do a lot of tests. Of course not everyone has the same scientific approach to the disease, and some people do, in fact, suffer disabling consequences. But with good control, you will probably finally realize that you haven't gone blind, your kidneys are fine, and you still have your feet. Your life may not be that much different from what it was before your diagnosis. In fact, with good control, you may even have more energy and feel healthier than you have in years.

Some people have met spouses as a result of being diagnosed with diabetes. Others have seen new careers open up. Some have discovered an interest in medical matters and have become certified diabetes educators, helping others deal with the disease. Some have even written books.

Venting helps

The best way to overcome the initial depression is first of all to understand that it's a normal part of the mourning process and second to get in touch with other people who really do understand what you're going through, and this means other people with type 2 diabetes. As is true with other depressing situations like being widowed or losing a child, people who have never been in that situation can never really understand. Venting, expressing your anger or your frustration or your depression to other people who understand, can be much more helpful than attending workshops run by well-intentioned health-care people who usually don't have a clue about what it's actually like to live with diabetes.

Interestingly, some people who have pancreas transplants and suddenly cease being diabetic also go through a mourning process, in this case mourning the diabetic person they were. Apparently, dealing with diabetes had become so much a part of who they were that even though they'd always wanted their diabetes to go away more than anything else in the world, when it actually did go away, they mourned their "loss."

Like any kind of mourning, mourning for your formerly nondiabetic self will eventually pass. In the meantime, remember that feeling blue after any major life change is normal. Don't worry that something is wrong. It's OK to be sad for a while. As is true after the death of a friend, it's better than pretending you don't care. Mourning helps with healing. You go through it, and then you come out the other side and get on with your life.

IN A SENTENCE:

Mourning the loss of your nondiabetic self is normal after you're diagnosed, but after you work through this stage, you may feel better than you have in years.

What Treatment Should I Get?

You've probably started out trying diet and exercise, maybe with an oral drug, as the first treatment of your disease. Now you may begin to wonder if this is the best treatment for you.

The best treatment for type 2 diabetes is the one that gets *your* blood glucose (BG) levels as close to normal as possible. This will minimize glucotoxicity (see Week 2) and reduce the chances you'll ever develop diabetic complications. Today, there are many choices available, and what works best for someone else might not be the best choice for you.

The classic treatment of type 2 diabetes started off with a trial diet and exercise plan. Then you came back in a few weeks or months, and if your BG levels hadn't come down, you would be given a sulfonylurea (see Week 3). If this didn't bring your BG levels down sufficiently, you would be given a big lecture about the importance of sticking to your diet and getting more exercise or you'd have to take insulin shots. Then you'd come back in a few months, and if your BG levels still hadn't come down, you'd be told you had to give yourself shots of insulin.

Oral drugs may work for you

Just with the brief review in Week 3, you can see that today there is a huge choice of treatments, with many different classes of drugs and different drugs within each class. Because of the multiple effects of the diabetes drugs and because people have different flavors of diabetes, the choice depends on your particular medical needs as well as your lifestyle, personality, and budget.

If your insurance covers the cost of drugs, the prices of the drugs won't matter. But if you're on a very limited budget and have to pay for your own drugs, make sure you know what the various drugs cost before you and your doctor make a final choice. There's a wide range of prices. In 2015, you could get a month's supply of generic metformin for $4, or even free at some places. A month's supply of one of the newer incretins was $546 list price, although discounts can usually be found. If you're on a Medicare Part D drug plan, generics are often "free," although they add the list price to your total drug costs, which means you may reach the "doughnut hole" sooner if you take a lot of other drugs.

If you're paying for your own drugs and your budget is tight, it might make sense to start with one of the cheaper drugs and use the money you've saved to spend on nutritious, tasty food that will help you stick to your diet.

Quite often, you will be started out on one oral drug, and then if this doesn't bring the BG level down enough, another drug that works in a different way (see Week 3) will be *added*. For example, you might take metformin to keep your liver from producing too much glucose and a glitazone to try to reduce your insulin resistance (IR).

You can see now why something like the C-peptide test (see Day 5) might be useful. If you find you produce a lot of C-peptide, it means you're producing a lot of insulin, which means you've got a lot of IR. Thus starting off with a glitazone drug that reduces IR might make more sense for you than a sulfonylurea that would just make your insulin levels even higher.

But glitazones often cause weight gain. If weight loss is a major goal for you, metformin might be a better choice. If you're not seriously overweight and a C-peptide test shows that you're not producing a lot of insulin, then a drug that helps your sluggish beta cells out might be a better choice for you. If your C-peptide level is low, you might want to start right off with insulin.

Insulin is another choice

Insulin? Some people think that insulin is used only for type 1 diabetes and that if you take insulin you've converted from type 2 into type 1. This is not true. Many people with type 2 diabetes take insulin, either because none of the other options have worked for them or because they prefer using it.

Doesn't that mean painful shots? Why would anyone want to do that when all these oral drugs are available? Well, first let's try to understand the rationale for the classic approach to treatment: diet and exercise, then oral drugs, then insulin.

Fear of needles. Most doctors assume that patients just diagnosed with diabetes aren't really champing at the bit for a chance to give themselves shots with hypodermic needles. There is some justification for this view. Some people are scared of shots of any kind, not to mention having to inject themselves. In the old days, needles were large and used over and over again until they got dull and hurt. And some type 2 patients do, in fact, burst into uncontrollable sobs when told their oral drugs aren't doing the job and they'll have to start injecting themselves with insulin. In many cases their sorrow comes not only from their fear of giving themselves shots but also from a sense that because they didn't succeed with the oral drugs, they are failures.

Unfortunately, because of the common fear of needles, some doctors use the idea of insulin injections as a threat. "If you can't lose at least five pounds by next month, I'll have to put you on insulin." This simply reinforces the idea that injecting insulin is a form of punishment and a horrible fate.

But remember glucotoxicity and beta cell "exhaustion." They mean that **the longer your beta cells are exposed to a high-glucose environment, the greater the chance they will suffer irreversible damage.** Say you are started on a diet and exercise program for a couple of months and the BG levels are still too high, so you take oral drug A for another few months. If this doesn't work, you take a combination of drug A plus drug B. This approach means your beta cells are going to be exposed to high BG levels for months until you find a treatment plan that works for you.

Starting on insulin. For this reason, some people feel that the best solution is to *start out on insulin* to bring the BG levels down to normal right away and to maintain them there for a while. This reduces glucotoxicity and gives the beta cells time to rest and recover a bit from the stress they've been under for however long you've had diabetes without knowing it.

Then after the BG levels have been normal for a while, in many cases you can stop using the insulin and use only oral drugs or just diet and exercise. It may be scary to think about using insulin right from the start, but ironically, it might be the best way to ensure that you won't have to use it for long.

Injecting insulin isn't the painful and time-consuming procedure that it used to be (see Month 5). Syringes these days are disposable, and the needles are extremely thin. You can even get "insulin pens" with the insulin already in a syringe so you can dial up the amount of insulin you need at a particular time.

There are some advantages to insulin therapy. Insulin is a natural substance, and there is less likelihood of unknown long-term side effects, which are always possible with new drugs. If you lack good insurance, it might be important that insulin is cheaper than many of the oral drugs, especially when you need several different drugs.

There are also some disadvantages. Like the sulfonylureas, insulin has the potential to produce *hypoglycemia*. In addition, many people say their appetite increases when they take insulin, and they gain weight, just as they do when they take the sulfonylurea drugs, which make your own pancreas produce more insulin. If you're overweight to start with, and if this is contributing to your IR, then insulin might not be the best way to start. However, this effect on appetite is not universal: "It was certainly my experience that before I went on insulin I was *ravenously* hungry, and after I started, my appetite went *way* down, and twenty-five pounds melted off like ice in a firestorm!" said Natalie S.

If you have polycystic ovary syndrome (see Month 2), in which high insulin levels may cause high levels of male hormones, it would not be a good idea to start on insulin.

Hyperinsulinemia. Another controversial aspect of insulin treatment is the question of **hyperinsulinemia**, or high levels of insulin in the bloodstream. Some people think that high insulin levels cause heart disease. When you have type 2 diabetes, you are usually insulin resistant, and if you inject insulin, you might have to use a lot more than the normal amounts that people with type 1 diabetes, and no IR, would use.

Other people think that high insulin levels do not *cause* heart disease. They say that it is the underlying problem, IR, that is associated with heart disease. People who are insulin resistant but have well-functioning beta cells produce more insulin than people without IR. Thus the high insulin levels that have been associated with heart disease may simply be a sign that these people have IR. This question has not yet been resolved.

Demanding insulin. Some people think the benefits outweigh the disadvantages. "The idea of sticking needles into my body didn't thrill me, but I wanted to control the disease and not have it control me!" said Carol M. "Since going on insulin, I feel so much better! I feel like I have 'me' back again! I was in a fog all the time on the pills, and now I feel so much clearer and with more energy." Some people actually *ask* to be allowed to use insulin because they are not satisfied with their quality of life when using diet and exercise or some of the oral drugs. Sometimes they actually have to argue with their doctors, who still believe that insulin is a last resort, something to inflict on a patient who has failed to control the diabetes by any other way.

"I asked for insulin back in 1991, and it took me several months," said Ehlonna H. "My doc kept hemming and hawing, wanting me to 'wait a little longer,' try a different sulf, etc. So I went doc shopping. I found a young gal, recently out of med school, and I looked her square in the eye and said that I would hire her if she would prescribe insulin for me. She said, 'OK.' It has been smooth sailing ever since. I love not having to take a bunch of pills and having direct control over my BG."

My control was good without insulin, but I wanted to have better control and even occasionally to eat some fruit or a piece of bread. It took more than a year for me to find an endocrinologist who agreed to prescribe it, and even then he did so reluctantly.

Resting beta cells. You may not be as eager for insulin as Ehlonna was, but even so, you should never look at insulin as a punishment for your sins. Insulin is just one of many kinds of treatment available for type 2 diabetes today. In some ways, it's easier to use. The many different kinds of insulin available today make its use very flexible, and once you learn how to count carbohydrates, it gives you a lot more choices of what to eat. Insulin is not expensive. A vial of one type of human regular insulin (the kind you inject before meals) can be purchased for about $24 in 2015, and each 10-milliliter vial contains 1,000 units, so if you don't have much IR and need a total of 30 units a day, a vial would last about a month. If you have a lot of IR, the cost would be greater. Unfortunately, manufacturers are discontinuing their cheaper insulins and replacing them with more expensive insulin analogs (see Month 5), which can cost $250 or more per vial.

Perhaps the best reason to think about using insulin right away is that insulin is kind to your beta cells. Even though there is now little concrete evidence that other types of treatment wear out the beta cells, we know that glucotoxicity is not good for them. If you can get your BG levels down to normal with diet and exercise, or with one of the other drugs, that's good. But if this doesn't happen quickly for you, going right to insulin might be something you should consider.

If you *do* decide to try insulin, don't settle for one of the old once-a-day injection routines, in which you have to eat even when you're not hungry. This can make you gain weight. Like oral drugs, insulins now come in many varieties, and their usage can be customized for you. Month 5 describes using insulin in more detail.

Insulin may not be best for everyone with type 2 diabetes. For instance, if you have a tremendous amount of IR and need to lose a lot of weight, a glitazone that reduces IR or metformin, which reduces appetite, might be better choices.

Just remember that insulin doesn't mean you are too weak to conquer your diabetes without it. Insulin means you are strong enough to take charge of your diabetes and take care of your beta cells. Someday you may be glad you did.

IN A SENTENCE:

■ *No single diabetes treatment is best for every patient, so you and your doctor have to figure out which one matches your own particular needs.*

First-Month MILESTONE

It's now a month after your diagnosis, and you're beginning to get a handle on controlling your diabetes:

- You know that you must be in charge.

- You understand more about why it's important to keep your blood glucose levels close to normal.

- You have been introduced to the main classes of diabetes treatment and their pros and cons.

- You understand that it's normal to be a little depressed at first, but this phase should pass.

living

Diabetes
ABCs

You may wonder why I'm waiting until your second month with diabetes to give you the diabetes ABCs. Well, I'm assuming the basics summarized in this chapter were described to you by your doctor, or a nurse, or a certified diabetes educator (CDE), or in some of the many pamphlets they probably gave you right after your diagnosis. What I've tried to do so far is to discuss some of the things these people *didn't* talk about.

But now is a good time to take stock, go back, and review some of the basics and make sure you understand what they are. You may have been in too much shock in those first days to take it all in, or maybe you were still in denial and thought it didn't apply to you. In any case, it never hurts to review the basic stuff in case something was left out in your initial training.

If you want more basic information, one good source is the National Diabetes Information Clearinghouse (800–860–8747; see Resources). They offer a plethora of free publications on all aspects of diabetes care, many in both English and Spanish. They will no longer mail you the booklets, but you can read them online or print them out.

Keep your blood glucose levels as close to normal as possible

I may sound like a broken record, but this is just about the most important thing you can do to control your diabetes. Keeping your blood glucose (BG) levels in the normal range will almost ensure that you'll never develop diabetes complications. If you already had early complications when you were diagnosed, it can even reverse some complications like neuropathy.

Test as much as you can afford

Everyone is different. As described in the Learning section, there are many different kinds of diabetes. Furthermore, everyone has a different personality, lifestyle, and budget. What works for someone else might not work for you. YMMV (Your Mileage May Vary). Don't take anyone's word for it. The best way for you to find out how your diabetes responds to various factors is to use your meter and test.

Keep records of your BG numbers (see Month 9 for a discussion of sophisticated record-keeping systems), along with brief descriptions of any unusual events in your life, so you'll learn how these events affect your BG levels.

Stick to your diet as closely as possible, but don't be afraid to modify it based on your test results

This is probably not something your CDE would have told you. The basic diabetes books usually say, "Discuss this with your health-care team, who will work out a plan that is right for you." Many people don't really have a "team"; doctors in health maintenance organizations are often allowed to spend only five to fifteen minutes with a patient. Your insurance won't allow you to see them every week, and some of them don't really know much about nutrition.

I don't mean you should throw away your pills and suddenly adopt a wacko "Lose 20 pounds in three days" weight-loss plan that involves eating only grapefruit and coffee grounds if the readings on your meter tell you that your initial diet is not controlling your BG levels.

But it never hurts to try small modifications, one at a time, to see if you can improve your BG readings. For example, if you find that the half a banana approved on your diet makes your BG readings go high but straw-berries do not, substitute strawberries for bananas. Then if you make a lot of modifications and your BG levels improve significantly, make an appointment with your doctor and see if you can reduce or eliminate any drugs you may be taking.

Jennifer's Advice—Test! Test! Test!

Sounds like you're planning a move to take control of your diabetes. Good for you.

There is so much to absorb—you don't have to rush into anything. Begin by using your best weapon in this war: your meter. You won't keel over today; you have time to experiment, test, learn, test, and figure out just how your body and this disease are getting along. The most important thing you can do to learn about yourself and diabetes is *test, test, test*.

The single biggest question a diabetic has to answer is: **What do I eat?**

Unfortunately, the answer is pretty confusing. What confounds us all is the fact that different diabetics can get great results on wildly differing food plans. Some of us achieve great blood glucose control eating a diet high in complex carbohydrates. Others find that anything over 75 to 100 grams of carbs a day is too much. Still others are somewhere in between.

At the beginning all of us felt frustrated. We wanted to be handed *the* way to eat, to ensure our continued health. But we all learned that there is no one way. Each of us had to find our own path, using the experience of those who went before but still having to discover for ourselves how *our* bodies and this disease were coexisting. Ask questions, but remember that each of us discovered on our own what works best for us. You can use our experiences as jumping-off points, but eventually you'll work up a successful plan that is yours alone.

What you are looking to discover is how different foods affect you. As I'm sure you've read, carbohydrate (sugars, wheat, rice—the things our grandmas called "starches") raises blood sugar the most rapidly. Protein and fat also raises it but not as high and much more slowly. So if you're a type 2, generally the insulin your body still makes may take care of the rise.

You might want to try some experiments.

First: Eat whatever you've been currently eating . . . but write it all down.

Test yourself at the following times:

- ✓ Upon waking (fasting)
- ✓ One hour after each meal
- ✓ Two hours after each meal
- ✓ At bedtime

That means eight times each day. What you will discover by this is how long after a meal your highest reading comes—and how fast you return to "normal." Also, you may see that a meal that included bread, fruit, or other carbs gives you a higher reading.

Then for the next few days, try to curb your carbs. Eliminate bread, cereal, rice, beans, any wheat products, potato, corn, fruit; get all your carbs from veggies. Test at the same schedule as above.

(continues)

(continued)   ## Jennifer's Advice—Test! Test! Test!

If you try this for a few days, you may find some pretty good readings. It's worth a few days to discover. Eventually, you can slowly add back carbs until you see them affecting your meter. The thing about this disease—though we share much in common and we need to follow certain guidelines—is that in the end, each of our bodies dictates our treatment and our success.

The closer we get to nondiabetic numbers, the greater chance we have of avoiding horrible complications. The key word here is *aim*. I know that everyone is at a different point in his or her disease, and it is progressive. But, if we aim for the best numbers and do our best, we give ourselves the best shot at health we've got. That's all we can do.

Here's my opinion on **what numbers to aim for**; they are nondiabetic numbers.

Fasting BG Under 100
✓ One hour after meals: under 140
✓ Two hours after meals: under 120

Or for those in the mmol parts of the world:

Fasting Under 5.5
✓ One hour after meals: under 8
✓ Two hours after meals: under 6.5

Recent studies have indicated that the most important numbers are your after-meal numbers. They may be the most indicative of future complications, especially heart problems.

Listen to your doctor, but you are the leader of your diabetic care team. While his or her advice is expert, it is not absolute. You will end up knowing much more about your body and how it's handling diabetes than your doctor will. **Your meter is your best weapon.**

Just remember, we're not in a race or a competition with anyone but ourselves. Play around with your food plan. *Test, test, test*. Learn which foods cause spikes, which foods cause cravings. Use your body as a science experiment.

You'll read about a lot of different ways people use to control their diabetes. Many are diametrically opposed. After a while, you'll learn that there is no one-size-fits-all around here. Take some time to experiment, and you'll soon discover the plan that works for you.

Best of luck!
Jennifer

Jennifer has type 2 diabetes, and her "test, test, test" advice on various Internet lists and websites has helped many patients normalize their BG levels.

Move as much as you can

Unfortunately for those of us who hate it, exercise is something that seems to benefit everyone. Not everyone is able to do strenuous exercise. But move as much as you can. It really will help you feel better and control your BG levels.

Be alert for low blood sugar incidents

If you aren't using insulin or taking sulfonylurea drugs that make you produce insulin all day, you probably don't need to worry about hypoglycemia (low BG levels). Drugs like metformin or the glitazones (see Week 3) aren't supposed to cause hypoglycemia. However, some people have reported incidents of hypoglycemia when they were taking only metformin, and sometimes even when taking no diabetes drugs at all. So you should be aware of its existence, even if its likelihood is low.

If you sometimes go low, it's wise to wear a diabetic identification bracelet so people won't think you are drunk if it happens in public. Sources include MedicAlert (800–432–5378) and American Medical Identifications (800–363–5985).

Hypoglycemia is usually defined as a BG level below about 70 mg/dL (milligrams per deciliter). However, the symptoms depend more on the *rate* at which the BG level is falling than on the actual BG level itself. This makes sense. If you were several yards away from a child who was starting down a slide that would dump her into a pile of broken glass, you'd want to start running toward the slide to catch her *before* she reached the bottom. If you started when she was at the bottom of the slide, it would be too late. So too, the body is pretty smart, and if it senses that your BG level is falling rapidly, it wants to start correcting it *before* it's gone so low that you pass out. If the body waited until the BG level hit 70 mg/dL, you might have gone dangerously low before the corrective measures had taken effect.

Thus if you've just been diagnosed with BG levels in the 400s and you suddenly drop down to 200, you might feel symptoms of hypoglycemia even though your BG level is still way above normal. As your body gets used to lower BG levels, you won't feel symptoms until you reach the usual levels in the high 60s or below.

Symptoms of hypoglycemia vary slightly from person to person. Because some of the BG correction is a result of the production of adrenaline, many of the symptoms are similar to the fight-or-flight reaction described in Day 7: shakiness, sweating, rapid heartbeat, anxiety, and a feeling of nervousness or impending doom. Some people also feel hungry or irritable or act confused.

Because hypoglycemia means the brain isn't getting enough glucose, when you go very low your thinking may be impaired. When Amal K. had hypoglycemia, she saw an orange candy wrapper on the kitchen table and concluded that the world was going to end in fire. When Karen G. had hypoglycemia while traveling in France, she looked out the window and asked her husband why they were in Russia. He knew she was low and handed her a candy bar.

Learn how much correction you need for hypoglycemia

If you *do* get hypoglycemia, you need to eat some fast-acting carbohydrate to bring your BG levels back to normal, and you should keep some with you at all times. Don't overdo it. Because of the feeling of panic that sometimes accompanies hypoglycemia, some people eat and eat until their BG level is back to normal. And then it keeps going up and up and up. Remember, it takes a few minutes for anything you eat to get into your bloodstream.

One way to deal with this is to follow the 15/15 rule: eat about 15 grams of carbohydrate, wait 15 minutes, and then retest. If you still need more correction, eat another 15 grams and test again. Glucose gets into the bloodstream the fastest, and you can buy glucose tablets or gels and know exactly how much glucose you're taking.

A better way is to test yourself *before* you have hypoglycemia to find out how much correction you need. Sometime when your BG level is stable and not high, eat one glucose tablet and see how much your BG goes up. If it doesn't go up much, try two, and then three, until you find out how many you'd need to take to raise your BG level by a certain amount.

When you have hypoglycemia, don't eat something with a lot of fat or protein, like ice cream. The fat will slow down the emptying of the stomach and delay the effect of the carbohydrate. If you're taking an alpha-glucosidase inhibitor (see Week 3), starch or sucrose won't be able to help with hypoglycemia (the inhibitor keeps the carbohydrate from being broken down into sugars) and you'll have to rely on glucose.

Liquids are usually digested faster than solids, and some people find that skim milk raises their BG level faster than anything else. The protein in the milk also adds some staying power.

If you have really serious problems with hypoglycemia, you can get a prescription for glucagon, the hormone that counteracts the effects of insulin, and someone can inject it when you need it.

Learn the signs of high blood glucose levels

Different people react differently to **hyperglycemia** (high BG levels). Some people get very sleepy, but others do not. Blurred vision is common, but it may come hours after a high BG episode. Thirst and frequent urination are symptoms of sustained high BG levels.

Symptoms of high BG levels in one person might indicate low BG levels in another, so it's important to learn what your own symptoms are. Test, and even if you can't bring the BG level down right away, you'll know that whatever you did before the episode of hyperglycemia is something you should try to avoid.

Be especially careful when you're sick

Illness is a stress that increases insulin resistance (IR) and may make your BG levels go up. In addition, if you're vomiting and have diarrhea, you may get dehydrated, and dehydration also causes IR. Thus you shouldn't stop taking your medication when you're sick. In fact, if you're seriously ill, you may need to take insulin on a temporary basis to keep your BG levels from going too high.

But you also don't want to risk going too low from insulin or sulfonylureas if you're having trouble keeping any food in your stomach. In this case, work out ahead of time what kinds of foods you can usually tolerate when you're feeling sick and how much you'd need to keep you from going low. Make sure you keep them in the house, and instruct others in the family not to eat them because they're emergency rations for you. Maybe you can keep them in a special place.

If you don't live near a drugstore, you should also stock sugar-free versions of any standard cough or cold remedies that you expect to take. Most cough syrups and drops contain a lot of sugar. One regular cough drop probably won't cause much harm, but many could.

Even if you're not treating with insulin or sulfonylureas and don't need to worry about hypoglycemia, vomiting and diarrhea can also cause problems with dehydration, which can be serious if severe.

People with type 1 diabetes have to worry about something called diabetic ketoacidosis (DKA), which can be very serious. In the absence of insulin, the body burns fats and produces very high levels of ketone bodies, often known as ketones. Because the ketones are acidic, the blood becomes too acid, hence the name *ketoacidosis*.

When you have type 2 diabetes, you're not apt to get ketoacidosis, even though your body can produce some ketones when you don't eat at all, you eat a lot of fat, or you go on a low-carbohydrate diet. The level of ketones that the body can produce depends on the amount of fatty acids in the blood. High levels of ketones stimulate the production of insulin, and it takes only tiny amounts of insulin to slow down the production of these fatty acids. Thus as long as you can produce any insulin at all, you can be in **ketosis** (high levels of ketones in the blood) but your body has a fail-safe mechanism to protect against ketoacidosis. Many people, even some dieticians and doctors, confuse the two terms.

If you have type 2 diabetes, you can most always produce enough insulin to stop ketoacidosis, even if you can't produce enough to deal with a lot of carbohydrate in your diet.

With type 2 diabetes, however, a related problem called *hyperosmolar hyperglycemic nonketotic syndrome (HHNS)* can occur. It's rare, but when it does occur, the fatality rate is high, so you should know about it and become familiar with the symptoms.

HHNS can happen when you let your BG levels go very high. Your body tries to get rid of the excess glucose by dumping it into the urine. This makes you lose a lot of fluid, and you get dehydrated and thirsty. Thus the beginning of HHNS is very similar to what may have happened before you were diagnosed.

This condition becomes much worse if you are sick, especially with vomiting and diarrhea, and may not be able to drink a lot of fluids to rehydrate your body. Maybe you're sleeping a lot or maybe you can't even keep liquids down. So your BG levels go even higher, you get more dehydrated, and as a result you may get confused or even go into a coma. If not treated, HHNS can be fatal.

Unlike DKA, HHNS usually has a slow onset, over several days, and occurs mostly in elderly people, especially when they're in nursing homes and not getting the attention they need. But if you're sick, make sure you keep track of your BG levels. If you're too sick to test, ask someone else to do it for you. If your BG levels go high (over 300 mg/dL) and don't come down, call a doctor for advice.

Have regular medical checks

Toughing it out without any medical care is not a good idea when you have diabetes. A penny spent today may save thousands of dollars tomorrow. The American Diabetes Association (ADA) recommends that you have *at least* the following checks for diabetes control:

Every six months (every three months if you're on insulin):
Doctor's visit
Hemoglobin A1c test

Every year:
    Lipid tests
    Kidney function test
    Dilated eye examination
    Examination of feet
Every two to three years:
    Lipid tests if you're in a low-risk category.

In the first year, you should visit your doctor more often than six months until you have a treatment plan that works for you. Many people have an A1c test every three months. Medicare will pay for this.

Control your blood pressure and cholesterol

Having diabetes means you're at greater risk for heart disease. So make sure your blood pressure and cholesterol levels, as well as your BG levels, are tested and take corrective action if necessary. The National Diabetes Education Program calls this the "ABCs of diabetes" for A1c, Blood pressure, and Cholesterol.

Take care of your feet

When they hear about diabetes, some people think it means you're going to lose your feet. It can happen if you don't keep your BG levels under control. But it's not inevitable.

One problem with some books about diabetes is that they don't distinguish between different types of diabetes, different degrees of severity within the types, or the length of time you have had diabetes. They just lump everyone together as "diabetics."

Thus some people will say diabetics should never go barefoot. Diabetics should use a mirror to examine their feet every day (diabetic supply places carry special mirrors designed to do this). Diabetics should wear special padded socks. Diabetics should call a doctor whenever they have cuts on their feet.

These admonitions *do* make sense if you have any signs of neuropathy or impaired circulation to the feet. If you have no feeling in your feet, you can easily let a small stone in a shoe, or even a callus, cause an abrasion that will turn into an ulcer and take forever to heal. Such ulcers can cause gangrene, which may result in an amputation.

If you think the feeling in your feet is impaired, make sure your doctor checks your feet for any problems at every visit. You can also get a small filament to check the feeling in your own feet at home. The filament is designed to produce an exact amount of pressure when it is pushed against the foot. As long as you can feel the filament, you should have enough sensation left to feel small cuts and bruises. The Lower Extremity Amputation Prevention (LEAP) Program (888–275–4772) will no longer mail free filaments to individuals, although they'll send ten filaments to health professionals. However, the filaments are not expensive if you wish to buy one. You can ask a health-care worker to show you how to use the filament.

So do be careful with your feet. If you get a sore, keep an eye on it and see a doctor if it doesn't heal quickly. Use a filament to see if you have any loss of sensation. But if the feeling in your feet is still normal, don't go overboard with the mirror routine every morning. Do something you enjoy instead.

Keep track of your total health

Remember, you're chairman of the board. **Keep track of all your health records yourself and know where you stand.** This makes it easier if you move or have to change doctors. Good record keeping also gives you a better sense of where you are with your health, and understanding all this may help indicate if it's time to change health-care providers.

Stop smoking

If you smoke, you're already quite aware that you shouldn't. Everyone is already nagging you about it.

You may feel you've had to give up enough already. You're trying to eat less of your favorite sugary, starchy, and fatty foods. You're trying to sacrifice precious free time so you can exercise more. If you have high blood pressure, you've probably been told to cut out the salt.

Now they want you to stop smoking too? It may seem like a lot to ask but it's really important. Smoking causes some of the very same problems that high BG levels do. If you've got diabetes, your chances of having a heart attack are already two to four times higher than normal. If you add smoking to the diabetes, you're really asking for trouble.

Sure it's hard. But if there's any way you can do it, dump the cigarettes. According to the ADA, almost all diabetic people who need amputations are smokers.

IN A SENTENCE:

■ *Basic diabetes care means learning how to keep your blood glucose levels as close to normal as possible using diet, exercise, and medication if necessary; making sure you get regular medical checkups; taking care of your feet; and being alert for high or low blood sugar levels, especially when you're sick.*

Types of Diabetes

As you learned in Day 1, diabetes comes in many forms. The main distinction is, of course, between type 1 diabetes, the *autoimmune* kind that always requires insulin, and type 2 diabetes, which can sometimes be controlled with diet and exercise alone. Some types of diabetes, for example gestational diabetes, are now considered neither type 1 nor type 2. However, because such patients can often control their diabetes with diet and exercise, in some ways they are more similar to type 2.

Overweight type 2 is the most common

The most common form of type 2 diabetes (almost 90 percent have this form) involves insulin resistance (IR). (Some people used to refer to this as type 2R for *resistant*, but this term is not in general use today. You may come across it when reading older books.) When you have this kind of diabetes, you tend to be overweight when you are diagnosed, and losing weight may help you control your blood glucose (BG) levels, especially if you are diagnosed at the very early stages, while you still have a lot of beta cell function remaining.

In the early stages of this kind of diabetes, the body tries to compensate for the IR by producing more insulin than normal. Thus your C-peptide levels (meaning also your insulin levels; see Day 5) are usually higher than normal. However, if you have had this kind of diabetes for a long time without knowing it, glucotoxicity and beta cell failure (see Week 2) may have destroyed enough beta cell function that your C-peptide level is normal, or even below normal, as I illustrated in Figure 2 in Week 2.

The important thing is to keep track of your BG levels, and if they don't come down pretty quickly with whatever treatment you start with, don't wait. Try something else. There are a lot of choices today.

Some thin type 2s don't produce enough insulin

Not everyone with type 2 diabetes is overweight when diagnosed. Some (a minority) are even quite thin, and their IR is normal. (Some people used to call this type of diabetes type 2S for *sensitive*, or 2D for *deficient*, but this terminology is uncommon today.) If you have this kind of type 2 diabetes, it means that for some unknown reason, and probably for many different reasons in different people, your beta cells simply aren't producing enough insulin, especially after meals. In this case your C-peptide levels would be in the normal range.

Some people initially diagnosed with this kind of type 2 diabetes turn out to have *LADA*, a form of type 1 diabetes.

LADA is really type 1

LADA stands for *latent autoimmune diabetes of adults*. Like type 1 diabetes, it seems to be an autoimmune disease in which your own immune system destroys your beta cells, so it is really a form of type 1 diabetes that occurs in older people. For some unknown reason, LADA usually proceeds much slower than typical type 1 diabetes in children, and because LADA occurs in adults, many people with LADA are initially diagnosed as having common garden-variety type 2 diabetes. Thus some people call it "type 1.5."

If you have LADA and your doctor thinks you have type 2 diabetes, you may be prescribed various oral medications and told to diet and exercise, but the medications won't work very well or very long. Don't feel bad. It's not your fault. It's just a different kind of diabetes.

One way to see if you have LADA is to test your C-peptide level. If the level is close to the bottom of the normal range, that's a good indication. Another way is to test for anti-GAD (see Day 5) antibodies. If you have the antibodies, you probably have LADA.

If you have LADA, eventually all the oral drugs will stop working entirely, and you will have to start using insulin. You're better off going right to insulin to give your pancreas a rest and help preserve the beta cells you have left. Type 1 diabetes is easier to control when you still have a little bit of beta cell function remaining, as many people with type 1 do.

Gestational diabetes may be an early warning sign

Gestational diabetes is not really type 2 diabetes but a form of diabetes that may occur in a pregnant woman and usually goes away after the baby is born. However, a woman who has had gestational diabetes is at much higher risk for developing type 2 diabetes later in life: between 40 and 70 percent of such women eventually do.

In a sense, gestational diabetes is an early warning sign that tells you that you don't have much pancreatic reserve. What this means is that for genetic reasons, your pancreas is able to cope just fine as long as you don't make extra demands on it.

During pregnancy, IR normally increases because of increases in the levels of various counterregulatory hormones that are necessary for the growth of the baby. In a person with a strong pancreas, this is no problem. But if you don't have much pancreatic reserve, this extra stress may be just enough to push you over into diabetes. When the baby is born and the hormones abate, the IR becomes normal and the diabetes usually disappears.

However, if other stresses occur in the future, for example, surgery or a bad infection, or extra IR from being overweight, that may be enough to push you into a diabetic state again.

Thus if you've had gestational diabetes, it is important to work hard to keep active and keep your weight at a normal level to reduce the chances that you'll ever become diabetic again.

Because the effect of some of the oral diabetes drugs on the fetus is not known, if you have gestational diabetes you will be asked to control with diet and exercise or, if that doesn't work, with insulin.

Type 2 diabetes in children is increasing

Unfortunately, type 2 diabetes is being diagnosed more and more frequently in children. The most common form of type 2 diabetes in children is associated with extreme overweight, often in populations that recently adopted a high-calorie, low-physical-labor lifestyle. Such children sometimes have signs of *acanthosis nigricans*, which is a soft, velvety darkening of the skin, especially on the neck and under the arms. Sometimes parents think it's dirt and try to scrub it off. Acanthosis nigricans is a sign of severe IR. Anyone with such signs should try hard to lose weight and get more exercise to avoid getting overt diabetes.

MODY stands for *maturity-onset diabetes of the young* and refers to a very specific type of diabetes that is inherited as a dominant gene. This means you only need to inherit a gene from one parent to get the disease.

There are a lot of subtypes of MODY, for example MODY1, MODY2, and so forth, and more is known about the genetics of some of these MODY subtypes than is known about common garden-variety type 2 diabetes. Different genes that cause MODY have been identified in different families with MODY.

MODY is not common, and it is no longer considered type 2 diabetes Some people have used it to refer to all children who don't have type 1, regardless of the cause.

Steroids can cause diabetes

Steroids like cortisone or prednisone cause IR and if taken for long periods of time can cause *steroid diabetes*. If you stop taking the steroid drugs, the diabetes usually goes away. But if you let your BG levels remain high for long enough, the resulting glucotoxicity and beta cell failure may mean that your diabetes will be permanent.

Technically, steroid diabetes is no longer considered type 2 diabetes, but because it's not type 1 and you may not need insulin, many people group it with type 2.

Hemochromatosis causes diabetes

Hemochromatosis is a genetic disorder that makes you accumulate iron. It's also called *iron overload disease* or *bronze diabetes*. It is especially common in people with a Celtic background. The huge stores of iron that accumulate in the organs damage various organs, including the pancreas, and diabetes can be one result.

If untreated, this disease can be serious, even fatal. If detected, it can be controlled simply by giving blood periodically to get rid of the excess iron in your system. Lab tests for an iron-carrying protein called *ferritin* can diagnose the problem.

Polycystic ovary syndrome causes infertility

Polycystic ovary syndrome (or *disease*) (*PCOS*), also called *Stein-Leventhal syndrome*, is a disease of women characterized by IR and resulting in high insulin levels, irregular monthly periods and infertility, acne, excess body hair and thinning hair on the head, and abdominal obesity, but as with type 2 diabetes, not everyone with the syndrome is overweight. It seems that in women with a genetic predisposition, high insulin levels stimulate the formation of too many male hormones (androgens), and these cause the symptoms.

More than a quarter of women with PCOS develop diabetes by age thirty. The treatment is weight reduction (to reduce the extra weight-induced IR) and insulin-sensitizing drugs such as metformin or the glitazones (see Week 3). Some suggest low-carbohydrate diets to reduce insulin levels. Sometimes the drugs can restore fertility, which is listed as a side effect of these drugs, so if you have PCOS and take one of these drugs, be prepared.

Ketosis-prone type 2 diabetes is less well known

Ketosis-prone type 2 diabetes (KPD), also known as *Flatbush diabetes* because of the location of the area where it was first described, or *idiopathic type 1 diabetes (type 1B),* has some characteristics of type 1 diabetes (diabetic ketoacidosis, or DKA) and some characteristics of type 2 diabetes (not always requiring insulin).

It is found primarily in nonwhite populations, especially those of sub-Saharan African descent, although it is also sometimes found in Asians, Hispanics, and Caucasians.

The hallmark of Flatbush diabetes is presenting in DKA with sudden onset of extremely high BG levels (BG levels of 700 mg/dL and hemoglobin A1c levels of 12 to 14 are not uncommon). Because DKA used to be considered a hallmark of type 1 diabetes (in older terminology, type 2 diabetes was sometimes called *ketosis-resistant diabetes*), people with KPD were originally considered to be type 1.

However, people with KPD don't have antibodies against beta cells; unlike "regular" type 1 diabetes, it's not an autoimmune disease.

People with KPD are also often overweight, as in type 2 diabetes, and have relatives with type 2 diabetes, and they may have some IR.

A major distinguishing feature of KPD is that when the very high BG levels on diagnosis are brought down with insulin, people can often do quite well with oral drugs, or even just diet and exercise, for months or even years. People with "regular" type 1 diabetes often have a "honeymoon period" in which their insulin requirements are fairly low, but they always progress toward insulin dependence, and if they stop taking insulin, they go into DKA.

KPD is becoming more and more common in Africa, and in America, it now accounts for up to 50 percent of the cases among African Americans who are first diagnosed with DKA. No one is sure exactly what causes it, but it has been suggested that people with KPD are extremely sensitive to temporary damage to the beta cells by glucotoxicity and lipotoxicity, and when those conditions are reversed with insulin and diet, the beta cells are able to recover.

There may turn out to be several subtypes of KPD. Some people are *not* able to control without insulin after their diagnosis, whereas most are.

If you had DKA and you've never been tested for antibodies, the results of such a test would give a clue. If you have the antibodies, you're probably "regular" type 1, not type 2, and you'll have to stay on insulin. If you don't have the antibodies, there's a chance you could do well on just oral drugs.

Prediabetes is the first step on the way to diabetes

Today, what used to be called *impaired glucose tolerance* and *impaired fasting glucose* are both called *prediabetes*. Impaired glucose tolerance means that your fasting BG levels are within normal limits, and at the two-hour point in a glucose tolerance test, your BG levels are not at diabetic levels (200 mg/dL [milligrams per deciliter] or more), but they don't fall below 140 by that time.

It's really the first step on the way to full-blown diabetes, and anyone who has impaired glucose tolerance should work like the dickens to do whatever is necessary to improve the BG levels. At this stage of the disease, you usually have a lot of beta cell function remaining, and sometimes just losing some weight and exercising more can keep you from ever developing diabetes. If you wait until your BG levels are quite high, it may be too late.

Impaired fasting glucose means your fasting BG level is above the normal limit (99 mg/dL) but not high enough for a formal definition of diabetes (126 mg/dL). As with impaired glucose tolerance, this is a warning sign that you'd better do something quickly to avoid progressing to diabetes.

Some health-care organizations spend a lot of time defining limits for these various stages of disease. So if Toby has a fasting BG level of 125 and Ben has a fasting BG level of 127, they'll say that Ben has diabetes but Toby doesn't. In fact, they probably have just about the same level of BG control and should take the same precautions to keep the condition under control.

This is the stage of diabetes that some used to call "a touch of sugar" or "borderline diabetes" so patients didn't take it seriously and usually progressed quickly into officially diagnosed diabetes.

There are many other kinds of diabetes

Many different diseases, especially those that cause abnormal levels of the various counterregulatory hormones like growth hormone (increased in acromegaly), cortisol (increased in Cushing's disease), and adrenaline (increased in pheochromocytoma), can cause forms of diabetes. Other diseases that disrupt the delicate balance between various hormones, or tumors that cause increased secretion of hormones like glucagon, can also cause diabetes. Most of these conditions are uncommon.

Damage to the pancreas from accidents or other diseases can also cause diabetes. In addition to steroids, some other drugs can also cause diabetes.

Defects in other BG-controlling substances, some of which are known and some of which have probably not yet been discovered, can also cause forms of diabetes.

Diabetes is really a symptom

As you can see from this brief discussion, diabetes is really not one disease but many diseases. In fact, *diabetes is really not a disease as much as a symptom of many diseases*. And there are many people who don't fit neatly into any of the official categories, for example, a thin person with or an overweight person without IR. What diabetes really means is that your BG level is too high. Many different diseases can make your BG level go too high, so it's not really surprising that different people react differently to different diets and treatments. They may have different types of type 2 diabetes.

Most treatments of type 2 diabetes today are aimed at controlling the main symptom of this spectrum of diseases: high BG levels. This is, of course, extremely important. High BG levels are lethal.

The glitazone drugs (see Week 3) are the first type of drug aimed at controlling the cause of one type 2 subtype: insulin resistance. Researchers are studying other causes of type 2 diabetes, and many different genes have been suggested. Unlike MODY, which is caused by a mutation in a single gene, many kinds of type 2 diabetes are probably caused by more than one gene. As the research continues, more underlying causes of the other subtypes will undoubtedly be discovered and drugs will be developed to treat them more specifically.

Until then, don't despair if your particular type of diabetes doesn't react like someone else's. You're not nuts. You may just have what Natalie S. calls "type weird." The cause of your diabetes may be slightly different from the cause of someone else's. Test your BG levels and find out how your diabetes reacts. No one can ask for more.

IN A SENTENCE:

■ *There are many different types of diabetes, so you may react differently to a diet or a treatment than someone else does.*

living

Will Supplements Help My Diabetes?

Shortly after you've been diagnosed with diabetes, you'll probably begin to notice all sorts of articles about **vitamins** and minerals and other supplements that are supposed to help control blood glucose (BG) levels. Do they work? Should you try them? Which ones?

Controlled trials provide evidence

As is true with most "complementary" or "alternative" medicine, opinions about some vitamins and minerals, as well as herbs, vary widely from people who swear they couldn't control their BG levels without them to people who say they're useless and maybe even harmful in excess. In many cases, the supporters are backed by anecdotal evidence, without controlled scientific trials.

When doctors prescribe any medication to a patient, they need to be extremely careful. Hence mainstream doctors usually recommend only drugs that have been shown to be effective through randomized controlled clinical trials published in *peer-reviewed* journals. This is called *evidence-based medicine*.

A **controlled trial** means you don't just give a drug to a bunch of people and see if they get better. They might have gotten better anyway, or maybe they got better because of the *placebo effect*, the psychological effect that a fake (placebo) pill or "sugar pill" can have on a patient who thinks it's really medicine. In a controlled trial, half of a group of randomly chosen patients are given a study drug and the other half (carefully matched by age, sex, health, and so forth) a placebo. The patients aren't told if they are getting the drug. A **double-blind** controlled trial is even more rigorous. In this case, even the doctors and nurses don't know which patients actually got the real drug so they won't unconsciously communicate their hopes or fears to the patients.

When the trial is concluded, the researchers write up the results and submit the paper to a medical journal. The journal, in turn, sends it out to other doctors in the field (so-called peers) to ask whether they think the paper's methods were valid. If the reviewers say the research seems good, then the journal publishes the results.

Usually just one study, even if it's in a peer-reviewed journal, doesn't prove something works. Sometimes different research groups get different results or come to different conclusions, so several studies showing an effect or lack thereof mean more.

Doing controlled drug trials is expensive and time consuming, and the trials are usually financed by drug companies. Drug companies don't want to spend money doing trials of drugs they can't patent. So the effect on diabetes of many of the supplements that some people say help have never been studied in such trials. There are usually more studies of vitamins and minerals than of obscure herbs from faraway places.

The other type of evidence for and against various alternative remedies is what's called *anecdotal evidence*. This means your aunt Agnes told you that honey and vinegar make a good cough syrup and cinnamon helped your uncle Albert keep his BG levels down. Some people call such treatments *folk remedies*. Sometimes folk remedies turn out to have a basis in fact. For example, aspirin is closely related to a drug found in the bark of the white willow tree, which Native Americans used for pain and fever, and metformin is closely related to a drug found in goat's rue (also known as French lilac), which has been used as a folk remedy for diabetes since the Middle Ages.

Decisions about using supplements are complex

When supplements haven't been studied in controlled trials, most doctors won't recommend them. Does this mean they don't work? No. Does this mean they do work? No. In many cases we simply don't know.

You've got to decide for yourself how much risk you're willing to assume. If you're the supercautious type, you may want to wait until studies show that a remedy is safe and effective. If you enjoy experimenting and are willing to risk damage to your own body, you may want to try every alternative drug on the market and see what happens. As some people say, "My body, my science experiment." Most people fall somewhere between these extremes.

If you do decide you want to try a supplement to help control your BG levels, the best way is to try one thing at a time and carefully keep track of your BG levels as well as your general health while you do. If you suddenly start taking twenty-seven different vitamins and minerals and find that your BG levels go up or down, you'll never know which ones were responsible for the change, and you may be paying for a lot for stuff you don't need.

Read as much as you can about each one before you make up your mind. One way to get a somewhat balanced view is to read all the promotional material provided by the peddlers of vitamins, minerals, and herbs and then read the diatribes against them by conservative medical people and make up your own mind. If you have access to the Internet, you can visit a site called Quackwatch that discusses alternative treatments they think are particularly bad.

Keep in mind that studies *in vitro* (in glass, meaning they are done outside the body) are not always applicable to situations *in vivo* (in the living body). Similarly, studies done with mice do not always translate into human cures. Remember *leptin*? Certain strains of mice were found to be deficient in the hormone leptin, and giving them the hormone made them slim down. Everyone hoped it would work with overweight people. A tiny number of leptin-deficient people were discovered, and leptin did work for them. But leptin deficiency turned out not to be the primary cause of obesity in humans. However, it may be a major player in controlling hunger, and some people think that leptin resistance may be more important than insulin resistance in causing diabetes.

Supplements can be like Dr. Jekyll and Mr. Hyde

When you're reading about the effects of supplements on the human body, remember that the body is a masterpiece of balance. Sometimes a substance that works miracles when given in small amounts can be toxic when given in large amounts. For example, you need iron to transport oxygen to your tissues, but too much iron can kill you.

Sometimes substances that help one condition harm another. For example, some anti-inflammatory drugs that help arthritis may harm the kidney or liver or give you a heart attack. It's a trade-off. Usually your doctor studies the published reports and decides if the benefits from a drug are worth the risks of harm in your particular case. If you supplement on your own, you'll have to make those decisions yourself.

An example of possible good and bad effects is the **antioxidants** that many people take to fight **free radicals**. There is some evidence that when you have type 2 diabetes, you have more free radicals and fewer antioxidants than other people. The process of producing energy from food produces free radicals, and many people with type 2 diabetes have huge appetites, so metabolizing all this food might cause some of the extra free radicals. High BG levels have also been associated with increased free-radical levels, even in people without diabetes.

What are free radicals? Free radicals are highly reactive compounds with unpaired electrons. If you don't remember the details from a chemistry course, it's not important. What is important is that the free radicals, and we're especially concerned with *oxygen free radicals*, also called **reactive oxygen species (ROS)**, are highly reactive and can be toxic.

You can think of free radicals as little bombs. When they hit other molecules they "explode" and, like molecular werewolves, not only damage the other molecules but turn the other molecules into free radicals themselves, thus starting a chain reaction. Free radicals can cause **plaques** on arterial walls, contributing to atherosclerosis, or mutations to your genes, causing cancer.

Oxidation is also important

One way to lower your level of free radicals is to eat less. In order to produce energy from your food, you must *metabolize* it (break it down into its constituent parts). The end stage of this process involves cell organelles (little organs within cells) called *mitochondria*. The mitochondria react with oxygen to produce ATP (see Month 8). Unfortunately, this process is not 100 percent accurate, and the mistakes can result in ROS. This means that the more you force your mitochondria to produce ATP by eating more food, the greater the chances for ROS formation.

As we age, our mitochondria become less efficient and produce more ROS. These may attack the mitochondria themselves, making them even less efficient, and a vicious circle ensues. There is also some evidence that when you have diabetes, your mitochondria are less efficient to begin with. Even the nondiabetic children of people with diabetes tend to have deficient mitochondria.

The body contains a lot of antioxidants designed to keep the free radicals under control. Fruits and vegetables also contain antioxidants. Unfortunately, modern living, including polluted air, cigarette smoking, and other toxins, seems to increase the number of free radicals we normally have. And if you're limiting your intake of calories, you may not be able to eat a lot of fruits and vegetables, especially fruits. Thus extra antioxidant vitamins seem like a good idea.

But here's one problem. The cell uses free radical bombs to get rid of some unhealthy invaders of the body, including bacteria and cancer cells. In fact, some anticancer drugs and radiation treatments work by producing free radicals that damage rapidly dividing cancer cells. Thus some researchers say people undergoing such cancer therapy should avoid taking antioxidants during the therapy. Others say the opposite, that the antioxidants actually help destroy the cancer cells and protect the healthy cells. In one study in mice, removing antioxidant vitamins A and E from the diet slowed the growth of tumors.

How about when you're not taking anticancer drugs and you don't have cancer? Are antioxidants good or bad? Some are probably good. At this point in our knowledge, no one really knows the exact amounts that are best. It undoubtedly depends on your own individual physiology, diet, lifestyle, and so forth. Taking a supplement containing antioxidants doesn't guarantee that they'll reach the particular tissues or cells that need them. You'll just have to decide whether you're going to be conservative or go out on a limb and spend a lot of money on antioxidant pills.

Read as much as you can about each one before you decide to take a lot of it. You'll find that opinions not only differ but change from year to year, sometimes from week to week, it seems. Sometimes study A says a supplement is beneficial and study B says it has no effect. This can happen because different studies use different populations, different methods, or different time periods or have different definitions of "beneficial." For example, one study of the effect of a supplement on cardiovascular events could measure its effect on deaths from heart attacks in a twenty-year period, or on the incidence of nonfatal heart attacks during a five-year period in men thirty-five to sixty years old with no previous heart disease, or on the rate of second heart attacks in elderly women during a three-year period, or on many other "end points." News reports tend to oversimplify. Whenever possible, try to read the original reports of studies that interest you.

You can take too much

If you take several supplements that have the same effect, the total dosage may be too high. This can happen with some supplements that "thin" the blood, a popular term meaning they make it less likely to clot.

Heart attacks are caused by clots that clog a blood vessel in the heart, and strokes can be caused by clots that plug up vessels in the brain (*ischemic strokes*). In both these cases, so-called **blood thinners** are help-ful because they discourage the formation of clots.

But strokes can also be caused by ruptured vessels that let the blood leak out. In these strokes, called *hemorrhagic strokes* (or "bleeds"), if the blood doesn't clot to plug the hole, you will bleed to death. If you have this type of stroke, blood thinners would be harmful. Too many blood thinners can also increase the severity of preexisting diabetic retinopathy.

Popular nonprescription blood thinners include aspirin, vitamin E, fish oils, fenugreek, ginger, garlic, and *Ginkgo biloba*. Taking one of these sup-plements might seem like a good idea, because when you have type 2 dia-betes, your **platelets** may be "stickier" than normal, meaning they're more apt to form clots. But if you take them all, you may be getting too much of a good thing and increasing your chances of stroke and worsening retinopathy.

Supplements can interact with prescription medications

Another potential problem with supplements is that they could interact with prescription medications you're already taking. For this reason, if you do decide to take supplements, tell your doctor exactly what you're taking. If your doctor isn't familiar with the supplements, ask your pharmacist. It's a good idea to get all your prescriptions filled at the same place, so the phar-macists there can keep track of all the medications you're taking and be alert for possible interactions. If you're also buying your supplements there, the pharmacist should be willing to take some time to discuss them with you. It's not easy to find a pharmacist who has time to explain things to custom-ers. If you do find such a person, make that your regular pharmacy.

If you have access to the Internet, there are sites where you can plug in the names of the supplements and drugs you're taking to see if there are known interactions. Search on "drug-supplement interaction" to find cur-rent sites (see Month 12 for tips on Internet searching).

There are no easy answers when deciding whether or not nonprescrip-tion supplements are for you. It's your body, your science experiment. But be cautious.

IN A SENTENCE:

■ *There is often less published evidence about the effectiveness of supplements than there is about prescription drugs, but learn as much as you can about a supplement before you decide to take it.*

Learning More About Testing: Blood Glucose Meters

By now you should be comfortable using your first blood glucose (BG) meter, and it's time to go beyond the basics of BG monitoring.

Plasma readings are higher than whole-blood readings

The first thing to understand is the difference between plasma levels and whole-blood levels of glucose. *Whole blood* means the blood just as it comes out of your body, what you get when you stick your finger and get a drop of blood. Whole blood contains a liquid plus *red blood cells*, *white blood cells*, and *platelets* (small disk-shaped structures in the blood that are required for clotting). When you remove the blood cells and platelets, the liquid that is left is called *plasma*. (When you let the blood clot and then remove both the blood cells and the clot, what's left is called *serum*, but we don't need to worry about that.)

The concentration of glucose in the red blood cells is a little lower than the concentration of glucose in the plasma. So when you remove the red blood cells, the resulting plasma gives a slightly higher BG reading than you get from whole blood, usually 10 to 15 percent higher, depending on how many red blood cells were in your blood in the first place. People who are anemic have fewer red blood cells.

When you read various books and pamphlets about diabetes, you'll probably find that they give different values for "normal" BG levels. Some books may say normal BG levels are between 60 and 100 mg/dL (milligrams per deciliter). Others might say between 70 and 130 mg/dL. Part of this is simply a matter of definition. Sometimes an official medical committee gets together and redefines things. As I noted earlier, in the 1990s the definition of diabetic fasting levels was changed from anything over 140 to anything over 126 mg/dL, thus giving a huge number of people diabetes with a stroke of the pen (and actually doing them a favor in the process, because the best treatment is early treatment). In 2003, the upper limit of normal fasting BG levels was reduced from less than 110 to less than 100 mg/dL. Some writers may be reporting the officially defined upper limit of normal, and others may be referring to the most common levels. In addition, some may be using plasma levels (which are higher) and others referring to whole-blood (lower) values. They usually don't bother to say.

Most labs test the BG levels in your plasma. The home meters use whole blood. But today's meters convert the BG levels measured on whole blood into plasma values. So unless you are using an ancient meter, you don't need to worry about doing conversions yourself. The old meters read about 12 percent below lab values.

Venous blood can read lower than capillary blood

It gets more complicated. There is sometimes a difference in the BG level of blood from your veins and blood from your capillaries. Your blood flows out of your heart in blood vessels called **arteries** This blood is bright red because it contains a lot of oxygen, and if you've just had a meal, the blood also contains a lot of glucose from the meal. This blood flows into smaller and smaller arteries and finally into tiny arteries that are called **capillaries**. The capillaries have thin, permeable walls and, like a combination of a grocery delivery and a garbage pickup, easily give oxygen and glucose to the cells that need them, picking up carbon dioxide and other waste products at the same time. Then the oxygen-depleted (bluish), glucose-depleted blood flows into larger and larger blood vessels called **veins**, goes through the liver to pick up more food, and goes back to the lungs to drop off the carbon dioxide and pick up more oxygen.

What this means is that *after a meal* the blood in the veins may have a lot less glucose in it than the blood in the capillaries, which dumped a lot of their glucose off to feed the cells. When you do home BG testing, you use blood from the capillaries. When you give blood at the doctor's office, they take blood from a vein. As long as you're testing fasting samples, there's not much difference in the BG concentration, so it won't make much difference where you get the blood. But if you were measuring after a meal, you might see a large difference, up to about 70 mg/dL, between capillary and venous blood.

Accuracy and precision mean different things

If you want to know how accurate your home meter is, the best way is to take it with you when you have your BG level measured by a lab. Do your testing right before they draw your blood. Don't be tempted to use a drop of the blood the technician takes from a vein. The chemical reaction used by many home meters depends on oxygenated blood, and sometimes the venous blood doesn't have enough oxygen for an accurate test. Do this testing several times and average the results. If you find your lab gives readings about 14 percent higher than yours, then multiply your results by 1.14 to estimate the lab values.

Home meters are not guaranteed to be as accurate as lab tests. Most meters guarantee accuracy only plus or minus 20 percent, although the American Diabetes Association would prefer that this was 10 percent. This means that if you get a reading of 100 mg/dL, the true BG level could be between 80 and 120 mg/dL, and the manufacturer would consider the meter was just hunky-dory. In practice, most meters seem to be more accurate than the acceptable limits.

The term *accuracy* means how close to the true value your meter measures. There's another possible variation in results called *precision*. This refers to how close several readings taken one after the other will be. For example, a meter that gave readings of 97, 99, and 96 would be very precise. A meter that gave readings of 97, 120, and 80 would not be precise. Note that a meter can be very precise but not accurate. For example, if the blood being measured by the first meter had a true BG level of 120, the meter would be precise but inaccurate.

Don't try to measure the precision of your meter at a time when you think your BG level might be changing quickly. It takes a certain amount of time to do the test, and if the BG level is changing very fast, you might think it was imprecise when it was actually reflecting changing levels of glucose.

There are different types of meters

Meters have two slightly different methods of measuring your BG level. One type (which I'll call *colorimetric*; another name is *color reflectance* meters) measures a color change. The other type (which I'll call *electrochemical*; another term is *amperometric*) measures an electrical current. One way to tell which kind you have is to see if your meter has little flashing red lights when you turn it on. If it does, it's the colorimetric type of meter.

The strips in BG meters use *enzymes* to measure the glucose. Different brands of strips use slightly different measuring systems. In one of the most common ones, when you add blood to the strip, an enzyme called *glucose oxidase* oxidizes the glucose in the blood, producing peroxide. In the colorimetric meters, in the presence of a second enzyme, *peroxidase*, the peroxide oxidizes a dye to form a blue color. The intensity of the color is proportional to the amount of the glucose. In the "old days," a similar procedure was used, but you had to compare the color of the strip with a chart, which gave only an approximation of the glucose level. You can still buy such strips, which you use without a meter, but they are no longer common and may be difficult to find. Most people use meters that read the intensity of the color and give you a numerical value.

The electrochemical meters start off oxidizing the glucose in a similar way. But then, instead of measuring a color change, the small electrical current released in a couple of additional steps is measured, and you get a numerical reading from the meter.

The glucose oxidase method requires oxygen, and venous blood sometimes doesn't contain enough oxygen for an accurate test unless the sample is shaken before testing. If for some reason you need to test venous blood, check the package insert that comes with your strips to see if the method they use is accurate with venous blood.

With older meters, some people found the electrochemical meters more sensitive to temperature variations. When they used their meters in cold places, for example, on ski trips, they said they found the colorimetric meters to be more accurate. Even so, it's important not to let the meters freeze but to keep them underneath some clothing, although not right next to the skin, where they could get too hot and damp. BG meters have been used successfully even on expeditions up Mount Everest, so don't let problems with temperature control keep you from skiing or hiking or mountain climbing if that's something you enjoy.

Because they depend on measuring the intensity of the color formed on the strips, the colorimetric meters can be sensitive to variations in light intensity. So you shouldn't move your meter or drastically change the amount of light falling on the strip during the test. Some colorimetric meters don't work well in bright light and may have warning signals if you try to measure in sunshine or under a bright lamp. The electrochemical meters aren't affected by light, so if you need to measure under a tropical sun, you might prefer that type of meter. Today's meters are almost all electrochemical.

Many factors can affect test results

Humidity. All test strips are sensitive to light and humidity. Some brands come in individual foil packages that you unwrap just before you do a test. Others come in special dark vials that contain a desiccant (a substance that removes moisture from the air) to keep the strips dry. It's important to take out a strip quickly and then reclose the vial to avoid getting moisture on the strips. For the same reason, it's not a good idea to do a lot of testing in a humid room such as the bathroom.

Temperature. Most of the meters are guaranteed accurate only within a certain temperature range, and some of them have warning signals if you're out of range. Although the lower end may seem low (around 55 degrees F; slightly different for each meter), if you're testing outside or live in a drafty old house heated with wood as I do, the temperature in the morning can sometimes be below the minimum given for the meter. So too, the high limit (around 95 degrees F; this also varies with the brand of meter) can be a problem during heat waves when you have no air-conditioning. The humidity during a heat wave can also be greater than the maximum recommended for testing (about 85 percent). You can still test under these conditions and get an estimate of your BG level, but don't expect superaccurate results.

Technology is constantly changing, and some of the newer meters are less temperature sensitive than the older ones. If you're apt to use your meter under extreme conditions, look for one with the largest temperature range.

Strips can also degrade at high temperatures. This means it's not a good idea to leave your strips in a closed-up car on a hot summer day. Sitting in direct sunlight isn't good for the meters either. If you need to travel with your meter and strips in hot weather, put them in an insulated box. Don't add ice. When you take something from a cold place and put it in a hot place, you get condensation, and the condensation could dampen the strips and make them ineffective. If you're in such a hot place that some kind of cooling is needed, the trick is to make sure the vial of strips is warmed up to ambient temperature before you open the lid. A few minutes at 100 degrees F won't cause the same damage as several hours or days.

Even if you're very careful to keep your strips in temperature-controlled rooms, you have no control over what happened to the strips while they were in transit between the factory and the store where you bought them. They might have sat in the hot sun or in subzero temperatures while they were being shipped. So if you get a reading that really doesn't seem right, first retest using another strip from the same vial. If it still seems odd, try using a strip from a new lot. If you're still getting readings that don't seem right, use some control solution if you have it. If not, call the technical support number that should be in your instruction booklet. It might be that your meter is out of order. Most companies are very good at helping you find out what is wrong and sending free replacement strips or a new meter if there's any possibility that could be the problem. They want you to keep on buying their strips.

Altitude. Extremes of altitude can also affect meter readings. At high altitudes, the amount of oxygen in the blood is lower, and this can cause erroneous readings. One study found that at altitudes above ten thousand feet, one electrochemical meter read high but a colorimetric meter read low.

If you live at a high altitude or plan to visit high mountainous areas—or if you want to climb Mount Everest—check your meter instructions or call customer service to find the limits for your meter.

Common problems. With all the meters, common problems causing incorrect results include not using enough blood, using old strips (check the expiration dates), using strips that have been exposed to high or low temperatures, not matching the code on the strips with the code on the meter, using a meter with a weak battery (some warn you when this happens), or adding a second drop of blood after the test has begun. It's also not a good idea to use a cell phone or similar device in the area while you're testing.

Sometimes, if your blood is very thick, it won't flow into the strips at a fast enough rate, and this can cause bad readings. Thus, severe dehydration may give falsely low results. Other potential problems include extremely poor circulation, so your capillary blood doesn't reflect the BG levels in the rest of your blood vessels, and a low or high *hematocrit*, meaning too few red blood cells (anemia) or too many red blood cells (polycythemia), respectively. Readings can vary from 4 to 40 percent for each 10 percent change in hematocrit. In general, a low hematocrit will result in a reading that is too high, and a high hematocrit will result in a reading that is too low.

Various other factors, for example, extremely high levels of lipids or vitamin C, can affect the readings on your meter. Read the slips that come with each batch of strips carefully to find out which ones affect your meter's tests. If they don't say, call the manufacturer.

Know your meter. Because of all these variables, it's a good idea to stick with one kind of meter most of the time. Even if the results don't match lab values exactly, you'll learn to feel comfortable with the readings on your meter, and you'll know what they represent for you. My main meter reads low, but I know it reads low. And it's easier for me to compare my readings now with my readings several years ago without having to correct for a different meter. On the other hand, if you find a meter you like better, then switch. But unless you've done tests to show that two meters read the same all the time, don't go back and forth a lot.

From all this, you can see that the results you get from home BG meters can vary considerably depending on the type of meter, the freshness of the testing strips, the particular physiology of the person doing the testing, and testing technique. So don't ever accept anyone else's BG levels as absolute numbers. If someone tells you they keep their postprandial readings under 140 and yours always go up to 180, don't feel they're necessarily doing better than you are. It could be they have a meter that reads lower than yours.

The important thing is to use your meter to tell whether you're doing better or worse than you were last week or last month, whether potatoes make your BG level go higher than lentils, whether starting or stopping a new drug helps or hinders your control. If you use your meter and modify your lifestyle as a result of what you find, you can control your diabetes instead of letting your diabetes—and complications—control you.

IN A SENTENCE:

■ *Blood glucose numbers depend on the type of blood you are testing (plasma or whole blood), and the readings you get on your meter depend on the type of meter, the strips, and your technique.*

Should I Take Vitamins and Minerals?

Dieters may need extra vitamins

Some people think extra vitamins are not necessary for anyone who eats a lot of fruits and vegetables, but almost no one will tell you that it's harmful to take vitamin pills that provide only the RDI (reference daily intake) amounts, or slightly more. (The RDI is a relatively new term used instead of the old USRDA, or recommended dietary allowance.) A lot of research has been done to determine the amounts of vitamins and minerals needed in both humans and animals in order to avoid deficiency diseases. What is sometimes controversial is taking vitamins or minerals in much larger amounts, sometimes ten or even one hundred times the RDI, or the role of vitamins and minerals in controlling blood glucose (BG) levels in people with diabetes.

For people without diabetes, eating a lot of fruits and vegetables is probably the best way to get enough vitamins and minerals because the produce may contain nutrients that haven't been added to vitamin pills yet, and the fiber is good for you. But if you have type 2 diabetes, you are probably trying to limit your total intake of food. Furthermore, fruits and even starchy vegetables can raise BG levels when you have diabetes, so you may not be able to eat a lot of them without sacrificing good BG control. Thus you should consider taking at least a multivitamin pill.

If you prefer to get your vitamins and minerals from foods, any standard book on nutrition will tell you which vitamins and minerals are found in which foods. Or ask your dietician for help with this.

There is also some evidence that people with type 2 diabetes have more free radicals than other people, so some people take a lot of extra antioxidants, including vitamins A, C, and E and alpha-lipoic acid. Be careful with vitamin A. Too much can be toxic. The precursor to vitamin A, beta-carotene, is much safer and has the same effects.

Vitamins C and E. People with type 2 diabetes tend to be low in *vitamin C*, which also protects against damage caused by the sugar alcohol **sorbitol** (see the box in Day 3). High levels of sorbitol are thought to contribute to the formation of diabetic cataracts. Both vitamins C and E are antioxidants. Vitamin C is water soluble and works in the liquid portions of the body. Vitamin E is fat soluble and works in the membranes.

Observational studies (meaning you look at a bunch of people who do one thing and compare their rates of some result you're interested in with the rates in another bunch of people who do something different, but you don't intervene to tell some people to change a behavior or take a pill) suggested that people with high intakes of vitamin E had lower rates of cardiovascular events.

However, some recent studies suggested that vitamin E supplements of about four hundred units a day were not beneficial in middle-aged and elderly persons, many of whom had diabetes. This is similar to a study of beta-carotene (a vitamin A precursor) supplementation. People with high beta-carotene intakes in their diets seemed to have lower cancer rates, but the formal study showed that the supplements actually increased the rates of lung cancer in smokers and asbestos workers.

All these studies are limited by the fact that they were conducted in a limited patient population for a limited time with only one dose of the vitamin. So the conclusions are not carved in stone. It may be that people who eat foods high in certain vitamins tend to eat other healthy foods. Or it may be that other substances in food are acting *synergistically* (meaning that some unknown substance makes the vitamins work better) with the vitamins. In the case of vitamin E, some people note that the supplements used in the studies contained only one form of vitamin E (alpha-tocopherol). Foods contain several kinds of vitamin E, and perhaps the other kinds are the beneficial ones. Taking high doses of alpha-tocopherol might even reduce the body's production of the other forms of tocopherol.

Supplemental vitamin E has also been shown to reduce the beneficial effects of statins and niacin on cholesterol levels.

Folic acid. Another vitamin often recommended for people with diabetes is *folic acid*. This vitamin, which is found in green leafy vegetables, seems to reduce the concentration of a compound called *homocysteine*, which is associated with higher levels of heart attacks, for which people with diabetes are at higher risk. If you eat a lot of green vegetables—as you should unless you are taking **anticoagulants**—you should have plenty of folic acid, but it's not expensive and might be worth adding to your list of vitamins.

Vitamin B12. If you've been taking metformin (see Week 3) for several years, you should consider taking *vitamin B12* supplements. In some people (about 10 percent), metformin inhibits the uptake of vitamin B_{12} from food. You can get vitamin B_{12} shots, to make sure it actually gets into your system. There are also sublingual pills that are supposed to be taken up more efficiently than the regular oral pills. There is one report that taking more calcium increases vitamin B_{12} levels in people taking metformin.

Unless you're a vegetarian, this is not an immediate problem, as most people who eat meat have enough vitamin B_{12} stored in the liver to last several years.

B vitamins. Some people with type 2 diabetes say the vitamin *biotin* helps control their BG levels. Others say it has no effect. Some say extra B vitamins help with their control; although again, this effect is not universal. Biotin is usually produced by bacteria in the gut, so most people are not deficient in this vitamin.

Alpha-lipoic acid. *Alpha-lipoic acid* has been used for decades in Germany to treat diabetic neuropathy. It's also a powerful antioxidant that is both fat and water soluble, and it recycles vitamins C and E after they have reacted with free radicals. When infused into the veins, alpha-lipoic acid can also reduce insulin resistance (IR). Unfortunately, oral preparations seem to lack the latter effect to any great degree, and the lifetime of the lipoic acid in the bloodstream is very short. However, some people report that their fasting BG levels decrease when they take the supplement, and today one can buy continuous-release alpha-lipoic acid supplements. The relatively low amounts in some vitamin pills probably won't have that effect.

N-Acetylcysteine. N-Acetylcysteine (NAC) is a precursor of glutathione, which like alpha-lipoic acid and vitamins C and E is an antioxidant.

A recent study has shown that oxygen free radicals, or *reactive oxygen species*, may be a cause of IR, and adding antioxidants including NAC to cell cultures reduced the IR. NAC also improved insulin sensitivity in obese insulin-resistant mice. (Mice seem to get better treatment than we do: they're always getting cured of their diabetes.)

Some studies have shown that supplementing with NAC reduced IR in women with polycystic ovary syndrome (see Month 2).

However, NAC dos not have the long history of clinical use that alpha-lipoic acid does.

Minerals can be both good and bad

With some minerals the body is in a delicate balance between too much and too little. I'll illustrate this with the situation in sheep, which I raise.

Sheep, as well as people, need the mineral *selenium*, which like vitamins A, C, and E is also an antioxidant. Without selenium, lambs may get something called *white muscle disease*, in which the heart muscle is defective. In the Northeast, where I live, soils tend to be selenium deficient, and many farmers supplement their sheep with selenium to make sure they get enough.

In the West, however, soils tend to be high in selenium. During periods of drought, the plants in the West sometimes concentrate the selenium in their leaves. The famished sheep eat the high-selenium plants and die from selenium toxicity. Thus both too little and too much selenium can be fatal in sheep. The same is true with copper. If you give your sheep grain formulated to have the proper amount of copper for cows, the sheep may drop dead from copper poisoning. Without copper they'll also die. It's a delicate balance.

Humans are likely similar with respect to a lot of minerals. We need them to live, but too much can be toxic. We get our food from all over the country, even all over the world, so it's hard to know whether it's from soil that was high in a particular mineral or mineral deficient.

Iron is a good example of a mineral that we need but which can be toxic in excess. *Hemoglobin*, the molecule that carries oxygen in the blood, needs iron to function. Older people used to be told to take extra iron for "tired blood." More recently, it has been suggested that too much iron actually *increases* the risk of cardiovascular problems by producing free radicals, and older people seem to have more difficulty getting rid of excess iron, so geriatric vitamins usually contain less iron than the others. As noted in Month 2, the inherited iron-overload disease *hemochromatosis* can be deadly.

Chromium and vanadium. Two minerals you'll most likely hear about after you're diagnosed with diabetes are *chromium* and *vanadium*, both of which are heavy metals reported to help with BG control. There is no doubt that a deficiency of these minerals can cause problems with BG control. The real debate is whether most Americans are deficient in them and whether larger-than-RDI amounts can be toxic. Some people say that many Americans, especially the older ones who tend to get type 2 diabetes, tend to be deficient in chromium because of marginal diets with too few fruits and vegetables. They say soils all over the world are becoming depleted of minerals, so even when you eat plenty of fruits and vegetables, you may be deficient in some nutrients. Others say hogwash to that and worry that large amounts of heavy metals can harm the kidneys.

One study in China showed that chromium supplements improved BG control in people with type 2 diabetes. Critics say the Chinese who were studied were chromium deficient to start with. Some other studies have shown benefits and others have shown none. One possibility is the ever-present YMMV (Your Mileage May Vary). People who are chromium deficient may benefit from chromium supplements. Others may not. Eating a lot of sugar and other carbohydrate may deplete the chromium from your system. If you think chromium may help you, try it for a while and see if it has any effect on your BG levels. If it doesn't, stop taking it.

Note that the *trivalent* (meaning it has three positive charges) *chromium* used in dietary supplements is different from the *hexavalent* (meaning it has six positive charges) *chromium* you can get from industrial exposure to chromium metal dust. The latter is toxic, another example of how a mineral can be beneficial in certain states and lethal in others. So don't think you can help your diabetes by gnawing on the chrome bumpers of old cars.

The situation with vanadium is slightly different. There are controlled studies that show that vanadium can reduce BG levels. The problem is that you have to use huge amounts to see an effect, and such large amounts cause side effects. The tiny amounts found in vitamin pills shouldn't be any problem. Taking a lot of vanadium can hinder your absorption of chromium, yet another example of the delicate balance your body must maintain for optimal health.

Magnesium and zinc. Two other minerals that some people say are deficient in people with diabetes are *magnesium* and *zinc*. As with the other minerals, without actually measuring the levels in your blood, it's difficult to know if you need extra magnesium or zinc or not. If you decide to supplement, be sensible; don't overdo it. Too much magnesium causes diarrhea, and too much zinc can be toxic.

Note that some summaries of studies showing mineral deficiencies simply refer to "people with diabetes." This includes many people who are not well controlled, whose bodies are producing extra urine in an attempt to get rid of the extra glucose in their blood. Along with the glucose, they are losing minerals. The same applies to people taking **diuretics**. So, for example, high BG levels could cause low magnesium levels by increasing its loss in the urine, instead of low magnesium levels causing high BG levels. If your BG levels are well controlled and you're not taking diuretics or drinking huge amounts of beer or coffee, you're less likely to be deficient in minerals.

Calcium. Finally, *calcium* is a good idea for most people, especially if your diet requires you to limit your intake of dairy foods.

Reasonable amounts. In reasonable amounts, most vitamins and minerals shouldn't harm you. The problem is deciding what is reasonable. Water-soluble vitamins can usually be taken in much-larger-than-normal amounts without any side effects because they are simply eliminated from the body in the urine. One group reported that in very high doses, vitamin C might be a pro-oxidant (producing free radicals) instead of an antioxidant, but others say that study was flawed. Vitamin E has been reported to be a pro-oxidant in smokers. All the fat-soluble vitamins, which means vitamins A, D, E, and K, can be toxic if you take large amounts.

People with healthy metabolisms who don't smoke and who live with clean air and water and eat diets rich in organic fruits and vegetables grown in healthy soil probably don't need any vitamin or mineral supplements. But having type 2 diabetes means your metabolism is out of whack. In addition, you may be on a diet that restricts your consumption of some healthy foods. Thus some supplementation with vitamins and minerals may be a good thing for you. Just don't go overboard. More is not always better.

IN A SENTENCE:

▪ *Because you're probably limiting your total food intake, you might want to take reasonable amounts of common vitamins, minerals, and antioxidants.*

How About Herbs and Stuff?

Herbal remedies are usually more of an unknown than vitamins and minerals, because even less research has usually been done on them. In some cases, especially with exotic herbs, there's been almost none.

That doesn't mean they don't work and aren't safe. That just means no one has conducted controlled trials to show that they do work. Sometimes a study was done that showed that the herb helped people with diabetes, but the study was done in some foreign country and published in an obscure journal almost no one in the United States has ever heard of. Some people reject that evidence as something you shouldn't trust. If the journal in question is a legitimate one in some foreign country, that attitude is elitist. On the other hand, if the journal is one published by a group affiliated with the people who sell the supplements, then that attitude is valid. When the country is far away, it may be difficult to know the difference.

When deciding whether or not to try various herbal supplements, read as much as you can about them first and consider the following points.

Learn what is in the supplement

Most dietary supplements tell you what they are supposed to contain. The problem is that some of the supplements contain plants that many of us are not familiar with. Unless you're an herbalist, you probably won't even be familiar with the names of common American herbs, much less obscure plants found only in Siberia or Sri Lanka.

There are a few sources that will tell you more (see For Further Reading). Herbs are used more frequently by physicians in Europe, especially Germany, and the German Commission E's report on herbal medicines is one of the most complete, but it hasn't been updated lately. The entire report is quite expensive; see if you can find a copy at your local library or health-food store. *The Physicians' Desk Reference* series now includes a volume on herbal medicines, including a paperback designed for popular use. These books are good places to start when you're trying to find out if medical authorities consider that the ingredients in some supplements are safe. If you have access to the Internet, you can find information there. However, be aware that most articles found through standard Internet searches are written by people who sell these supplements and naturally tout their safety and effectiveness and ignore any indications they might cause harm.

Ask how many ingredients it contains

Many herbal preparations sold to help with blood glucose (BG) control contain many ingredients. When they do, it's difficult to know which particular one is helping with your BG control, if the preparation does work. There might be one useful ingredient and ten others that are doing nothing at all or maybe even doing harm. Of course the people who sell the supplements will say you need the exact balance found in their preparation to see any results. Maybe they're right. But probably not. Sometimes they're just trying to make their own particular brand of a supplement seem better. Remember the old ad for the painkiller that said, "Contains not one, but a combination of ingredients," as if that were somehow a good reason to buy it.

It's better to try things one at a time, so you can find out which ones really work.

Try to find out how it works

Just because you don't know how a drug works is no reason it shouldn't be used. People used aspirin for years before scientists discovered at the end of the twentieth century how it works.

Nevertheless, if you can find out as much as possible how an alternative supplement is supposed to work, you'll have a better idea of whether it might be a good idea for you. For example, some people don't want to take sulfonylurea drugs because they're worried that they might burn out the pancreas. Let's say you decide instead to take an obscure "miracle supplement" from Myanmar that contains a plant you've never heard of. How do you know the plant isn't simply a natural form of one of the sulfonylureas you didn't want to take in the first place?

Again, do as much research as you can before making a decision. A good place to start is an article in *Diabetes Care* called "Traditional Plant Medicines as Treatments for Diabetes" (see For Further Reading). This article lists dozens of plants that are supposed to have BG-lowering qualities with summaries of their proposed mechanisms of action and references to any research that had been done on them by that time (1989).

There are also journals devoted to medicinal herbs and foods. If you have Internet access, search on "journal medicinal food" and "journal medicinal plants" to find them.

Consider the purity

One problem with supplements is that they are not as regulated as drugs are, so the active ingredients in the supplements can vary greatly from brand to brand and from the amounts stated on the labels. The composition of active ingredients in plants can also vary greatly depending on the soil conditions, growing conditions, and time of harvest. So if someone grows a plant, dries and pulverizes the leaves, and sells it as a supplement, its active ingredient might vary a lot from batch to batch. If the active ingredient is not very potent, this might not make much difference. In other cases it could. This is also a problem with studies of herbal remedies. The activities of the herbs used in different studies may not have been the same.

A perhaps greater concern is the inadvertent or even purposeful addition of contaminants. There have been reports of poisoning from lead and other heavy metals in herbal preparations from India and China. Even worse, some from China were found to contain manufactured sulfonylureas; phenformin, which was banned in the United States; or steroids. No wonder they worked. The companies just advertised their miracle herbs and added a cheap drug. Because supplements aren't controlled, there's no way to be sure this won't happen.

Consider the cost

Some herbal diabetes treatments are extremely expensive; they cost more than some prescription drugs, and even if your insurance pays for prescription drugs, it won't pay for herbal supplements. If you're convinced the supplement helps you, maybe it's worth the cost. Otherwise, you might be better off spending the money on some very good food that would help you stick to your diet, or enrolling in some kind of exercise club, or joining a golf club, or buying a brand-new mountain bike.

Make sure it's not snake oil

Some herbal remedies are sold by well-meaning people who really think they work. And some of them do. Unfortunately, others are sold by get-rich-quick snake-oil salespeople who are out to get a quick buck from desperate people. How can you tell the difference?

One difference is in what they're charging. If a friend says he's found that cinnamon really helped him with his BG control, I'll probably try it. He's not selling me anything, cinnamon is cheap, I like the taste, and it's not likely to hurt me. But if Sleeze E. Bague mails me a brochure advertising a Diabetes Miracle Cure and says he's willing to let me have a month's supply for only one hundred dollars, my rubbish-detecting antennae will go up.

Another tip-off that you're dealing with snake oil is if the product contains a lot of "mystery ingredients" and you can't find them listed in any references you consult. Another is if the product was discovered by some exotic means. Maybe the ingredients were dictated from another world while the maker was in a trance. Or maybe a mysterious manuscript with a formula for a lost diabetes cure was discovered in an ancient monastery in Tibet. Diabetes has been with us for a long time, and you can be sure that if anyone had ever found a cure, it wouldn't have been lost.

The decision is yours

You might think from all these concerns that one should never, ever even consider taking any kind of herbal supplement. But remember that some of the same concerns I've mentioned may apply to prescriptions approved by the Food and Drug Administration (FDA) and over-the-counter drugs as well.

We often don't know exactly how prescription drugs work. They're supposed to be pure, but everyone makes mistakes, and sometimes they have to be recalled because of errors. Manufacturers in France sold blood products without testing for the AIDS virus, and children with hemophilia died as a result.

Even carefully controlled, FDA-approved medications can be lethal. More than sixty people died from taking the drug troglitazone (Rezulin). People die from allergic reactions to prescription drugs. People die from taking prescription drugs during FDA trials. Many drugs cause kidney or liver damage. Even painkillers like acetaminophen can be harmful, even fatal in combination with a lot of alcohol.

On the other hand, one must remember that just because a supplement is "natural" doesn't mean that it is safe. Strychnine is all natural. So is poison hemlock.

So how do you decide? The first question you should ask before taking either a prescription drug or an herbal supplement is "Can this drug harm me?" Try to find out the likely cost-benefit ratio of taking the drug. With a prescription drug, the *Physicians' Desk Reference* or the leaflet that should come with the drug (if you don't get one, ask the pharmacist for it) should tell you what percentage of people during clinical trials showed what side effects. Every drug has some side effects. Most people are happy to live with the side effects of drugs like caffeine or alcohol or nicotine or too much chocolate pie. What you have to decide with a prescription drug is whether a 2 percent risk of headache is a reasonable risk to take. Probably yes. A 5 percent risk of fatal liver damage would be another matter indeed.

With herbal remedies you don't usually have such statistics, so you have to make the judgments yourself. If you're interested in trying herbal remedies, probably the best place to start is with common herbs and spices.

Some common foods are supposed to help

Many common foods have been reported to help with BG control. A lot of them contain a lot of soluble fiber, so it's possible that the fiber is what is doing the job. Fiber-rich remedies include prickly pear cactus (nopal), fenugreek, guar gum, barley, oat bran, and flaxseed. Note that eating a lot of fiber can inhibit the uptake of some drugs, so try to take your medications when you are not eating huge amounts of soluble fiber. Other common foods and herbs that have been reported to help are cinnamon, onion, garlic, mushrooms, bay leaves, sage, allspice, and thyme.

Studies have shown that eating vinegary foods reduces the *glycemic index* (see Day 4) of the meal. It seems to be the acetic acid in the vinegar that has this effect. Lemon juice (which contains citric acid) doesn't work.

It's unlikely that any of these foods will cause you any harm in reasonable amounts. Don't go overboard, as huge amounts of common spices can be dangerous (for example, large doses of sage oil can cause convulsions; infusions are less toxic). If you want to test the effect of foods and spices, try them one at a time. Measure your BG levels before and after eating them (along with a meal whose effect on your BG level you've already determined if you don't want to eat bowls of garlic or tablespoons of cinnamon alone) to see if they have any effect on your BG levels, or add a spice to all your meals for a week and see if your average BG levels change. If not, don't bother with it unless you like the taste.

Many other herbal remedies have been reported

Diabetes has been known around the world for centuries, and many countries have folk remedies. The following are some of the ones you'll hear mentioned most often.

Gymnema sylvestre. This is an Ayurvedic remedy used in India, where it is called *gurmar*. When the leaves of the plant are chewed, the sweetness of food is blocked, so people stop eating sweets because they have no taste. There is also some evidence that it may reduce the uptake of sugar in the intestine.

However, the most controversial aspect of *Gymnema* is its reported ability to cause the regeneration of beta cells. Research showing this was published in the *Journal of Ethnopharmacology* in 1990. Critics say if there were any truth to it, the research would have been repeated elsewhere by now. Supporters say drug companies don't want to do the research because they can't patent it. Many "miracle cures" you'll see advertised contain *Gymnema*.

Momordica charantia. This is a cucumber-shaped melon called *bitter melon* or *karela*, used in Asian cooking. It is (surprise) bitter, and it is used in Asia to lower BG levels. Many preparations that contain *Gymnema* also contain *Momordica*. You can buy the vegetable at Asian grocery stores. Extracts are usually used to control BG levels.

Ginseng. Ginseng has been reported to lower BG levels. The problem is that there are many different varieties of ginseng, and the active ingredients can vary a lot even within the same variety and depending on whether the product contains extracts of roots or leaves. Some types of ginseng have been reported to *increase* BG levels. If you decide to try ginseng, make sure the kind you read about is the same kind you try, and test your BG levels when you take it. Some preparations of ginseng have been reported to interfere with warfarin and diuretics.

Bilberry. Bilberry (*Vaccinium myrtillus*, not the same as blueberry, with which it is often confused) leaves have been reported to help with BG levels. Bilberry is also supposed to aid with night vision. But be careful: too much is toxic.

Fenugreek. In addition to its soluble fiber, fenugreek (*Trigonella foenum-graecum*) may contain compounds that help to lower BG levels. Unfortunately, taking a lot of fenugreek can give you a rather odd odor. It may also "thin" the blood and should be used with caution by anyone taking other anticoagulants ("blood thinners") including aspirin.

Ginkgo biloba. *Ginkgo* has been shown to increase the circulation and is used primarily to increase circulation to the brain. It may also help with circulation to the extremities, which is often poor in people with type 2 diabetes. Because it is also a blood thinner, it should be used cautiously if you're also taking other blood thinners.

Evening primrose oil. Some people with diabetes find that *gamma-linolenic acid (GLA)* helps reduce the pain of neuropathy. It is also supposed to be synergistic with alpha-lipoic acid. Evening primrose is high in GLA. Another source of GLA is borage oil; there are reports that borage leaves can damage the liver, but borage oil is probably OK. GLA forms prostaglandin E_1, which is a blood thinner. Both GLA and alpha-lipoic acid are relatively expensive.

Banaba leaf. Banaba (*Lagerstroemia speciosa*; a type of crepe myrtle) leaves have been used to treat diabetes in the Philippines. A major active principle is thought to be corosolic acid, but the intact leaves show greater effect, so other compounds, including tannins, may be involved.

Pterocarpus marsupium. The dried resin of *Pterocarpus marsupium*, or the Indian kino tree, looks like dried blood and is sometimes called *dragon's blood*. It is reported to lower BG levels in both animals and humans and has been used in India to treat diabetes.

There are also reports that it protects the beta cells from destruction by toxins and, like *Gymnema*, even promotes beta cell regeneration. Other studies say it has no effect. It is often found in diabetic herbal combination medications along with *Gymnema*.

Interestingly, one active component, a flavonoid antioxidant called *epicatechin*, is also found in chocolate and green tea.

Berberine. Berberine is found in some plants such as goldenseal, goldenthread, and barberry. It is used in traditional Chinese medicine as an antiseptic.

It also reduces blood sugar, and the primary mechanism seems to be similar to that of metformin, lowering the liver's production of glucose. Some studies have shown that its effects on the hemoglobin A1c are about the same as those of meformin.

Some studies in rodents show that berberine increases the amount of brown fat (the fat that burns fatty acids to produce heat and energy) and thus might help with weight loss. But some of the studies on berberine were not well controlled, and hence the results should be considered suggestive and not definitive.

Berberine also reacts with substances in the liver that detoxify drugs, so taking berberine can affect the levels of other drugs you are taking. Thus if you choose to try berberine, it's essential that you tell your physician you're using it and check for possible drug interactions.

Also, as it's antimicrobial, berberine can change the bacterial composition of your gut. If it kills off unhealthy bacteria, that would be good, and some have hypothesized that this is how it works. If it kills off beneficial bacteria, that would be bad. Research into human gut microbiota (bacterial populations) is just starting to take off, so we may soon have a definitive answer to this aspect of berberine.

It's your body, your science experiment

Because herbal remedies are often unknowns, many doctors won't be thrilled if you say you want to use them. Some don't know much about herbs, and others go ballistic if you mention them, especially if you say you got the information on the Internet. So if you have a personality that needs a pat on the back from your physician, herbal remedies are probably not the way to go.

But if you're the adventurous sort who likes taking risks, you might want to try some of the herbal remedies. If you do, just be cautious. Read all you can about them before you try them. Try one at a time. Keep records to help you decide whether or not they work. If they don't, save your money.

Be on the lookout for possible drug interactions. As I mentioned before, sometimes too many supplements that might help individually can cause problems when taken together. Your pharmacist will probably know more about possible interactions than your physician, but it's also a good idea to tell your doctor which supplements you're taking.

Herbal and other folk remedies sometimes are the starting point for so-called miracle medications. Some of the herbs may turn out to be beneficial, and some may work only by the power of suggestion. Until well-controlled studies of herbal medications are done and published, we won't know for sure. If they can't hurt you, the only thing you have to lose is your cash.

If they don't have much effect on your control and your budget is tight, it would make sense to spend your money on something that would help you stick with your diet or exercise instead.

IN A SENTENCE:

Many different herbs are used to treat diabetes in different parts of the world, and some of them may turn out to be good treatments, but there have not yet been controlled studies of most of them.

living

Using
Insulin

Injecting yourself with insulin may sound scary, a last resort that you wouldn't want to try unless you had no alternatives. But as discussed in Week 4, some people actually prefer to go right to insulin when their blood glucose (BG) levels are high. Current guidelines also recommend using insulin in type 2 diabetes at earlier stages than previously, when many people considered insulin to be a last resort.

If you're considering this, here's what you should know. Injecting with insulin is not difficult. It's almost painless. It's cheaper than using several of the new oral drugs. And it works. I know, because I've used insulin myself.

For me, the most difficult part about taking insulin was remembering to do it. I'm a little absentminded, and when my watch alarm went off and I was out in my barn office, I'd plan to take the insulin when I went into the house to get a cup of coffee in ten minutes. Then I'd forget.

For people with type 1 diabetes who are producing almost no insulin of their own, working out a proper insulin regimen can be complex, and timing is critical. If they don't take their insulin, they risk going into ketoacidosis (see Month 2). They have to be on constant alert for low blood sugar. After some years of type 1 diabetes, some people stop producing the counterregulatory hormone *glucagon* (see Day 7 and the Learning section of this chapter) and lose their sensitivity to lows, and this makes things even more complex.

However, when you have type 2 diabetes, you can elect to start using insulin when you still have beta cells left and hence are still producing some insulin yourself. This gives you a certain amount of buffering capacity. So, for example, if you don't inject quite enough insulin, your insulin response will eventually kick in and bring your BG levels back to baseline. If you inject a little too much insulin, you'll be able to produce glucagon, as well as *adrenaline* (see Day 7), both of which will help to bring your BG levels back up again. If you inject too much insulin for your glucagon and adrenaline to compensate, at least you'll be able to sense that you're low so you'll be able to treat the low.

Today there are many different insulins on the market. Older insulins are being phased out, and new ones are being developed all the time. Each insulin has its own profile of action: when it starts working, when it peaks, and when it stops working. You and your health-care team will try to match the profile of your insulins with your own particular physiology and lifestyle. Because the response to the different insulins can be different under different conditions, or in different people, a lot of this individualization is by trial and error. What works in José may not work in Josiah.

I won't describe the detailed profiles of the various insulins available today—which may not be what is available when you read this book. If you do decide to go the insulin route, you probably won't want to grab some insulin and start injecting without any initial supervision. Your physician, nurse, or certified diabetes educator will help you get started. Then, if you want to read about the details, you can try some of the books devoted to insulin use. Several are listed in the section For Further Reading. Magazines and Internet searches will get you up to speed on what's available at the time.

If you want to try modeling what might happen to your BG levels with different insulins before you start, you can use the free AIDA program (www.2aida.org), although it hasn't been updated with current insulins.

Basal insulins work on premeal BG levels

What you should understand is the difference between two basic types of insulin. One is called a **basal insulin**. A basal insulin is designed to keep your BG levels in the normal range when you're not eating: between meals and overnight. Basal insulins available in 2015 include glargine (Lantus) and detemir (Levemir). The new basal insulin degludec (Tresiba) was rejected by the Food and Drug Administration (FDA) because of lack of evidence of cardiac safety, but the company has resubmitted its application to the FDA, which should make a decision in fall 2015. If it's approved, the company hopes to launch it soon afterward.

Your body, and especially your brain, needs some glucose to function all the time, even when you're fasting. Thus when your BG levels drop below a certain point and no more glucose is coming in from food, your blood insulin levels also drop, your glucagon levels increase, and your liver starts producing glucose from the **glycogen** it has stored there (see the Learning section of this chapter). If there's not enough glycogen, it will start converting some protein and some other compounds like glycerol from fat (see Day 3) into glucose.

But just making the glucose isn't enough. After the liver releases the glucose into the bloodstream, you need some insulin to help that glucose get into the muscle and fat cells (brain cells can take up glucose without insulin). Even when you're sleeping, these cells are using some energy to keep their basic machinery running.

People who don't have diabetes are constantly releasing small pulses of insulin into the blood, just enough to cope with the small amounts of glucose that your liver is shipping out into the blood. When you inject a basal insulin, you're trying to mimic as closely as possible those small pulses of insulin a nondiabetic pancreas would produce.

Hence, the best basal insulin is one that has a very flat profile, meaning that it is released slowly in about the same amount every hour. Different long-acting basal insulins use different mechanisms to make them get absorbed slowly.

When you use a basal insulin, you start at a low dose and keep increasing it slowly until your fasting and premeal numbers are at satisfactory levels. It's best to wait several days after increasing a basal dose before trying another increase. This is because when you start injecting the basal insulin, it's not all dumped into your bloodstream right away. Some of it is temporarily stored in what is called a **depot**.

The size of the depot varies with the amount of insulin you inject, but it acts as an insulin buffer. When the insulin in your system goes down, the depot can release some insulin. This is like a boiler furnace. First you have to heat up the water in the system (fill the depot), and then the hot water releases heat into the house. Even after you've stopped heating the water in the boiler (stopped filling the depot), the remaining hot water will continue to give off heat.

Bolus insulins cover meals

The other type of insulin is called a **bolus insulin**, sometimes called a *mealtime* or *prandial* insulin. This type of insulin is injected before meals and is designed to cover the postprandial (after-meal) BG peaks you get when you eat carbohydrate foods. Thus the best bolus insulins start working quickly, so you can inject them right before you start a meal, and don't last very long, so you don't go low when you're through digesting the meal. Bolus insulins available in 2015 include regular (the kind your body produces), lispro (Humalog), aspart (Novolog), and glulisine (Apidra).

When you use a bolus insulin, you first calculate how much carbohydrate you're planning to eat for that meal and then calculate how much insulin you need to cover that much carbohydrate. When you're starting, you can use ballpark estimates of your *insulin:carbohydrate (I:C) ratio*, that is, how many units of insulin you need to cover X grams of carbohydrate.

Different people can have quite different I:C ratios; the ratio depends on how much you weigh and how much insulin resistance (IR) you have. As you get more experienced, you can refine that number to find what works for you, using various formulas or actually measuring your own ratios. With practice, many people can estimate the carbohydrate content of a meal and inject very close to the correct amount of insulin to cover that meal. Even children can become proficient at this.

When you have type 2 diabetes, you may find that you don't need to use a bolus insulin for meals. A basal insulin may be able to keep your premeal BG levels low enough that the mealtime excursions will not be high, especially if you're on a low-carbohydrate diet. When your beta cells don't need to work all day pumping out the basal insulin, they may be able to store enough insulin between meals to cover a limited-carbohydrate meal.

One approach is to use a basal insulin and oral drugs to cover the meals. Or, conversely, you might want to use oral drugs to reduce your IR and keep your baseline BGs down and use a bolus insulin to cover high-carbohydrate meals.

Other approaches can be used

In addition to very slow basal insulins and very fast bolus insulins, there are also some insulins that have an intermediate action. Some people inject one of these insulins at night to cover the dawn effect the next morning. Or they inject them at breakfast; the insulins peak around lunch-time and cover that meal.

You can also inject mixtures of several insulins designed to give peaks at the approximate times you plan to eat. You can actually mix several types of insulin in a syringe (but never mix Lantus) or you can buy pre-mixed insulins. A common premixed combination is 70:30, 70 percent in-termediate-acting NPH (see later) and 30 percent regular.

The problem with this older approach is that it ties you down to eating your meal at the time of the insulin peaks. If you don't, you risk going low. It also means that to avoid these lows, you may have to eat even if you aren't hungry, and this can cause weight gain, not something you're apt to want.

You should also know that one of the intermediate insulins, called *NPH* (for *neutral protamine Hagedorn*, after the man who devised it) contains a protein called *protamine*. This protein is sometimes used to reverse the actions of anticlotting drugs used in heart surgery, and in a very tiny mi-nority of people who have used NPH, a serious allergic reaction can occur when they're given protamine. For this reason, some people say this insu-lin should be avoided. Others say the risk is so low you shouldn't worry about it. Whatever you decide, you should be aware of this.

Some of today's basal insulins have a very flat profile. This means you're much less likely to go low than with the older, peakier insulins. It also means it's possible to skip meals if you don't want to eat at a particular time. Then, when you do eat, if you need a bolus insulin, you can inject it right before the meal. Another approach that uses the basal-bolus method is the *insulin pump*. The pumps are used primarily when you have very few beta cells left and are producing almost no insulin of your own. You wear the pump twenty-four hours a day, and it releases short pulses of fast-acting insulin all day and all night to cover your basal needs. Before meals, you dial up the amount of insulin you want for your bolus and pump it in. Because insulin pumps are expensive, your insurance com-pany may not cover them unless your own insulin production is almost gone. Some people call the basal-bolus system used with traditional sy-ringes "the poor man's pump."

Rates of absorption vary

Insulin can be injected in different places, including the fat in the legs, the arms, the buttocks, and the stomach area (and most of us type 2s don't need to worry about running out of the latter). It can be absorbed at dif-ferent rates depending on a number of factors. These include where you inject (insulin injected in the stomach tends to start working faster than insulin injected into the arm); how deeply you inject (insulin injected into muscle starts working faster than insulin injected into superficial fat, which works faster than insulin injected into deeper fat layers); how much blood is flowing where you inject (exercise of a muscle you've injected into increases the rate of absorption, as does massage and even a hot shower or sauna); and how much you inject (with most insulins, larger doses start working faster, peak later, and last longer).

Your personal physiology as well as your own injection technique may also affect how quickly the insulin is absorbed, which is one reason so much of working out insulin dosages is by trial and error. The charts and graphs of insulin profiles that you'll find in various sources are only very general guides. For example, a new basal insulin that lasts more than twenty-four hours in some people might only last fifteen hours in others. Note that different sources may tell you that the identical insulin has a different starting time, peak, and length of action. This is because different authors are using data from different studies to illustrate their point, and the insulin profiles can vary in different groups.

Because different parts of your body absorb insulins at different rates, it's a good idea to stick to one area, for example, either the stomach or the legs, when you're working out the dosages that are correct for you.

But how about the problems?

But doesn't all this injecting hurt? Mostly no. Mostly you won't even feel it. Today's needles are so thin that injecting insulin is a lot less painful than stabbing your fingertips to test your BG levels. Some acidic insulins may occasionally sting after they've been injected, but then, so do mosquito bites. Some people gently tap their skin with the point of the needle until they find a spot that has less sensation and inject there, reducing the potential for stinging.

Isn't injecting insulin embarrassing when you're out in public? It shouldn't be. Wiping your skin with alcohol doesn't sterilize; it just cleans a bit, and the alcohol dries out your skin. Unless you've been rolling in dirt, there's no need to clean your skin with alcohol before injecting. Many people simply inject through their clothing when they're out and about. If you inject through your clothing under the table, your tablemates may not even notice, especially if you're using an insulin pen (see later).

Isn't injecting insulin inconvenient? Yes, it can be inconvenient to remember to bring along your insulin and your syringes when you're going to be away from home. If you travel through a very hot climate, keeping the insulin cool may be a problem. But the advantages of keeping your BG levels normal should outweigh the inconvenience. And most insulins can tolerate reasonable room temperatures for a certain number of days.

How do I inject?

Today, with many insulins you have a choice of using syringes and bottles of insulin, or pens. With the syringes, you use a fresh syringe every time; you puncture the bottle with the needle, inject an amount of air equal to the amount of insulin you want to use, then invert the bottle and withdraw the insulin into the syringe. The air exchange is so you don't build up a vacuum in the bottle, which would make removing the insulin more difficult.

If you see a lot of bubbles in the needle, you can push the insulin back into the bottle and slowly withdraw the insulin again. Air bubbles aren't dangerous. You'd need to inject an awful lot of air directly into a vein to cause problems. But they can make the measurements inaccurate, especially if you're using small amounts.

Then you pinch up some fat, quickly put the needle in with a dart-like action, and inject the insulin. If you find a drop of liquid appearing after you've removed the needle, you may want to leave the needle in for a few seconds the next time before removing.

When you're using clear insulins, you don't need to agitate the bottle before using the insulin. If you have one of the cloudy insulins, most people will tell you to roll the insulin between your hands and never to shake it. Others say this advice is based on older formulations that foamed, and you'll get much better mixing if you shake the bottle. As is so often the case, see what works for you.

Insulin is fairly stable, and once you've opened a bottle, you can keep it at normal room temperature for at least thirty days. Note that the expiration date on the bottle is the date up to which the manufacturer will guarantee that the insulin will be good. After the expiration date, some of the older insulins may continue to be usable, slowly losing potency with time. Newer analog insulins seem to be less stable. Even the older insulins shouldn't be used too long after the expiration date, as contamination with bacteria could occur. The vials do contain antibacterial agents, and these are actually more potent at room temperature, but the antibacterial agents may eventually become less effective.

However, although insulin will tolerate room temperature, it will not tolerate extreme temperatures or direct sunlight; some of the newer insulins should be kept in the dark. Never let the insulin freeze. And if local temperatures exceed 95 degrees F, you'll need some kind of cooling pouch. These are readily available. Never leave a bottle of insulin in the car during hot weather.

You can also use insulin pens, which come prefilled with insulin. You put on a new needle, dial the amount you want, and inject. Some pens are refillable with cartridges, and others are not. Whether you use a syringe or a pen, the shorter the needle, the easier it is to inject, and the thinner the needle, the less painful. A needle with a higher gauge is thinner (a 31-gauge needle is thinner than a 29-gauge needle).

Needle-free jet injectors are also available in case you really can't tolerate needles. But they are expensive, and some people say they are actually more painful than needles. Others say the opposite.

Note these caveats

Most of the insulin that is commonly available in the United States today is called *U-100*. This means that there are 100 units per milliliter (mL) in the bottle. The bottles contain 10 mL, so there are 1,000 units in the bottle. The insulin syringes that you get are designed to match the U-100 insulin, and they are marked with units, rather than by volume.

A new insulin, Toujeo, came on the US market in 2015. It is U-300 insulin glargine (Lantus), or 300 units-mL, so one would inject a smaller volume to get the same number of units as Lantus. It is also designed to release the insulin more slowly, so it may last longer.

If you travel abroad, you may encounter other concentrations of insulin, for example, U-40. This insulin has only 40 units/mL, that is, it is less concentrated. Make sure you *always* match the type of insulin with the type of syringe. If you're using U-100 insulin, make sure you have a U-100 syringe. If you're using U-40, make sure you have a U-40 syringe. If you don't use the right syringe, you'll inject way too much or way too little insulin.

A U-500 formulation (more concentrated) of regular insulin is also available in the United States for people with very extreme insulin resistance, but it is not often used and will most likely have to be special-ordered. If you do use U-500, make sure you use it with a syringe designed specifically for that insulin.

As with oral drugs, new insulins continue to be developed, and some of them may eventually replace the older insulins.

When you use insulin, just as when you use sulfonylureas, you will have to be alert for lows, and you should always carry your meter and glucose tablets with you in case of a low. Especially if you live alone, at night put your meter, some glucose tablets, and a glass of water next to your bed. See Month 2 to review how to deal with lows. Because you should still have the ability to produce the counterregulatory hormones glucagon and epinephrine, you shouldn't have a lot of extremely low BG levels, but too much insulin can always overwhelm the body's ability to cope, so you need to be alert to this.

You can inhale insulin

Until recently, the only way you could take insulin was by injection. This is because insulin is a protein, and intestinal enzymes in addition to the very acidic environment of the stomach break down almost all the proteins that you eat.

However, today you can also get your insulin through an inhaler. An inhaled bolus insulin called Afrezza was approved by the FDA in 2014 and marketed in early 2015. It peaks very rapidly and is then quickly cleared from the body (An earlier inhaled insulin called Exubera that had a bulky doser was pulled from the market because sales were low.) The inhaler produces a mist of fine particles that contain regular insulin. When you inhale them, the insulin is absorbed through the lining of the lungs, and the insulin works faster than if injected.

Some early adopters are reporting amazingly flat BG levels when they use Afrezza instead of an injected bolus insulin, but because Afrezza is cleared from the body so quickly, others find they have to use a slower-acting injected bolus as well, especially when they eat fat. Some people with type 1 report that Afrezza brings down highs much faster than injected insulin.

For people who are totally needle-phobic, inhaled insulin may be a blessing. However, the dosages you get from the inhaler are not as exact as the dosages you get from an injection. And the devices are new. No one knows what the long-term effect of inhaling these particles will be.

The clinical trials that preceded acceptance of the device by the FDA showed no significant lung damage, but they did show some small changes. Coughing was a problem for some people but decreased with time. The device is not recommended for anyone who smokes (smoking increases absorption) or anyone who has chronic lung disease. Taking Afrezza with a glitazone may cause heart failure because of fluid retention.

Other devices are in the pipeline

Because there are a lot of needle-phobic people in the world, drug companies are working hard to invent other methods of insulin delivery. One such device delivers a spritz of insulin into the mouth. This "buccal insulin" device has been approved for use in Ecuador but was not available in the United States at the time of this writing.

Other people are looking into nasal insulin delivery. The problem with this is that every time you suffered from a cold or an allergy, the absorption of the insulin would change, so the doses would not be very accurate.

Some researchers are trying to develop an insulin pill, something that could be coated with a substance that wouldn't dissolve until the insulin got past the stomach. But even then, the problem is that the intestines don't easily absorb entire proteins. Instead, they are generally broken down into the amino acid building blocks used to make them. Another approach is the insulin patch, with some kind of treatment to get the insulin molecule absorbed through the skin.

None of these alternative insulin-delivery systems is as accurate as injected insulin. So for now, insulin injections, with either syringes, pens, or pumps, seem to be the simplest and most accurate way of taking insulin. The injections are not difficult, and they hardly hurt at all.

Diet and exercise are wonderful ways to help your type 2 diabetes. The oral drugs can do amazing things. But some of the newest oral drugs are quite expensive, and because they're so new, no one knows what their long-term effects will be. People have been taking insulin since early in the twentieth century, some for more than sixty years.

Insulin isn't for everyone with type 2 diabetes. But if you think it might be for you, don't be afraid. Try it. You might like it. Remember: it works.

How Do They Do It?

You don't need to know how the drug companies make insulin before you decide to use it. But if you're curious, here's a quick rundown of how some of the insulins are made.

In the early days of insulin usage, the insulin was isolated from the pancreases of food animals, beef and hogs. Insulin is a protein, which means it's made up of long chains of protein building blocks called *amino acids*. Each protein has a specific number of different amino acids, in a particular order.

Insulin from different species is very similar, but not identical. Pork insulin is the closest to human insulin; it differs in only one amino acid. Beef insulin differs in two. However, these differences are small enough that the beef and pork insulins will function in the human body.

One problem with these animal insulins is that we develop antibodies against foreign proteins, even those that are very similar to our own. In most people, these anti-insulin antibodies do not cause harm. They simply slow down the absorption of the nonhuman insulins. In some cases, this slowing can actually be beneficial.

However, in a small minority, the insulin antibodies can cause problems. For a while, manufacturers started with pork insulin and used enzymes to convert it into human insulin. But quantities of pork insulin are limited by the number of hogs that are slaughtered every year.

Thus when recombinant DNA technology became available, the drug companies began using the technology to produce human insulin. They inserted genes for human insulin (or for parts of the insulin) into bacteria or yeast cells. Then they grew these cells and isolated and highly purified the human insulin. These human insulins contain a lot fewer noninsulin contaminants than the older animal insulins and don't cause as many allergic reactions.

Today, only human insulin is available in the United States; animal insulins are no longer produced here. However, in England, a few manufacturers still produce the animal insulins for those who prefer it and will export it for those who need it. Insulin is also produced in some other countries.

The human insulin that you produce in your own body is called *regular* insulin, often R for short. If you inject it directly into your bloodstream, it works very fast. But if you inject it into your fat or muscle, it doesn't work as fast because it has to be absorbed from the tissue into the capillaries in that tissue. Regular insulin is available without a prescription.

Insulin molecules tend to associate in groups of six, called *insulin hexamers*, and this association is stabilized by the addition of zinc. If you inject the hexamers into your tissues, before the insulin can be absorbed into the capillaries, it has to break apart into single insulin molecules (monomers), and this dissociation takes time.

Some time ago, researchers discovered that if they added more zinc to the insulin, the hexamers would associate into fine precipitates (powder-like particles). Adding even more zinc made the insulin form large crystals. After injection, the precipitates dissolved slowly (and the insulin was called *lente*), and the crystals dissolved very slowly (and the insulin was called *ultralente*). However, US drug companies recently stopped making these insulins in favor of newer, much more expensive insulin analogs.

Another intermediate-acting insulin is NPH. This insulin is formed by adding a basic (alkaline) protein called *protamine* to regular insulin in the presence of zinc (protamine is isolated from salmon sperm). This forms a precipitate that is intermediate acting. Like regular insulin, NPH insulin is available without a prescription.

The newer insulins are called *insulin analogs*. This means that although they are similar to regular insulin, the insulin has been modified in some way to give it the desired properties.

To make the rapid-acting bolus insulins (which currently include lispro [Humalog], aspart [Novolog], and glulisine [Apidra]), the scientists have changed a few amino acids in the insulin molecule. As a result of these changes, the insulins don't associate into the hexamer form as much, so they're absorbed much more rapidly.

To make one very slow basal insulin (glargine [Lantus]), the scientists have changed a few amino acids so that the insulin is soluble in acid but precipitates (becomes insoluble, so the solution is cloudy instead of clear) when you inject it into a neutral environment such as human tissues. This is also one reason one should never mix the acidic Lantus with another insulin, as it would precipitate in the syringe.

Another slow basal Insulin (detemir [Levemir]) is made by removing one amino acid from the insulin and adding a fatty acid. The fatty acid makes the insulin tend to bind to substances in the tissues, and this slows down its release into the bloodstream. The insulin also binds to albumin, a major protein in the blood, forming a kind of reservoir of insulin molecules that are slowly released as the insulin levels in the blood go down.

These new insulin analogs work very well for many people, and new insulin analogs will undoubtedly be developed in the future. One in the works is regular insulin with additives that speed up its absorption.

One problem with the analogs is the cost. A vial of regular insulin can cost as little as $24 in 2015, but the insulin analogs cost $250 a vial at the time of this writing, and the price is rapidly increasing. No wonder the drug companies like the insulin

(continues)

(continued) **How Do They Do It?**

analogs and noninjected insulin. If your insurance pays for your insulin, this is not a problem. If you don't have good insurance, it can be.

Some companies are working on "biosimilar" insulins, which are like generic drugs. As of this writing, none had been approved by the FDA.

The rapid-acting insulin analogs are supposed to be less immunogenic (producing an antibody response) than the animal insulins, but they are also "foreign" proteins, and foreign proteins tend to trigger the formation of antibodies, so like the animal insulins, they have the potential to cause insulin allergies. However, even regular human insulin can cause insulin allergies when injected, and no one yet knows which insulins will turn out to be the best for long-term use.

How Does Insulin Work?

Insulin is a *hormone* that helps the body take up glucose from the blood to either burn for energy or store for future use. This is a lot like what we usually do with money. We either spend it immediately or put it into the bank for later.

In order to understand what insulin does, first you need to understand a little about how glucose is stored in the body.

When glucose in the bloodstream is abundant, the body takes steps to store the extra glucose. The body can store energy in two main ways, either as *glycogen* in the liver and muscles or as *fat* (triglycerides) in the fat cells. Glucose is the source of quick energy. Glycogen is used for short-term storage. Fat is used for long-term storage.

Exercise depletes your glycogen stores

Glycogen is a *polysaccharide*, or a string of many glucose molecules linked together. You can think of glucose as cans of food and glycogen as cans of glucose taped together with duct tape so they won't fall apart and then set on a shelf in the pantry for future use. This is analogous to the long chains of glucose molecules stored in the "pantry" of the liver and muscle as glycogen.

In a well-fed person who eats carbohydrate, up to 10 percent of the liver may consist of glycogen granules. (This is why you'll see in nutritional tables that animal liver contains some carbohydrate.) Only 1 to 2 percent of the muscle is glycogen. However, because our muscle mass is so much greater than our liver mass, the average person has more than twice as much glycogen in muscles than in liver.

This is one reason exercise is so important for people with diabetes. When you eat and then lounge around in front of the computer, as I'm doing now, the glycogen pantry fills up. Just as you stop putting cans of food in the pantry when the pantry is full (and store your food somewhere else), the body stops making more glycogen when the glycogen stores are full. The extra goes into fat, where it's stored for future use. Think of this as boxes of butter that you store in the basement. The basement is larger than the pantry, and you can store more food there. But it's quicker to get food from the pantry.

Because so much glycogen is stored in the muscle, and because the major way the muscle can deplete those stores is by exercise, exercising is (alas!) very, very important in type 2 diabetes control.

This also explains why the effects of exercise last beyond the period of exercise itself. Let's say you start with a full pantry of glycogen in the muscles. As you exercise, some of the glycogen gets broken down to produce the required energy. This breaking down of glycogen is called **glycogenolysis**. But then when you stop and collapse on the sofa wishing you had another disease instead, the muscles start rebuilding their glycogen supplies. The way they do this is to extract glucose from the blood and "tape it" together to make more glycogen. So until the pantry is full again, the muscles, which have twice the storage capacity of the liver, help keep the blood glucose (BG) levels down. This also explains why muscle-building exercises are good. The larger your muscle mass is, the larger your pantry and thus your capacity for taking up BG and storing it as glycogen.

The liver is altruistic

Although most of the glycogen in the body is stored in two places, liver and muscle, the liver is more "altruistic." When the BG level starts getting low (*hypoglycemia*), the liver goes into its pantry to get glycogen, breaks it down, and ships it off into the bloodstream so it can be used by other organs that need it, for example, muscles and brain. The muscles are more selfish. They use their glycogen pantry stores only for themselves. This is because they lack an enzyme that is needed in order to export glucose from cells.

The liver can make new glucose

Just to complicate things, the liver (and the kidneys) can produce glucose from protein when glucose needs are high. This involves breaking proteins down into their parts (*amino acids*; see Day 3) and converting the amino acids into glucose. This process is called **gluconeogenesis**, or making new glucose. This is analogous to finding that your pantry was low on cans of glucose and putting more glucose into cans.

Remember I said that the muscle cells are "selfish" and can't export glucose to other tissues when the BG levels are low. Well, maybe they're not completely self-centered. When the rest of the body needs glucose badly, the muscle cells break down their protein into amino acids and export them and other substances to the liver, where they are converted to glucose by gluconeogenesis. This is one reason that undiagnosed or un-controlled type 1 diabetes was originally described as "melting of the flesh." In the total absence of insulin, the muscles "melt" down to provide glucose for the brain (which doesn't need insulin to use glucose).

The end product of both glycogenolysis and gluconeogenesis is the same: they both produce glucose. The words also look alike, and some people get them confused (see the box Confusing Terms). In general, you don't need to know when your body uses glycogenolysis and when it uses gluconeogenesis. You really just need to know that a particular activity will increase or decrease the glucose levels in your blood. However, there is one instance in which the distinction is important. Alcohol inhibits the process of gluconeogenesis. It doesn't affect glycogenolysis. Also, if you're on a low-carbohydrate diet or you've just done a lot of strenuous exercise, your glycogen reserves may be depleted and glycogenolysis rates would be low. But gluconeogenesis could still occur.

The main players are insulin and glucagon

The two main hormones that control the storage and breakdown of glucose are *insulin* and *glucagon*. Insulin tells the body that food supplies are abun-dant and it's time to store the energy from food as glycogen or fat. In general, glucagon does the exact opposite of insulin. Glucagon tells the body that food supplies are scarce, so it's time to break down glycogen in the liver and fat in the fat cells and use them to produce energy. Levels of both insulin and glucagon fluctuate, depending on how recently you've eaten, and it's the ratio of the two that determines whether energy is produced or stored.

When you've eaten a meal containing carbohydrate, insulin levels rise. This tells the body that glucose and energy are abundant and it should shift from a mode of energy production to one of energy storage. Thus insulin inhibits reactions that produce glucose and those that produce fatty acids (see Day 3) from stored fat, both sources of energy, and stimulates reactions that store them (storage of glycogen in the liver and dietary fatty acids in fat cells).

When there's nowhere else to store glucose (the glycogen pantry is full), insulin also tells the liver cells to convert glucose into fatty acids and ship them off to the fat cells, where they're slurped up and stored as fat. As usual, glucagon has opposite effects.

This is one reason that high insulin levels can stimulate weight gain (stimulating the storage of fat and inhibiting its breakdown). This fact is emphasized by authors of low-carbohydrate diet books. However, other factors also affect the gain or loss of weight, including how hungry you are, how many calories you consume in relation to your own particular caloric needs (which can vary a lot depending on your genetic makeup), how active you are, and other factors discussed in Month 8.

Between meals, insulin levels fall and glucagon levels rise. This tells the body that it needs to get its energy from storage sites. Reactions that produce glucose and fatty acids are stimulated, and reactions that store them are inhibited.

Most diet books that discuss insulin focus on carbohydrates. But fats are important too. Many tissues in the body can burn fat as well as glucose for energy. In fact some tissues, for example resting muscle, actually prefer fatty acids to glucose. (Unfortunately, this doesn't mean you can lose a lot of fat by resting more often; it's the amount of energy you burn, not its source, that is important.) Other types of cells burn fat when their preferred food, glucose, is in short supply.

The fat stored away in the fat cells is broken down into its parts: mostly fatty acids with a little bit (about 10 percent) of glycerol (see Day 3). The glycerol is shipped off to the liver to be turned into glucose. Thus fat can raise your BG levels a little, but only a small amount of the glucose actually comes from the fat. When fat raises your BG levels a lot, it may actually be raising your insulin resistance (IR). In this case, your insulin is less effective, so any carbohydrate you eat along with the fat will raise your BG levels more than it would have without the fat. The fatty acids from the fat are taken up by the muscle cells and any other cells that need them and burned for energy.

Insulin is also needed for cells to take up the amino acids that come from the breakdown of proteins, and protein as well as carbohydrate stimulates the formation of insulin. However, protein stimulates the formation of glucagon as well as insulin, and because it's the ratio of the two that controls the BG level, the insulin stimulated by eating protein doesn't affect your BG levels very much, if at all. If you produce almost no insulin, then the glucagon resulting from eating protein can make your BG levels rise.

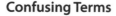

Confusing Terms

One problem when you're learning about diabetes is all those words that look alike, for instance, *gluconeogenesis* and *glycogenolysis*. The best way to decipher these terms is to understand the etymology.

Both *gluc* and *glyc* come from a Greek root meaning "sweet," but different people coining new words transliterated the Greek differently. Some of them used *glu* and others used *gly*. Very confusing.

> *gen* or *gon* means "generates"
> *lysis* means "breaks down"
> *neo* means "new"

So now we can decipher the words.

Glucose: You should be familiar with this by now. Glucose is the sugar that the body breaks down for energy.

Glycogen: Glycogen means "sweet generating." It's a polysaccharide composed of many molecules of glucose (or cans of glucose taped together with duct tape if you prefer a picture). When it breaks down, you get glucose.

Glycogenolysis: Glycogenolysis means "breaking down glycogen" to produce glucose. Taking a knife and cutting the duct tape that holds the cans of glucose together.

Glycolysis: Glycolysis means "breaking down glucose" to produce energy. (Getting a can opener to open those cans of glucose to get the energy out. Why didn't they call it glucolysis?)

Gluconeogenesis: Gluconeogenesis means "generating new glucose." In other words, you're building glucose out of building blocks from other types of food, like proteins. (A factory packing the glucose into the cans.)

Glucagon: Here's the tricky one. Unlike glycogen and glucose, glucagon isn't a carbohydrate. It's a protein and a hormone. Like glycogen, glucagon means "sweet generating," but it does it indirectly by stimulating both glycogenolysis and gluconeogenesis in the liver. In general, whatever insulin does, glucagon does the opposite.

Once you get these words unconfused, understanding all the literature gets a little easier.

As the protein is slowly converted into glucose, it can cause a rise in BG levels in people with very little insulin production of their own. When you have type 2 diabetes and are able to produce some insulin, quite often your pancreas is able to deal with the slow release of glucose from the protein you eat, and you won't see much of a rise in BG levels as a result.

No one knows yet exactly how insulin works

Insulin works primarily on three main types of tissue: muscle, liver, and fat. It used to be thought these were the only places that insulin had any important roles. But recent work has revolutionized the way people look at insulin. Researchers found evidence that insulin also plays important roles in the brain and beta cells as well.

There is evidence that IR in the brain keeps your appetite from being turned off by rising insulin levels, which normally seem to turn the appetite off. Injecting insulin into the brains of animals makes them eat less. This means that if you have IR, you would continue to be hungry after eating, when a person without IR would feel full. IR in the brain could keep your appetite turned on all the time, contributing to obesity. If you've always thought you were hungrier than other people, you were probably right.

So far, I've told you *where* insulin works, but not *how* it works. One reason is that no one really knows how insulin works. What is known is that insulin binds to receptors on cells called **insulin receptors** that are partly outside the cell (where they bind the insulin) and partly inside the cell. The insulin binding somehow changes the shape of the receptors so that the parts inside the cell activate enzymes that activate other molecules that activate other molecules and so forth in an incredibly complex chain of reactions that is not yet fully understood.

The end result of this chain is that *glucose transporters*, the little "ferries" I mentioned in Day 1, are moved to the cell membrane, where they carry glucose molecules across the cell membrane into the cell. The formal name of the ferries in muscle and fat cells is GLUT4. Other types of cells have slightly different transporters named GLUT1, GLUT2, and so forth. Some types of transporters, for example the GLUT2 found in liver cells, are present whether or not insulin levels are high, which means those tissues can take up glucose even when insulin levels are low.

At the moment, this information has very little practical use to you. I discuss it because if you later read books or articles that mention GLUT4 or GLUT2, you'll have a better idea of what they're talking about.

Your mileage may vary

You can see from this brief discussion why type 2 diabetes is such a complicated disease. Different people might have deficiencies in one molecule involved in this complicated chain of events and others might have flaws somewhere else. This situation has already been shown in people with the relatively rare form of diabetes called *MODY* (see Month 2). Mutations in several specific genes have been shown, with different families having mutations in a single different gene.

So far, such genes haven't been found for common garden-variety type 2 diabetes, which may be caused by variant forms of not just one but many genes. Depending on which molecule or molecules are involved and how much they are changed from normal, people might react differently to different situations and treatments.

Eventually, scientists will know how to tell where the defects are in the different subtypes of type 2 diabetes. Then they'll be able to develop treatments aimed at these specific defects. That time has not arrived. In general, certain approaches such as limiting calories and increasing physical activity, as well as BG-lowering and insulin-sensitizing drugs, seem to help the majority of people with type 2 diabetes, so until more is known, we'll have to stick with that. Diet and exercise aren't fun, but they work.

IN A SENTENCE:

■ *The relative amounts of insulin and glucagon in your bloodstream tell the body whether it should store energy as glycogen and fat (high insulin levels) or break down glycogen and fat to produce energy (low insulin levels).*

living

Eating Out and Traveling

If you need to eat out or travel for business, you've already had to deal with how to handle the difficulties that can arise when you're trying to stick to your diet plan in restaurants or even foreign countries where you may not be familiar with the food. If not, you may have put off facing the extra challenges of travel, or even just dining out at a local restaurant.

I've always loved to try new foods at ethnic restaurants that serve dishes I've never heard of. In fact, one of my main social outlets had always been meeting friends at interesting new restaurants and sampling their fare. With my restricted diet, however, I couldn't eat most of the food at these places, and because I loved it so much, I didn't want to be tempted. Easier to stay home. It was almost three years after my diagnosis before I trusted myself enough to go on a simple two-day trip to Canada.

Once you get over this initial hurdle of dealing with temptations, whether it's the week after you're diagnosed or several years, you'll find that traveling isn't that difficult if you do a little planning ahead.

Eating well when eating out takes practice

Unless you're just planning a trip to visit Auntie Em, traveling involves a lot of eating in restaurants, a sort of crash course in all the problems you face when eating out at home. I discussed some of these in Day 7. When you're traveling, however, you'll have to depend on others for all your meals. In foreign countries, choosing suitable meals can be even more daunting.

Thus it's probably not a good idea to take a five-week, twenty-one-city European bus tour before you've mastered the art of dining out at home. Start small and work up. Get used to finding things you can eat at restaurants in your own city, learning to ask about ingredients and asking for substitutions. Then try a weekend trip somewhere nearby. Then maybe you're ready to try the Big Leagues.

Don't be afraid to call ahead and ask if the hotel or bed-and-breakfast can accommodate your diet, whatever it is. If not, you might want to try another. When I did this on my Canadian trip, it turned out the innkeeper's father had type 2 diabetes, so she was very sympathetic and cooked me eggs for breakfast instead of the bread pudding and maple syrup she served to everyone else.

If you're traveling with other people, don't be afraid to be assertive. You don't want to deprive your traveling companions of the pleasures of trying interesting restaurants just because they're not ideal for you. But you also shouldn't have to go to bed hungry. If you're not on a tour but are traveling with another person, you could try alternating restaurant choices. "You pick the place for lunch, and I'll pick the place for dinner." That way you'll get at least one meal a day that will fill you up. Or buy food you can eat and bring it with you to restaurants that are going to be totally unsuitable for your diet.

If you're on a tour that includes all your meals, you'll have to check with the tour sponsors before you sign up to see whether they'll be able to accommodate your diet. If you're taking a sulfonylurea or insulin and need to eat at certain times to avoid going low, ask the tour sponsors before you sign up if meals will be regular. But try not to ruin things for everyone else by insisting that you all leave an interesting site before the others are ready just so you can reach the restaurant at the dot of noon. **Carry snacks with you at all times to deal with situations like that.**

Cruises usually have such a vast array of food that you should be able to find something you can eat no matter what kind of diet you're on. The problem will more likely be temptation from too much delicious food being offered too often than a lack of anything you can eat.

Planning ahead is important

Traveling with diabetes, like traveling without diabetes, is best done with a little advance planning. You need to plan for your health care as well as your itinerary. If you're going abroad, you need to do a little more.

The amount of extra planning you'll need depends on how you're controlling your diabetes. If you're controlling well with diet and exercise and you never have problems with low blood sugar, then you won't need to make quite as many extra plans as you would if you were using insulin and also might need to have other medications changed sometime during the trip.

Since 9/11, as we all know, security measures for travelers have not only increased but keep changing depending on the level of alert against possible terrorist attacks. So the regulations today may be different from what you'll find next year or next week. If you use insulin, the best approach when you're planning to travel by air is to telephone the airline well before your departure to find out exactly what you'll need to take in order to prove that it's OK for you to carry syringes on board, if asked. Then telephone again shortly before you leave just to make sure the regulations haven't changed.

Sometimes customer service people give incorrect information on the telephone, and you have no proof that they've done so. Hence, it's a good idea to telephone at least twice, at different times, when you'll likely speak with two different people. If they both say the same thing, it's probably true.

If you're going abroad, one of the first things you should do is to make an appointment with your doctor. The doctor may know if you need any special immunizations for the trip and if there are any special conditions in the countries you're planning to visit that would affect your diabetes. Otherwise, you can contact the International Association for Medical Assistance to Travellers (IAMAT) (716-754-4883). You have to join to use its services, but membership is free, and the association can provide a lot of useful information.

If you'll be crossing borders, it's important to ask your doctor for a letter, preferably in duplicate, explaining that you are diabetic and noting the medications you need, listed by their generic names. Also get prescriptions for the drugs. Guard the prescriptions as closely as you guard your passport. The letter is just in case a customs official asks about the drugs or syringes you are carrying. The list of drugs and prescriptions is in case you need hospitalization or run out of a drug or lose it. The trade names in foreign countries may be different, so it's important that the generic names be used. Keep your medications in their original containers, if possible.

If you don't already have one, this would be a good time to get a diabetic identification bracelet just in case you need medical care and can't communicate your condition because of language problems or you're unconscious.

You may also want to get from IAMAT a list of doctors in the countries you're visiting who speak English. If you didn't do this ahead of time and you're in Europe, you can call the International Diabetes Federation in Brussels (32-2/538 55 11) or ask at an American embassy.

Find out from your health insurance company whether or not hospitalizations are covered in the countries you're going to. If not, make plans for some kind of temporary foreign coverage just in case.

If you're going to a non-English-speaking country, it's a good idea to memorize a few phrases before you leave, for example, "I have diabetes," and "Please give me some sugar," and "I need a doctor." Write the phrases down and keep them in your wallet in case you go low and forget how to pronounce them.

Take extra supplies

Make a list of all the medications and blood glucose (BG) testing supplies you would normally use during the period of the trip. Take twice as many as you expect to use. Pack half in a carry-on bag with one copy of the prescriptions and letters from the doctor and put the other half in a purse or a baggy jacket. The duplication is so you'll have a backup if one of the items is lost, stolen, or damaged. Don't put your meters or any drugs in your checked-in luggage. The temperature of the baggage compartment can get extremely low; insulin could freeze, and meters and strips might get damaged. However, none of the meters are supposed to be affected by the X-rays used to check your luggage at the airport.

At the other extreme, if you're going to a tropical country and will be staying in places that have no air-conditioning, you should make some kind of plans for how you're going to ensure your meter is accurate (call the manufacturer for advice) and keep your strips or insulin from degrading. There are insulated packs designed to protect insulin from high temperatures. Remember not to keep meters or medications in a hot car.

If you have problems with hypoglycemia, make sure you have a good supply of glucose tablets and keep them with you at all times. Don't pack them in your luggage where you can't get them if the plane is delayed or your baggage is sent to Sierra Leone by mistake.

Take a supply of sugar-free medications for nausea and diarrhea in case they're not readily available where you're going. Both conditions are common when you're traveling, eating different foods, and drinking water with different mineral contents. If such illness does strike, remember to check your BG levels frequently, as dehydration can cause serious problems, as described in Month 2.

Remember to take extra batteries for your meter. Some people take BG strips that are read visually as a backup in case the meter breaks. If you use urine-testing strips, of course you'll need to take those as well. A box of glucose-testing strips for testing the sugar in drinks and food would be a good idea, especially when you're eating food you're not familiar with.

Take snacks to use en route

If you're traveling by air, you should bring something to eat if the flight is more than a few hours. Airlines today are apt to offer no food except crackers or nuts on domestic flights. If you're going abroad, you can usually get diabetic meals if you order them at least twenty-four hours in advance of the scheduled departure time. But be aware that the airline's definition of a "diabetic meal" might be quite different from yours. Some people with diabetes are following a high-carbohydrate and others a low-carbohydrate diet, and you can't expect the airlines to know what you want. You can try calling ahead and asking what kinds of special meals will be available and choosing one that sounds as if it would match your diet. One traveler finds that special Asian vegetarian meals tend to have the low-glycemic-index foods that are on his diet. Another recommends low-sodium meals, which tend to include fresh fruit and vegetables. Some people find they're better off just getting the regular meal and picking out the things they can eat.

No matter what kind of diet you're on, it's safer if you carry a lot of snacks as well. Meals may be delayed, or you may find there's almost nothing you can eat. Airport food tends to be fast food—greasy, starchy, and relatively expensive.

The same problems apply to train or bus travel. When possible, carry picnic meals and snacks with you, as the offerings on the train or at the bus terminals will probably be limited. Remember to use glucose test strips to check the sugar content of sodas unless they are served in the bottle.

Changing time zones may be a problem for people taking insulin. When you're flying from the West Coast to the East, you lose three hours. When you go from the East to the West, you gain three hours. With longer distances, the gains and losses are obviously greater. With oral drugs, this shouldn't be a big problem. Just take your next dose at the usual time. With insulin, check with your doctor before you leave to see how to adjust your doses.

Check your blood glucose levels often

Remember that your activity level affects your BG levels. If you normally walk for two hours after lunch but you've chosen to travel Europe by rail, or a twelve-city bus tour, your BG levels may be higher than usual. On the other hand, if you usually spend all day at an office job and you're walking from one museum to another, your BG levels may be lower than they normally are, and you can probably add a few treats to your menu.

Remember that stress makes BG levels go up, and happy stress such as excitement about a trip might affect your BG levels. So test more often than usual to see how the vacation is affecting you.

Take care of your feet

If you *do* plan to do a lot of walking during the trip, take along two pairs of well-broken-in shoes and alternate them to make sure you don't get blisters on the trip. This would be a good time to try some padded socks, or the special nonblister kind, even if you don't have any signs of neuropathy. You don't want to ruin a nice vacation with blisters.

Eating abroad may be challenging

Eating in restaurants abroad will have the extra challenge that you may not know the ingredients of various dishes. As when you're home, don't be afraid to ask. And if you can't eat part of the meal, ask if they can make substitutions.

If in doubt, go ahead and try a new food if you like adventurous eating, especially if you're normally in pretty good control. *Just control your portion sizes.* Part of the fun of traveling is trying new foods, and going a little high after a meal won't kill you as long as it's not your regular way of life. If you're embarrassed about asking for a doggie bag in a foreign country, where it might not be the custom, you can carry sealable plastic bags in your pocket or purse and squirrel away part of the meal inconspicuously. If you find you are *too* high after a mystery dish, do some extra walking to get your BG levels down.

If you're controlling with a low-carbohydrate diet and planning a trip to a country like China, where rice and noodles and sugared sauces will probably play a large part in most of the meals, you might think about learning how to use insulin, or one of the fast-acting insulin-releasing drugs that you take before meals, so you can enjoy some of these delicious high-carbohydrate meals.

Of course you don't want to just get a prescription for insulin and set off for foreign climes. Practice before you go on the trip. That practice might come in handy at other times, for example, if you ever get a bad illness or need steroid drugs that make your BG levels go up so much that insulin is the best temporary remedy.

If you're controlling with a low-fat diet and going somewhere like the Mediterranean, where everything is likely to be drizzled with olive oil, you'll just have to ask them to hold the oil, or you'll have to pick and choose. But remember that unlike saturated fat, the monounsaturated fat in olive oil isn't detrimental to insulin resistance and lipid levels (see Learning section).

Have fun

Diabetes can be draining because there are no vacations from the disease. But you deserve a vacation for yourself. So take care of your diabetes when you're traveling, but don't let it be the focus of your trip. If you plan ahead, you're less likely to find yourself stranded in Rome while your suitcase containing your snacks and medications heads for Tierra del Fuego.

Plan ahead so you can enjoy yourself. Focus on seeing new sights, meeting new people, tasting new foods. Above all, have fun.

IN A SENTENCE:

▪ *Eating out and traveling require a little more planning when you have diabetes, but there's no reason to limit such activities.*

Metabolic Syndrome

Here's some good news. Being diagnosed with diabetes may have saved your life. What's that? How can getting a potentially lethal disease be good for your health?

The fact is, type 2 diabetes is strongly associated with cardiovascular problems. By now, you've probably heard a lot about the *microvascular* (small blood vessel) complications of diabetes such as neuropathy, retinopathy, and nephropathy—the Three O'Pathy Sisters I introduced in Day 6. These complications are, in fact, possible if you let your blood glucose (BG) levels stay high for many years.

The main problem is cardiovascular events

In type 2 diabetes, although you should never forget that these microvascular complications could occur if you let your BG levels stay high, they are actually less of a concern than the *macrovascular* (large blood vessel) complications of heart attack and stroke, which can be lumped together as *cardiovascular* events. Most people with type 2 diabetes eventually die from cardiovascular disease. If you have type 2 diabetes, your risk for these problems is two to four times that of a nondiabetic person. Add smoking into the equation, and it's even higher.

What causes the cardiovascular problems? No one is sure, but there is some evidence that these macrovascular complications are caused not by the high BG levels themselves but by the underlying insulin resistance (IR) that contributes to the high levels of glucose in the blood, and the majority of people with type 2 diabetes have some or a lot of IR.

There seems to be a constellation of symptoms that go along with IR. These include high insulin levels; excess visceral fat (fat around your internal abdominal organs; the "apple shape"); high blood pressure; high levels of triglycerides; low levels of **HDL** (*high-density lipoprotein*); normal or only slightly elevated levels of **LDL** (*low-density lipoprotein*); high levels of **small, dense LDL**; and impaired glucose tolerance. This has been called **metabolic syndrome**, *insulin-resistance syndrome*, or *Syndrome X*. Many of these same symptoms are found in women with *polycystic ovary syndrome* (see Month 2), which is also associated with IR.

All these symptoms are *associated* with increased risks of cardiovascular events. This doesn't necessarily mean that all or any of them actually cause the cardiovascular problems. It just means that having the symptoms of metabolic syndrome greatly increases your risk of having cardiovascular problems.

The effect of hyperinsulinemia is controversial

One of the most controversial aspects of metabolic syndrome, and type 2 diabetes, is the role of *hyperinsulinemia* (high insulin levels in the blood) as a factor in causing heart disease. Some people say that the high insulin levels themselves are the *cause* of the cardiovascular problems. Some studies have shown that the only factor able to predict heart attacks in a group of people was their insulin levels. These studies are often cited by people promoting insulin-lowering dietary approaches.

However, it's also possible that it's not the high insulin levels themselves but the underlying IR that is in fact the cause of the cardiovascular problems. After all, if you have a lot of IR and your beta cells are able to increase their output, your insulin levels will rise to overcome the IR.

Another possibility is that another, as yet unknown, problem is causing both the IR (with its accompanying high insulin levels) and the cardiovascular problems. In this case they would simply be found together, but neither one would cause the other.

These questions have not yet been answered. What we do know is that metabolic syndrome is associated with a high risk of heart disease.

Heart Health Acronyms and Other Terms

When you read about heart health, you'll usually come across a passel of acronyms labeling all the different kinds of fats that are important for maintaining the health of your heart. The following are some of the most important acronyms and other terms that you need to know to understand heart disease and how to prevent it.

Cardiovascular. This is a general term referring to all kinds of issues involving your heart (*cardio*) or your blood vessels (*vascular*). Cardiovascular problems could include clogged arteries in your heart (leading to *heart attacks*), clogged or weakened arteries in your brain (leading to *strokes*), and clogged arteries in your legs and arms (**peripheral vascular disease**).

Cardiovascular event. This means an "incident" involving the cardiovascular system, for example, a heart attack or a stroke.

Arteriosclerosis and atherosclerosis. *Arteriosclerosis* means thickening and stiffening of arteries, regardless of the cause. It is popularly called "hardening of the arteries." *Atherosclerosis* is a more specific term referring to thickening of arteries as a result of plaques.

Lipid. *Lipids* are all types of molecules that don't dissolve in water and include *fats* (triglycerides), *steroids*, and *waxes*. When speaking of heart health, the most important lipids are the *triglycerides* and *cholesterol*, and when people refer to your *lipid levels*, they usually mean both these types. They don't care about your testosterone levels or how much wax you have in your ears.

Cholesterol. *Cholesterol* is a type of lipid that is chemically very different from triglycerides. Along with triglycerides, cholesterol is an important building block for cell membranes, and it is also the starting point for building important hormones, including *estrogen* and *testosterone*. Thus some cholesterol is essential for your body. If you don't eat enough cholesterol, your body will make it. What you want is for the cholesterol to be taken up by the cells that need it, rather than having a lot floating around in your bloodstream.

Plaque. A *plaque* is a deposit of cholesterol and other substances underneath the artery wall. It can grow and grow until it blocks the flow of blood in the artery. Also, a protruding plaque can trigger the formation of clots. With time, a plaque can take up calcium from the blood. Plaques can make the arteries stiff.

Lipoprotein. This means a particle that contains both fat (*lipo*) and protein. Cholesterol can't travel around in the bloodstream by itself because, like other lipids, it

(continues)

Heart Health Acronyms
and Other Terms

isn't soluble in water, and the blood is mostly water. So the cholesterol and other lipids hitch a ride inside particles that have protein on the outside. The protein is soluble in water, and the cholesterol and triglycerides are hidden inside.

Chylomicrons. The *chylomicrons* are the lipoproteins that transport the fats and cholesterol you eat from your intestine through the lymph to the bloodstream. Then the fatty acids can be dropped off at tissues that need fat for energy, taken to the liver for further processing, or taken to the fat cells to be stored.

HDL. This stands for *high-density lipoprotein*. It's supposed to be the good kind of cholesterol. I always got it confused with LDL until I started thinking of HDL as *Happy cholesterol*. Just to make things more confusing, there are also subfractions of HDL called *HDL2* and *HDL3*. HDL2 is supposed to be the best kind of HDL, and it's increased by exercise. Red wine seems to increase HDL3 levels. No one is sure if that's beneficial or not. Some people use the term *HDL-C*, meaning HDL-cholesterol. It means essentially the same as just plain HDL.

If you've ever wondered why it's called *high density*, it's because HDL contains less lipid, which floats on the top of water, than other lipid fractions. So when you spin down a solution in a centrifuge, the HDL ends up closer to the bottom of the tube.

LDL. This stands for *low-density lipoprotein*. This is the bad stuff. You can remember it by thinking of *Lousy cholesterol*. LDL, and especially *oxidized* and *glycated* LDL, contributes to the formation of *atherogenic plaques*, the deposits of lipids and other material in the arterial wall that lead to heart attacks and strokes. Again, LDL-C means essentially the same thing as LDL. As you can infer from the description of HDL, LDL contains more lipid and floats above HDL when centrifuged.

It is expensive to measure LDL directly, so many labs estimate the value using the formula LDL = total cholesterol − (HDL + TG/5), where TG is triglycerides.

VLDL. This stands for **very low density lipoprotein**. This contains a lot of triglycerides surrounded by protein and is the way the liver ships triglycerides out to the rest of the body to be burned for energy. When the VLDL drops off its triglycerides to the cells, it picks up cholesterol and turns into LDL.

Small, dense LDL. This is LDL that is in much smaller particles than usual. It is the worst kind of LDL we know of (so far). You can think of it as *Specially Damaging Lousy cholesterol*. Because the particles are small, they are thought to be able to get into the arterial walls more easily, starting the formation of plaques. Unfortunately, people with diabetes tend to have high levels of small, dense LDL.

Light, fluffy HDL and LDL. Some people have a form of HDL and LDL that is less dense, or lighter and "fluffier," than the average HDL and LDL. These lighter lipoproteins have been associated with longevity in an Ashkenazic Jewish population in New York City. Many of their children also have the light forms of the lipoproteins, suggesting that the characteristic (as well as longevity) is inherited.

Triglycerides. *Triglycerides* are fats. They consist of long chains of *fatty acids* (see Day 3) attached to a molecule of *glycerol* (see Day 3). They are often referred to as *TGs*. Some people call them *triacylglycerol (TAG)*. There are different kinds of fats, some more harmful than others.

Unsaturated fats. *Unsaturated fats* contain one (*monounsaturated fats*) or more (*polyunsaturated fats*) double bonds. Unsaturated fats are "kinky," and they can't pack closely together in cell membranes. They are usually liquid at room temperature.

Double bonds are chemically reactive, and unsaturated fats can be oxidized more easily than saturated fats. This is especially true of the polyunsaturated fats. When fats are oxidized, the popular term is *rancid*. Most plant oils contain lots of antioxidants, but they may be removed during the refining process. Olive oil contains an especially high level of antioxidants.

Monounsaturated fats aren't supposed to change cholesterol levels. Polyunsaturated fats decrease total cholesterol levels, but this decrease often includes the beneficial HDL as well as the LDL, and the ratio of the two may remain constant.

Monounsaturated fats are found in olive and canola oils, nuts, avocado, fish, chicken, and wild meats such as venison and kangaroo. Polyunsaturated fats are found in most vegetable oils and some nuts.

Saturated fats. *Saturated fats* have no double bonds, so they're less susceptible to oxidation. They are usually solid at room temperature.

Saturated fats are straight chains and can pack very tightly in membranes. Some people think that tightly packed cell membranes don't work as well as they should, but this is only a theory. A diet high in saturated fat can increase LDL cholesterol levels and cause IR.

Saturated fats are found in meat, dairy foods, and tropical oils such as coconut oil, palm oil, and cocoa butter. The saturated fats in some tropical oils have shorter chains, and some people say they're more apt to be burned for energy and hence are less dangerous than longer-chain fatty acids.

Trans fats. *Trans fats* are formed when chemists take polyunsaturated fats and partially saturate them with hydrogen gas. In this way they can turn polyunsaturated vegetable oils, which are liquid at room temperature, into partially saturated

(continues)

Heart Health Acronyms
and Other Terms

(continued)

fats, which are solid at room temperature and have been used for margarine and vegetable shortening.

During the chemical saturation process, some of the kinky polyunsaturated fats are turned into straight rods that pack tightly into membranes just like saturated fats, and some people think that trans fats are even worse for your health than saturated fats.

Small amounts of natural trans fats are found naturally in meat and milk. Certain natural trans fats that contain kinked double bonds elsewhere in the molecule, for example, conjugated linolenic acid (CLA), seem to be beneficial.

Chemically produced trans fats are contained in products that list *partially hydrogenated vegetable oils* in the ingredients list and are often found in cookies, crackers, solid margarine, and some salad dressings.

Apolipoprotein. *Lipoprotein* refers to the whole particle. *Apolipoprotein* means just the protein part of the lipoprotein. The prefix *apo* comes from the Greek "separated from." There are many different types of apolipoproteins. For example, apolipoprotein A (often called just *apoA*) is associated with HDL, and apolipoprotein B (apoB) is associated with LDL. Sometimes people call the apolipoproteins just apoprotein.

Lipoprotein(a). Just to make things more confusing, there's a special kind of LDL called *lipoprotein(a)*, or just *Lp(a)*. This LDL is attached to an extra glycoprotein (a protein containing some sugar) called *apolipoprotein(a)*. It's not the same as apolipoprotein A, which is associated with HDL. The amount of Lp(a) seems to depend primarily on your genetic background, although trans fats may increase it, and high levels are associated with increased cardiovascular risk.

Diabetes is an early warning sign

Metabolic syndrome sounds a lot like diabetes without the high BG levels. The difference is how much insulin your pancreas is able to produce. Imagine a bunch of people with metabolic syndrome, all at high risk for heart disease. A few of them will have diabetes genes that won't let their pancreas keep churning out insulin to overcome the IR that is part of the syndrome. Those people's BG levels will continue to rise until they're diagnosed with diabetes.

The rest of the group are "blessed" with strong pancreases that can keep cranking out more and more insulin. They can get quite obese, will never develop high BG levels no matter how much cotton candy they eat, and won't become diabetic. But they'll be just as much at risk for cardiovascular problems. Because they're not diabetic, they may not realize there's any problem until it's too late.

Having IR without getting diabetes can lead to heart attacks and strokes without the early warning sign of high BG levels. Being diagnosed with type 2 diabetes is thus in some ways a blessing. In most cases it warns you that you've probably got IR and gives you a chance to modify your diet and lifestyle before it's too late.

Keeping your BG levels low will help, but normal BG levels don't reduce the risks of macrovascular complications as much as they reduce risks of the microvascular complications of damage to the nerves, kidneys, and eyes. However, lower BG levels do matter. Even in people who are not technically diabetic, those with the lowest average BG levels have the fewest cardiovascular events. Postprandial BG levels may be more important than fasting levels. And some recent studies have suggested that *fluctuating* BG levels—going very high after meals and then coming down again—may be even riskier than sustained high BG levels in terms of oxidative stress, which is a risk factor for heart disease.

But there are other risk factors for heart disease in addition to high BG levels. Thus in addition to working on BG control, if you know or are pretty sure that you have IR (you can estimate this with a C-peptide test; see Day 5), you need to focus attention on the other aspects of metabolic syndrome—blood pressure, lipid levels, and trying to eliminate that apple shape.

Inflammation may play a large role

There is growing evidence that a chronic state of *inflammation* in the body may play a large role in cardiovascular disease. When you have an infection, your body produces an inflammatory attack against the invader. This involves specialized white blood cells as well as a barrage of chemicals that attempt to fight off the infection.

It is this inflammatory attack that causes the redness and swelling at the site of an infection. In such a case, inflammation is a good thing. It helps you to overcome the infection. When you are fighting infection, the levels of **C-reactive protein (CRP)** become increased, and testing for CRP gives an indication of this inflammation.

However, when, for reasons no one fully understands, your body becomes chronically inflamed, this is not a good thing, and it may contribute to cardiovascular problems.

With chronic inflammation, your CRP levels aren't usually elevated enough to show on the standard CRP test. However, recently a *high-sensitivity CRP (hs-CRP) test* has become available and may indicate that you're at higher risk of cardiovascular events.

Dietary recommendations are controversial

People with high lipid levels are often put on the American Heart Association (**AHA**) low-fat, high-carbohydrate diet. However, some think this is not the best diet for people with metabolic syndrome. If you have metabolic syndrome, you probably have high triglyceride levels, and high-carbohydrate diets often increase triglyceride levels even more.

In addition, it has been found that people with metabolic syndrome or type 2 diabetes often have high levels of the dangerous small, dense LDL particles. Low-fat, high-carbohydrate diets usually do reduce the total LDL levels, but they seem to produce even more of the small, dense LDL particles that may be more dangerous than the total amount of LDL.

Thus some think that low-fat, high-carbohydrate diets, although they may be beneficial for people who have no IR, actually increase the risk of heart disease in those who have metabolic syndrome. They recommend that anyone with metabolic syndrome eat less carbohydrate than the AHA diet recommends and substitute monounsaturated fat instead. Monounsaturated fat is the kind found in olive oil, avocado, and nuts. Unlike saturated fat, it seems not to increase IR or LDL levels.

Not everyone with type 2 diabetes has all the symptoms associated with metabolic syndrome. As usual, YMMV (Your Mileage May Vary). But if you do, make sure the treatment chosen to treat your high BG levels doesn't make your risk factors for heart disease even worse. And maybe you should thank your wimpy pancreas for giving you this early warning sign. Forewarned is forearmed. Take action now, and you should have years of healthy living ahead.

IN A SENTENCE:

■ *Insulin resistance can cause cardiovascular problems even without high blood glucose levels.*

Half-Year M I L E S T O N E

You're now halfway through your first year. You understand the basics of diabetes care and you're beginning to understand the more subtle and controversial aspects of diabetes and its control:

- You know there are many different types of diabetes.

- You've learned that supplementing with vitamins, minerals, and herbs is controversial.

- Your understanding of testing procedures and the physiology of diabetes is becoming sophisticated.

- You know that you must pay attention to your cardiovascular health as well as your blood glucose levels.

- You know you also need to enjoy life, and you're becoming confident enough about your diet to enjoy eating out and traveling.

As you enter the last half of the year, you understand that this learning process will always continue, but when you find a treatment and diet that work for you, your diabetes will gradually cease to be the focus of your life. In the coming months, you'll learn:

- The relation between weight loss and blood glucose control.

- How to evaluate various diets and find the one that works for you.

- How to calculate your personal glycemic index values.

- More sophisticated diabetes physiology, including the effects of exercise and the causes of type 2 diabetes.

- Where to go to continue this learning process.

living

Taking Stock

You've been dealing with diabetes for half a year, and some of the patterns of your diabetes care should be almost routine by now, although not all. There are still hurdles ahead, maybe your first Christmas on a diabetic diet if you were diagnosed in the spring, or your first summer vacation trip on a diabetic routine if you were diagnosed in the fall.

No one is perfect, and everyone slips off the wagon every now and then. Don't despair. If you *were* perfect, all your friends would hate you. So just pick yourself up and climb back on the wagon. It's your *overall* control that will matter in the long term, and 90 percent is so much better than no control at all.

Now might be a good time to sit back and reevaluate where you are, how far you've come, and where you want to go in the future. You should have had at least a couple of A1c tests by now, as well as a general idea of what your blood glucose (BG) levels are at different times of the day and after different activities like walking or watching TV.

Is your diet working?

The two most important things for type 2 diabetes are diet and exercise, so that's a good place to begin. If you need to lose weight, is your diet helping you to do that? Are you losing weight as fast as you expected to lose? How about your BG levels? Is your diet keeping them under control before meals? How about after meals? Recent studies have emphasized the importance of postprandial BG levels in your overall control.

If you aren't satisfied with the answers to any of these questions, this would be a good time to schedule another meeting with a dietician, unless you're the independent type who enjoys tinkering with diet on your own. If you started out on the American Diabetes Association exchange diet and you find that your overall control is just barely OK and your BG levels have been going high after meals, maybe you should consider trying a low-glycemic-index diet or a low-carbohydrate diet instead.

Before you *do* change your diet, it's ideal if you can get a lipid panel (see the discussion of lipids in Month 6) and an A1c test done. Then after you've been on the new diet for about three months, you can test again to see if there are any changes in your lipid levels or average BG levels as suggested by the A1c. Labs can test for many other factors in your blood, most of which won't be affected by diet. Before you start the new diet, ask your doctor if you should have any other blood tests done.

Are you exercising?

Now take a look at your exercise program. There's no point in having a fancy exercise program worked out if you never bother to follow it. If you're like me, you'll probably use every excuse under the sun to put it off. It's too hot. It's too cold. It's too rainy. It's too dry. I just bruised my rib. I've got the flu. I have to visit a sick friend. My library books are due.

When I find something I enjoy doing, I can somehow find the time even if the weather is a tad too hot or too cold or too wet or too dry. So if you've found some way of exercising that you enjoy enough that you actually do it, you're in real luck. Just keep it up.

But if you're honest with yourself and admit you've been putting the exercise on the back burner, now is the time to sit down and figure out why it is you don't enjoy it. Would it help if you found some other people to join you in your daily efforts to get moving? Maybe you could find a friend who could benefit from more walking, and you could think of it as helping a friend instead of a dreaded chore for you. Or maybe you could offer to rake leaves or do other calorie-burning chores for elderly people who could use the help.

Would it help if you found some new sport to learn or some team sport to join? Would treating yourself to a brand-new portable CD player inspire you to take a walk every day while you were listening to CDs?

Go to the library and browse around in the sporting section. Maybe there's some obscure sport you've never heard about that you could try and then introduce to all your friends. One woman took up belly dancing. Or would it help if you dumped the dreaded term *exercise*? Instead of staying inside to "exercise," tell yourself you're going out to "play" or "dance" or whatever it is that sounds like fun to you—and then do it.

Is your medication the best for you?

This might also be a good time to get together with your doctor and discuss your medications, if you're taking any. If your control is good, there's no reason to change. But if it could be better, maybe another drug or another combination of drugs would work better for you. By now you should have a good idea whether your main problem is high BG levels after meals, high BG levels in the morning, or high BG levels throughout the day. Different drugs treat different aspects of BG control, as described in Week 3. You may want to review how the drugs work so you can have a productive discussion about the options with your doctor.

Is your health-care team working with you?

You may also want to think about your diabetes "team," the medical professionals who are helping you achieve your control. Are you happy with them? Are they good listeners? Are they willing to take the time to explain things to you and pay attention to your concerns about your diabetes, or do they just rush you out the door as soon as possible after writing a prescription? Are they willing to accept A1c levels of 8 or 9 as "the best you can do," or will they try to work with you to bring those numbers down?

If you want to test a lot, do they tell you you're being compulsive? Do they say, "Once a week is fine for a type 2"?

If you work hard to get your BG levels close to normal and ask your doctor for help getting them down even further, into the normal range, are you brushed off with a comment like, "Oh, you're doing fine. I have patients who'd give their right arm for BGs like yours" and then told to come back next year while they spend more time with the really "sick" patients?

On the other hand, if you're not doing as well as they think you should, are your health-care providers trying to put the blame on you, by labeling you as *noncompliant* instead of considering that maybe the most popular drugs or diets aren't the correct ones for you?

Unfortunately, this labeling is not uncommon. Barbara F. had seen a dietician who told her to eat a lot of carbohydrate, even suggesting that she put raisins in her morning oatmeal to "get those carbs up." This didn't work for Barbara. Her BG levels, which were not terribly high when she was diagnosed, kept going up and up. But instead of considering that maybe the diet wasn't working, the dietician assumed that Barbara was noncompliant and blamed her. "After two weeks of eating the exact diet from their booklet," said Barbara, "my BGs were up, and I was told I really had to take my condition seriously and follow the diet. That's when I started testing after meals instead of before and discovered how high BGs were after eating all those carbs."

When Alex E. was diagnosed with type 2 diabetes, he asked his doctor if he should get a meter and test his BG levels. "She laughed disparagingly and said, 'Sure, an occasional test wouldn't hurt anything.' That's when I realized she didn't know how to treat diabetes, so I fired her on the spot." Some doctors accuse type 2 patients of being compulsive if they measure their BG levels a lot.

If you find that your health-care people patronize you like Alex's doctor, don't respect you as an intelligent human being, or blame you for "non-compliance" when a particular treatment doesn't work as Barbara's dietician did, don't waste your time seeing them again, if you possibly can.

Look around. Connect with other people who have diabetes and ask for recommendations. If there's a choice of potential doctors who are accepting new patients, ask for an appointment to interview them before you sign up for their care.

Explain that you want to understand your diabetes and what is being done to control it and want to be a partner in making decisions about your control. Ask if they're comfortable with this kind of approach. Ask how they feel about various drugs and diets used to control diabetes and make sure their views are compatible with yours. For example, if you want to try a low-carbohydrate diet and they tell you high-carbohydrate diets are the only way to go, or vice versa, you may not be able to work well together. If you want to try some insulin and they see insulin as a last resort for someone with type 2 diabetes, keep looking.

Remember, you're chairman of the board. You are hiring people to help you. You need these people. They know things that you haven't learned yet. But if you don't think they're doing the job you want them to do, don't hesitate to find someone else. There are some wonderful, caring doctors, dieticians, exercise therapists, certified diabetes educators, and ophthalmologists out there. You just have to find the ones that are the best for you.

IN A SENTENCE:

■ *Take stock of your diabetes treatment program and see if you need to make any changes.*

What Causes Diabetes?

Once you've been diagnosed with diabetes, it doesn't really make much difference what caused it. It's too late to go back and change.

Some medical people will tell you not to waste your time worrying about what caused your diabetes or what your C-peptide levels are or which variety of type 2 diabetes you may have. They're mostly interested in how to treat your diabetes and may treat different types the same, focusing on the A1c.

Of course keeping blood glucose (BG) levels down is just about the most important thing you can do to ensure a long and complication-free life. But if you're reading this, you're probably curious about your disease as well. You may want to know why you got diabetes and your overweight brother didn't or why your best friend can subsist on chips and doughnuts and never weigh more than 120 pounds when you just look at a pat of butter and you can feel your stomach expanding.

Both genes and environment are important

The cause of type 2 diabetes, as well as the cause of insulin resistance (IR), is not yet completely understood. What scientists do know is that for type 2 diabetes to develop, there are usually two requirements. First, your beta cells must have a genetic defect that makes them unable to cope with excessive demands for insulin. In other words, the first cause is genetic: not choosing your parents carefully. When one of a pair of identical twins gets type 2 diabetes, the probability of the other one getting it too has been reported to be 60 to almost 100 percent, depending on the study. A 2011 study found at least thirty-six gene variations linked with type 2 diabetes. Unexpectedly, most of these genes concerned beta cell function rather than IR. Many of the gene variations were common, but each one had a small effect. In other words, you'd need variations in many genes before your diabetes risk became significant. This is one reason it's so difficult to determine the genetic risk for type 2 diabetes.

The second requirement is that you must have conditions that require these excessive demands for insulin, especially when they persist for long periods of time. These conditions might include the IR associated with obesity; stress-induced IR caused by surgery, infection, certain drugs, or pregnancy; or many years eating more calories than you need, including a lot of saturated fat and high levels of processed "fast" carbohydrates that quickly dump a big load of glucose into your bloodstream. In other words, the second cause is environmental.

Under low-stress conditions such as a moderate or low caloric intake; a diet in which the carbohydrate is mostly unprocessed, with a lot of fiber, and the saturated fat intake is not excessive; lots of physical work that burns off the carbohydrates that are eaten; and no stress-induced IR, genetically "weak" beta cells may function just fine, and a person will never get diabetes.

Conversely, a person born with "strong" beta cells can undergo all these stressful conditions and just crank out more and more insulin to overcome them. Cranking out a lot of insulin is not necessarily a good thing, as discussed in Month 6. But such people will never develop high BG levels.

The Pima story illustrates environmental effects

The Pima Indians in Arizona, who have one of the highest rates of type 2 diabetes in the world (closely followed by the Sunni Arabs in Bahrain), and their close relatives in Mexico, who have low rates of type 2 diabetes, are often used to illustrate how environmental factors can influence the genes we are born with.

Arizona Pima Indians. Until the twentieth century, the Pima Indians in Arizona harvested wild plants and grew their own food in the harsh environment of the Sonoran Desert. They called themselves *Akimel*

O'odham, the "river people," and constructed a complex irrigation system to cultivate their crops. However, sometimes the irrigation systems failed, and periods of famine were not uncommon.

Their crops included wheat, tepary beans, cushaw squash, and Pima corn, which has a lower glycemic index than modern sweet corn. Other foods included acorns, cholla-cactus buds, honey mesquite, povertyweed, and prickly pears from the desert floor; mule deer, white-winged dove, and black-tailed jackrabbit; and squawfish from the Gila River. Thus their diet had foods that had very low glycemic index values and were high in fiber as well as low in fat.

The Pima Indians also expended a lot of energy in their farming and canal construction work and were lean, with diabetes almost unknown among them.

Then when whites moved West, they diverted the Gila River for their own farming enterprises, and the Pima Indians' way of life was destroyed. Starving, they were forced to accept government surplus food: lard, sugar, and white flour. In other words they ate high-glycemic-index, low-fiber, high-fat foods and had little physical activity to burn off the extra calories they took in. Today their diet is similar to that of other Americans. A favorite food is fry bread, made with white flour.

As a result, obesity became the norm and rates of diabetes soared. Today, more than 50 percent of the Arizaon Pima Indians have type 2 diabetes, which is appearing in younger and younger ages in children.

Some people feel that because of their periodic famines, the Pima Indians who survived were those with thrifty genes who were able to store fat easily in better times so they could survive the times of famine. Those genes served them well under those conditions. But with modern living and permanent plenty, the genes turned out to be a liability.

Mexican Pima Indians. The Arizona Pima Indians' close relatives in Maycoba, Mexico, who undoubtedly share those thrifty genes, have not yet abandoned their traditional lifestyles. They live in a harsh mountain environment where crops are difficult to grow, and they eat primarily beans, potatoes, and tortillas made from coarsely ground corn. They may have chicken once a month.

Interestingly, the Mexican Pima Indians actually take in more calories a day (about 2,200 calories) than their relatives in Arizona, but the Mexican Pima Indians also expend more energy with physical work. They lack modern transportation and still walk wherever they want to go. Often they run. They spend an average of more than twenty hours a week in hard or moderate physical labor, as opposed to the two hours a week spent by the average Pima Indian in Arizona. Most Americans have to be urged to exercise thirty minutes a day three times a week, or only 1.5 hours a week.

The Mexican Pima Indians almost surely have the same thrifty genes as their cousins in Arizona, but their lifestyle keeps diabetes at bay—at least for now. In the past twenty years, more grocery stores carrying processed foods have appeared in Maycoba, but economic limitations have kept the consumption of such foods low. In the future, they may face the same problems as the Arizona Pima.

Other ethnic groups that have recently changed from a lifestyle of lots of physical labor and little food to one of plentiful food and less activity are finding themselves in this situation. This often happens when rural residents move to a city. Rates of diabetes are soaring in these groups. Worldwide, high rates of diabetes are found among the Pima Indians (50 percent), Naurans (40 percent), Australian aborigines (25 percent), peninsular Arabs (25 percent), south Asians (20 percent), and West Africans (12 percent). For comparison, northern Europeans have a rate of 4 percent. In the United States, high rates are found among Native Americans, Hispanic Americans (rates in Cuban Americans are not as high), Arab Americans, African Americans, and Asian Americans. Populations with high rates of type 2 diabetes often have lower rates of type 1 diabetes than northern Europeans.

Many Americans of European descent follow a modern lifestyle that involves very little physical labor and a lot of processed foods, and they may gain weight, but they don't develop diabetes. They have the lifestyle but lack the genes.

No one knows if insulin resistance or beta cell defects come first

People who get type 2 diabetes usually show signs of both IR and defective production of insulin by the beta cells. As with the chicken and the egg, no one can yet agree on which usually comes first, the IR or the beta cell defects. Once you have diabetes, it doesn't really matter. Once the disease has progressed enough to be diagnosed, most people show signs of both.

There is no question that obesity, and especially what is called *visceral obesity*, is associated with IR. Visceral obesity means that there's a lot of fat around your viscera, or internal abdominal organs, and it usually means that your waist is a lot larger than your hips. Men who have "beer bellies" have visceral obesity. Another term for this is *apple shaped*. Women who have large thighs are called *pear shaped*, and this kind of overweight is associated with a lower risk of IR and diabetes.

There is also evidence that fat cells produce substances that cause IR. The hormone *resistin* seems to be such a substance. When mice get obese, the fat cells secrete resistin, which causes IR in other types of cells. The interesting thing is that the glitazone drugs, which reduce IR in humans, also inhibit the production of resistin in mice. Resistin exists in humans too, but its role in human type 2 diabetes is controversial.

Hormones secreted by fat cells are called **adipokines**. Some other adipokines are *leptin, adiponectin, tumor necrosis factor-alpha, chemerin, retinol-binding protein-4, 11-beta-hydroxysteroid dehydrogenase,* and *visfatin,* with more being discovered every year. Some of these have been discovered only recently. Don't think you need to learn all these names, but if you see them mentioned in news stories or journal articles, you'll know they're adipokines.

Adiponectin seems to be a "good adipokine" that reduces IR. Overweight people, people with diabetes, and people with heart disease have low levels of adiponectin, and treatment with the glitazone drugs results in increases in adiponectin levels along with reductions in IR.

Being overweight alone is not sufficient to cause diabetes. As mentioned before, people can be quite obese and have immense amounts of IR and their beta cells will just keep spewing out more and more insulin to keep the BG levels normal. Other people are quite obese but are very sensitive to insulin.

Nevertheless, the classic view is that obesity is the *cause* of type 2 diabetes—in other words, the IR comes before the beta cell failure. In this view, you eat too much and let yourself get overweight. The overweight causes IR. Because of the IR, the beta cells have to work a lot harder to put out extra insulin to cope. They are unable to keep up the pace, some of them become "exhausted" and die, and at that point the BG levels begin to increase and you are diagnosed with diabetes.

This view assumes that being overweight is caused by eating too much and not exercising enough and thus blames the patient for getting the disease. People with this viewpoint call type 2 diabetes a "lifestyle disease," implying that personal lifestyle choices caused your diabetes.

However, as one researcher said, "Nearly every major feature of this disease that we thought was true ten years ago turned out to be wrong." He was referring to the molecular mechanisms of the disease. But as understanding of the mechanisms at the molecular level changes, views of the causes of type 2 diabetes will undoubtedly change as well.

One possibility is that a genetically determined IR causes obesity when sufficient food is available. The obesity would increase the IR even more, and a vicious circle would ensue.

A second possibility is that an unknown factor causes both IR and obesity independently; in other words, neither one causes the other but they just go along together. This is analogous to drinking a lot of beer and becoming intoxicated and visiting the loo a lot. Intoxication doesn't cause you to visit the loo, and visiting the loo doesn't cause you to become intoxicated (at least it doesn't have that effect on me). A third factor, the beer, just happens to cause two different effects at once.

Studies in mice have shown that a high-calorie, high-fat, high-sugar diet causes IR in muscle before any weight gain; and studies in humans put on calorie-restricted diets have shown improvements in BG control before any weight loss. This suggests that the number of calories you eat affects both your weight and your BG control, but one doesn't cause the other.

Another possibility is that the beta cell failure comes before the IR. In this view, an inherited defect in the beta cells would make BG levels rise after meals long before anyone realized anything was wrong. The high BG levels after meals would cause glucotoxicity. The glucotoxicity would make the BG levels go even higher, and this would damage the beta cells even more. Another vicious circle would ensue.

A study in thin Japanese Americans has shown that their beta cells had a secretory defect *before* there was any increase in abdominal fat and before they were diagnosed with diabetes. Five years later, those with these beta cell defects had progressed to diabetes and had more abdominal fat.

Insulin is released in two phases

To understand beta cell defects, first you should understand what is called the *biphasic insulin response* (Figure 3). When a nondiabetic person eats, the cells almost instantly release a squirt of insulin into the bloodstream. This is called the *first-phase* or *phase-one response*, and it may be triggered just by tasting or chewing food. This insulin was probably already made by the beta cells and was sitting there in little packets waiting for a signal to be released. This short (usually about five to ten minutes) spurt of insulin is usually enough to keep the BG level from increasing a lot after the first bites of carbohydrate zip from the mouth to the bloodstream. The drugs nateglinide and the GLP-1 mimetics are said to restore this first-phase response, and the new inhaled insulin Afrezza, which peaks very quickly, is designed to mimic this response.

Then the beta cells produce a smaller but longer-lasting release of insulin called the *second-phase response*. This insulin release takes care of the rest of the carbohydrate from the meal, which is usually released over a period of time as the stomach slowly processes the food and releases it into the small intestine. The insulin release continues as long as the food keeps coming.

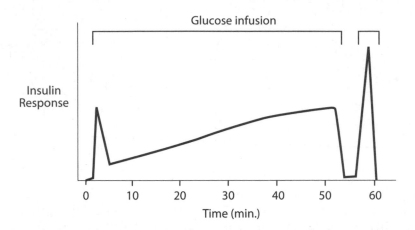

FIGURE 3. The two-stage insulin response. When you infuse glucose into the bloodstream, the beta cells produce a rapid burst of insulin that lasts about five to ten minutes. This is called the *phase-one response*. Then they produce a slow release of insulin (the *phase-two response*) that lasts as long as the glucose is given. If, after the first dose of glucose has been stopped, you give a second pulse of glucose, another phase-one insulin response occurs. Notice that this response is greater than the first one. This is called *priming* and means that a second carbohydrate meal may cause a smaller increase in the blood glucose (BG) level than the first one. People with type 2 diabetes lack the phase-one response.

People with type 2 diabetes usually lack the first-phase response. Furthermore, this lack of a first-phase response is sometimes found in nondiabetic relatives of people with type 2 diabetes, which suggests that the loss of proper beta cell function precedes the IR.

However, other researchers have also found IR in nondiabetic relatives of people with type 2 diabetes and say that the first-phase response is not lost until fasting BG levels reach about 140 mg/dL.

So the jury is still out on which comes first, the beta cell defects or the IR. One possibility is our old friend YMMV (Your Mileage May Vary). Some people may have lost beta cell function first and others may have acquired IR first. Regardless of the chronology, however, once the BG levels begin to increase, this increase is amplified by glucotoxicity.

Losing weight is difficult with thrifty genes

People who are overweight tend to have more fatty acids (see Day 3) in their blood whether they consume a lot of fat or not, and there is some evidence that fatty acids coming from the visceral (stomach) area into the liver are able to increase IR. This may be another reason visceral obesity is dangerous. Losing weight may help reduce lipotoxicity as well as IR and glucotoxicity and is therefore a good thing to try to do.

Unfortunately, losing weight is difficult when, like the Pima Indians, you have thrifty genes that tell your body it wants to store fat. Just remember, in most cases, *being overweight is not your fault*. You just got genes that would have been wonderful if you were living in a time of famine. In a time of plenty, they're a liability.

But those are the breaks. You've got those genes, and you can't give them back. So the only thing you can work on is controlling your environment, and that usually means losing some weight.

In a modern world filled with automobiles, convenience foods, and TVs, it's not realistic to expect anyone to adopt a lifestyle as rugged as that of the Pima Indians in Mexico. But the closer anyone who was born with the thrifty diabetes genes can come to that way of life, the less damaging the effects of those genes will be.

IN A SENTENCE:

■ *Type 2 diabetes is caused by an interaction between your thrifty genes and your food-filled environment and lack of strenuous exercise.*

living

Losing
Weight

When you were diagnosed, your doctor probably told you to lose weight and get some exercise. Sometimes that's all the doctor tells you.

The classic treatment is weight loss

Losing weight has always been a cornerstone of treatment of type 2 diabetes because being overweight increases your insulin resistance (IR). There is evidence that overfilled fat cells secrete substances that cause IR, for example, the hormone *resistin*. So if you have, in fact, managed to lose some weight, that's great. Your control will be easier because of it, and you may be able to keep your blood glucose (BG) levels down without oral drugs or insulin. But if you haven't lost weight, don't despair. Some people now think that controlling your BG levels is more important than losing weight.

You may have been told that if you would just lose ten or twenty pounds, your diabetes would go away. In some cases, especially if you're fortunate enough to be diagnosed in the very early stages of diabetes, when it's still just prediabetes (see Month 2), this may be true. Here's one success story:

"When I was diagnosed, I easily went over 180 postmeal," said Jim D. "But since I lost all the weight (ninety pounds) and exercise daily, my pancreas seems to have full control, again. I generally stay in a tight range, 80 to 95 mg/dL. Christmas dinner, I pigged out and also ate a half-dozen chocolate-chip cookies. I tracked my BGs, and the peak, at about 90 minutes, was 109, back to the 80s by 120 minutes."

Not always a cure. Otherwise, weight loss will reduce your IR somewhat and will make your diabetes easier to control, but it won't make it go away.

Kitty M. of Australia described her experiences: "When I was first diagnosed I read all I could, and losing weight and exercise seemed to offer the most promise of a cure, or at least regression/control. I lost 120 pounds on a low-glycemic-index diet and a lot of walking, and my fasting glucose fell from about 210 to 85 mg/dL. Most of the drop in blood glucose occurred shortly after I started walking regularly and losing weight.

"Five years later I still walk one to two hours a day, and my fasting blood glucose has remained about 85. I still get pronounced postprandial BG levels, and my hemoglobin A1c is slightly above normal, but I take no medication. A welcome side benefit was that my blood pressure returned to the normal range, and I was able to stop medication for that. The verdict: well controlled, but not cured."

One reason weight loss is not always curative is because once your beta cells bite the dust, they're not likely to come back to life. Some day scientists will figure out how to get the beta cells to multiply without causing uncontrolled multiplication (cancer), but we're not there yet. If you're diagnosed in the early stages, when your beta cells are still able to produce enough insulin to cope with normal demands but not enough to cope with the extra demands of IR or other stresses, then just reducing your IR may allow your still-vigorous beta cells to deal with the now-lower demands made on them.

If, however, you're not diagnosed until later in the course of the disease, or if you're diagnosed early but don't take the disease seriously and don't maintain good control, so glucotoxicity stresses the beta cells enough that many of them give up the ghost, then even with less IR, they won't be able to cope with the demand.

Another reason is that being overweight is not the only thing that causes IR. The diabetes itself also seems to cause IR; some have estimated that it causes about half. The additional IR caused by being overweight is sometimes just enough to overtax your beta cells. One man found that gaining thirty pounds doubled his basal insulin requirements.

Sometimes the promise that weight loss will reverse the diabetes makes you feel guilty if it doesn't happen. "I know that doctors are trying to be both motivational and encouraging when they say that if you lose a significant amount of weight, the diabetes may disappear," said Lyndy B. "But for me it turned into a statement of 'It's your fault you have diabetes' and 'If you would only behave, this would all go away.'"

The sooner the better. This possible beta cell exhaustion is also a reason to try to lose weight as soon as possible after you're diagnosed. The sooner you can get your IR down, the less stress there will be on your beta cells and the greater the chance that you'll be able to preserve a lot of them. If you haven't made efforts in this area by now, don't put it off any longer.

Studies have shown that if weight loss is going to help with your BG control, it's most likely to start showing results after a loss of five or ten pounds. If you've lost this much and can't see any difference in your BG control, then you may not see much improvement even if you become as thin as a pencil.

Of course this doesn't mean you should throw your diet plan in the trash and eat pizza and cupcakes all day. Remember that a diabetic diet is as much for controlling your BG levels as it is for losing weight. What it does mean is that if following your diet plan gives you good control of your BG levels but doesn't make you lose weight, you shouldn't beat yourself up about it. In the long run, controlling your BG levels is more important than losing weight.

Restricting calories helps

In fact, some of the benefits of weight loss may not be so much a consequence of the weight loss itself as of the fact that when you're losing weight, you're eating less food. Some studies of overweight people with type 2 diabetes have shown improvements in BG control even before any weight loss when the number of calories was reduced. In other words, simply eating less can help to control your diabetes even if you don't lose any weight. As an additional benefit, eating fewer calories seems to result in fewer damaging free radicals, and animals that eat less live longer.

Even if you've had your diabetes long enough that weight loss probably won't make it go away, don't give up. It will still have other health benefits. Weight loss will make controlling your BG levels easier, and it's good for your blood pressure and for your general health. When you weigh less, it's easier to exercise, and the exercise itself will reduce your IR.

Losing weight is difficult for anyone. It's often more difficult when you have diabetes and thrifty genes that are especially efficient at storing fat and especially reluctant to get rid of that fat once it's safely stored away. One study showed that when put on a similar weight-loss program, people without diabetes lost more weight than those with diabetes, even though adherence to the diet was the same in both groups.

Weight loss is usually more difficult for women than for men, because women normally have a higher percentage of fat and less muscle, and it's muscle that burns the most calories.

There's nothing more discouraging than sitting down to a meal of three peas, a tablespoon of hamburger, and a cup of spinach and still staying on a weight plateau while everyone else in the family is chowing down on cheeseburgers with french fries and creamed corn, followed by huge bowls of pie and ice cream, and they're all as thin as rails.

Bariatric surgery can reverse type 2 diabetes

If you're very overweight and find it extremely difficult to lose, *bariatric surgery* (or *weight loss surgery*) might be worth the risks, which are considerable. There are several types of bariatric surgery, which I won't describe in detail, but basically they reduce the size of your stomach to reduce the amount of food you can eat or reroute the plumbing in your intestines to reduce the absorption of nutrients, or both. *Gastric bypass surgery* does both.

With some types of bariatric surgery, not only do people lose weight, but their symptoms of type 2 diabetes disappear, even before they have lost significant amounts of weight. Some people think it's simply because of the massive decrease in food intake. Others say it suggests that intestinal hormones play a significant role in causing type 2 diabetes.

Bariatric surgery has risks. As with any surgery, you can suffer complications such as serious infections, or even die on the operating table. This is not something to be taken lightly. Furthermore, the surgery can't be reversed, and no one yet knows the long-term effects.

After most types of surgery, you won't be able to eat more than a half cup, or even less, of food at a time for the rest of your life. You also won't be able to tolerate certain foods. And you'll have to take vitamin supplements because your absorption of vitamins will be reduced.

Some people who have had this surgery do eat more than they are supposed to and eventually stretch their stomachs again, so they gain back the weight they have lost. Others stick with the program and lose incredible amounts of weight.

If you think this surgery makes sense for you, do a lot of research before you decide. It's important to find a surgeon who is experienced with the technique you choose, as mortality rates are higher with inexperienced surgeons. There are now numerous books devoted to this topic, as well as Internet discussion groups for people who are considering or have gone through the surgery.

Don't accept a "noncompliant" label

It's even more discouraging if you stick to a strict diet and don't lose weight and then when you see your doctor, the doctor says your diabetes isn't controlled because you're not losing weight, and that's because you're "not compliant," not following the diet the doctor or dietician gave you when you were diagnosed, implying it's all your fault. "I was very discouraged following the ADA diet because no matter how faithfully I dieted, my BGs were always high, and of course the doctor looks at you as if you are the biggest liar on the face of the earth," said Beth H.

Unfortunately, this kind of attitude is not uncommon, but it's not entirely the fault of the medical doctors. It's the way they were trained. A lot of medical books emphasize that the only important factor in losing weight is the number of calories the patient eats compared with the number of calories burned by exercise. The books say if the patient claims to be following the prescribed diet and doesn't lose weight, the patient is either lying or isn't aware of the number of calories actually eaten—for example, eating a large dish of something when the diet specifies a small dish or figuring "a few" peanuts aren't worth mentioning.

In addition, most doctors like to cure people. They like to write prescriptions or perform operations and solve all the patient's problems. That gives them a sense of accomplishment. Type 2 diabetes is chronic. It doesn't go away, and in most cases, especially when the disease isn't well controlled, it just gets worse. The doctors can't cure it. It may be frustrating for them to accept their inability to make you better. So unconsciously, they may shift the burden of blame onto you.

Another problem is that unfortunately some doctors simply don't like fat people. Overweight patients have more health problems, and they're harder to treat. So some doctors blame the overweight patient for any medical problems that arise, no matter how small. You go in for advice on getting rid of a hangnail, and they tell you to lose weight, as if you didn't already know you should.

So if you go back to see your doctor and you haven't lost any weight and your BG control isn't as good as you'd like it to be, don't be surprised if the doctor tells you the problem is that you haven't lost any weight. If this *does* happen to you, don't accept this explanation. If you're really doing everything you can to control your food intake and to exercise as much as you're able and you're still not losing weight, so be it. That doesn't mean you don't deserve excellent BG control.

Don't accept another lecture about "if you'd just lose a few pounds, your sugars would improve." Insist on a better treatment plan, maybe a different drug or a different combination of drugs, or ask for a referral to a dietician to see if some other diet plan would work better for you. By this time, you should have a good idea of whether your initial diet is working for you at all.

Remember that some of the diabetes drugs tend to *cause* weight gain, and they also make it more difficult to lose. It's not fair to tell a patient to lose weight, prescribe a drug that causes weight gain, and then blame the patient for not losing weight. This happened to Alex E.: "My doctor put me on glipizide. I gained thirty pounds, and she reprimanded me for eating too much." If you find your doctor simply can't understand the problems you're having with your weight, try to find another doctor.

Luckily, doctors' attitudes are changing, and if you look around, you may be able to find one who understands. As Carolyn M. said, "The new endo was a breath of fresh air. He said the fact that I'm fat is probably not my fault. At that point, I thought perhaps I'd somehow taken a hallucinogen, but he went on to say that in the 'old days' we didn't know about leptin and other hormonal factors in weight and doctors routinely blamed the patient for weight gain. He then said that it certainly doesn't help anyone to lose weight to have such a punitive attitude toward the problem." Look around and see if you can find an understanding doctor like this one.

There are many theories of weight loss and gain

If you're overweight, you probably don't need to be told what you need to do to lose. You've probably lost weight dozens of times. "I added up all the pounds I lost separately from the ones I gained back," said Edd A., "and I found I'd lost over four thousand pounds." The problem is, of course, that most people tend to gain the weight back again, usually within five years.

Set-point theory. One explanation for a difficulty with maintaining weight loss is called *set-point theory*. According to this theory, everyone is born with a "weight thermostat" that tells the body what weight it would prefer to be. If you're at your set-point weight and you eat a little extra food, you won't gain weight. If you eat a little less, you won't lose. If you force-feed rats or starve them, they get either too fat or too thin. If you then give them free access to rat chow, the fat ones will lose weight and the thin ones will gain weight until they all weigh the same as control rats that weren't either force-fed or starved.

This set point clearly only operates under certain calorie ranges. Anyone will lose weight on a starvation diet. The problem is, almost no one but an ascetic can maintain a 600- or 700-calorie diet for life. And if you do lose weight by such extreme means, when you return to a more normal caloric intake, your set point will try to return you to your former weight.

An additional problem is that you may lose weight as muscle and then regain the weight as fat. Because muscle burns more energy than fat, the next time you try to lose weight, it's twice as difficult. This loss and regain and loss again is called "yo-yo dieting," and it's something you don't want to do.

Uncoupling agents. Another explanation of why some people have weight problems and others don't involves uncoupling agents (proteins). These are chemicals or protein channels that uncouple the metabolism of food from the production of energy. When uncoupling agents are active, the body uses food to produce heat instead of energy that can be used to store fat. Some plants are able to use uncoupling agents when the temperatures get too low, thus sacrificing energy storage for heat.

The theory is that some thin people are also able to shunt some of their food energy into heat when they eat more calories than they need. These are the ones who can stuff themselves and never gain an ounce. Mice engineered to have more of one type of uncoupling protein (UCP-3) eat more than their littermates but weigh less. They also have less fat and lower BG levels.

In mice, at least, exercise seems to increase the amount of uncoupling proteins, yet another reason to try to get as much exercise as you can.

It's possible that people with thrifty genes aren't able to use the uncoupling agents to turn their extra food into heat. They turn it into fat instead. These are the people who eat almost nothing and still don't lose weight.

Some overweight people may just have huge appetites; their problem may involve faulty hunger mechanisms more than problems with uncoupling agents. Similarly, some thin people may be thin because they just have tiny appetites; if they ate a lot, they'd gain weight.

Another uncoupling protein (UCP-2) has been reported to be important in linking obesity, beta cell failure, and type 2 diabetes, at least in mice. In this case, too much uncoupling protein seems to be the problem. Obese, diabetic mice engineered to lack UCP-2 had their first-phase insulin secretion restored and had lower BG levels. In 2006, it was reported that an extract from a plant, *Gardenia jasminoides*, or cape jasmine, which the Chinese have used for thousands of years to treat diabetes, may reduce levels of UCP-2. The active compound is called *genipin*. However, there have been reports that genipin increases oxidative stress and suggestions that UCP-2 may protect the liver from damaging effects of fatty acids.

The details of how the uncoupling proteins are linked to a tendency to gain weight and get diabetes have yet to be worked out, but they may play an important role.

Do what works for you

Like type 2 diabetes, obesity has many causes. Scientists have found more than one hundred genes that may be associated with obesity. Thus YMMV (Your Mileage May Vary) applies to weight loss too. If you're overweight, you've probably already tried a lot of different types of diets throughout the years, and you should know which approach works best for you.

If you do think you eat more than you need, it may help to ask yourself why you overeat. Are you hungry all the time? It's possible that your IR or roller-coaster BG levels are contributing to your hunger. Focus on BG control instead of what the scale tells you. Some people find that once their BG levels are controlled, their appetite becomes more normal and the pounds start coming off without a lot of effort.

Are you eating because there's so much to choose from you have to try it all? Are you eating because you're bored? Because you're too polite to say no when offered food? Because you're unhappy? Because the food is put in front of you and you were raised to believe that wasting food is a sin? Are you eating even when you're not hungry because it's time to eat? Figure out what the triggers are and see if you can change them.

Enjoy your food. Think of your new diet regimen not as a temporary weight-loss plan that involves sacrifices but as a new pleasurable way of eating that you can live with for the rest of your life. *Enjoy your food.* Think of yourself as a gourmet who eats only the best kinds of food in small amounts. Buy only the best (rather than the cheapest) for yourself. You deserve it. Don't worry about the price. If you eat smaller quantities, you can get better quality. For example, eat only two ounces of filet mignon instead of the eight ounces of hamburger you serve to everyone else. Then enjoy every bite.

Remember that the first taste of everything always tastes the best. So savor a few bites of something—its sight, its smell, its texture, and its taste. Eat slowly and pay attention to what you're eating. Don't ever eat when you're doing something else like watching TV and can't really notice—or enjoy—what you're eating.

Buy the freshest food you can. Eat a fresh strawberry, preferably just picked, and imagine you'd never tasted fresh fruit and were trying to describe its taste. A really fresh, ripe strawberry has a symphony of flavors that is much more complex than the "strawberry flavoring" you'll get in processed or fast foods. If possible, go to farmers' markets and try different varieties of berries or vegetables. Try exotic new foods. Become a food connoisseur.

I think one reason Americans eat so much is that our food has so little taste, so the manufacturers add a lot of salt and sugar and fat to trick us into thinking it tastes good. We eat for quantity instead of quality. Avoid that kind of food. Remember, you're a gourmet. You eat for quality, not quantity. You spurn that junk.

Also—yes, I've mentioned this before—try to exercise as much as you can. Studies have shown that people who are able to keep their weight off after losing tend to be those who make exercise a routine part of their lives. Remember that muscle weighs more than fat, so don't worry if the scales don't budge even though you've taken your belt in a few notches.

Even though you probably know what kind of diet makes you lose weight, now that you have diabetes you also have to focus on the effect any weight-loss diet will have on your BG levels as well as on your weight. A wacko diet that makes the pounds come off but makes your BG levels go into the stratosphere is not a great way to go.

New way of eating. In the long run, wacko diets aren't good for you anyway. So in this respect look at your diabetes as an ally, not an enemy. Having diabetes makes you look at any kind of diet in terms of a lifelong way of eating, not a temporary torture that will be over when you can fit into a new pair of slacks. Having diabetes may give you the incentive to lose that weight you've probably been trying to drop for years. In the past, losing weight was simply a question of vanity. Now it's more than that.

Losing weight in a society that is replete with tempting food is hard. If the only way you can keep weight off is to stick to an eight-hundred-calorie diet for the rest of your life and you decide that's simply too much to deal with, then let it be. But don't make that an excuse to give up on your BG control. Controlling your BG levels is more important than losing weight. Don't give up on that.

IN A SENTENCE:

▪ *Losing weight should reduce your insulin resistance, but it's not a panacea, and keeping your blood glucose levels close to normal may be more important than losing weight.*

Understanding Exercise

"My blood sugar goes up when I exercise," says Tekastiaks. "My blood sugar goes down when I exercise," says Clover. What's going on? Which person should you believe?

The fact is, the effect of exercise on your blood glucose (BG) levels is very complex and depends on many factors including the length of the exercise, the intensity of the exercise, your BG levels when you start to exercise, your insulin levels when you start to exercise, the amount of insulin resistance (IR) that you have, your level of training, and other subtle variations in your own personal physiology.

Saying "Blood sugar goes down after exercise" is like saying "Diabetics don't produce insulin." Both statements are correct in particular cases, but they are too general to have much meaning overall. BG levels in a trained athlete after a hundred-yard dash may be quite different from BG levels in a sixty-year-old computer programmer after a three-hour walk in the woods.

As I've stressed before, in the long run, exercise is one of the most important things you can do to reduce your IR, increase the mass of your BG-reducing muscles, and protect your cardiovascular health as well. But the effects of exercise in the short run are quite variable.

To understand this better, you need to understand a few basic things about the physiology of exercise.

- To get energy, muscles can burn either glucose or fatty acids.

- Insulin becomes more effective when you exercise. Or, put another way, your IR decreases when you exercise.

- Muscles can take up glucose without insulin when you exercise.

- Exercise opens up small capillaries. This increases the surface area of muscle that is exposed to glucose-containing blood.

- *Prolonged* exercise depletes the glycogen levels in your liver and muscles.

- *Strenuous* exercise is a form of stress and causes the release of counterregulatory hormones that tell the liver to release glucose into the blood.

ATP is energy currency

Let's start with sources of energy. The immediate source of energy for the muscles is a molecule called **ATP** (adenosine triphosphate). ATP acts as a sort of short-term energy currency for the body. When you want to store energy, for example, in fat, you have to "spend" ATP to make the fats. When you break down the fats, they pay out some ATP.

Muscles need ATP in order to contract, but the muscles contain only enough ATP to work for a few seconds. Then another molecule, called *creatine phosphate*, gives up its energy to make a little more ATP. However, both these molecules combined can only produce enough energy to work the muscles hard for about ten seconds, enough for a short dash but no more than that. ATP is sort of like your petty cash account, or the money in your wallet. It's what you use to buy things, but it's not where you store most of your funds.

ATP isn't where muscle cells store significant energy. For any significant exercise, the cells have to get energy from other sources. The quickest source is glucose. Cells can quickly break down *glycogen* (the cans of glucose taped together with duct tape) to make glucose. Then they can break down the glucose (open the cans of glucose) to make more ATP.

They can even do this in the absence of oxygen, so this process is called *anaerobic*. It produces *lactic acid*.

However, even this process doesn't produce enough ATP to last very long, only about 1.5 minutes. After that, the cells need to rely on *aerobic* forms of metabolism, those that use oxygen. This it can do by oxidizing (breaking down and forming energy in the presence of oxygen) either glucose or fatty acids.

At rest, muscles use mainly fatty acids for their energy needs, and most of the glucose in the body is used by the brain. With mild exercise (about 25 percent maximum), most of the energy in the muscles continues to come from fatty acids.

With moderate exercise (about 65 percent maximum), the muscles begin to break down their glycogen stores and use about equal parts of glycogen, fat stored in the muscle, and fatty acids shipped in from the fat cells.

With a short burst of extreme energy (85 percent of maximum), glycogen supplies most of the energy to the muscle cells.

This gives you an idea of why it's sometimes difficult to predict how exercise will affect your BG levels: a lot depends on how rigorous the exercise is, and except in research settings, that's difficult to measure.

The more rigorous that exercise is, the more likely you are to start out burning glycogen and not fat. However, your muscle cells have another problem: the amount of glycogen in the body is limited. A 70-kilogram (154-pound) man has about 350 grams of glycogen in muscle and 80 grams in the liver, and about 20 grams of glucose in the blood and other extracellular fluids. After two hours of moderate exercise (swimming, skiing, running, or biking), the glycogen stores are down to less than 20 percent of their maximal level. That means that not only the intensity of the exercise but also its duration will affect your glycogen stores and your BG levels as well.

One study showed that after depleting the glycogen stores to 20 percent, it took a full two days to restore them to their maximal levels. This means that if you can do some moderate exercise for about two hours, your muscle cells will continue to take glucose from the blood to rebuild its glycogen stores for almost two days. In addition, a single bout of intensive exercise seems to decrease IR for almost sixteen hours. Seems like a good return on investment.

Exercise makes your insulin resistance go down

When you exercise, your insulin becomes more effective. This is true whether you have diabetes or not. In fact, although athletes often do something called *carbohydrate loading*, which is a way of increasing their glycogen stores so they will have more endurance, they are warned not to eat fast carbohydrates like sugar fifteen to forty-five minutes before they start an event. Why not? Because the carbohydrate makes their BG levels go up a little, and this triggers a release of insulin appropriate for the conditions at rest. When they start exercising, the insulin becomes more effective, and as a result their BG levels can go too low, as shown in Figure 4.

The same problem exists if you are injecting insulin or taking sulfonylurea drugs that can make your insulin levels go up. If before exercising you take a dose that would be appropriate for lounging around watching TV, it will probably be too high when you're exercising hard, and you too may go low.

On the other hand, this fact can be used to your benefit in some cases. If you find your BG levels increasing after whatever kind of exercise you usually do, try eating some carbohydrate fifteen to forty-five minutes before your exercise. This will make your BG levels go up, which will trigger an insulin response, and the exercise will make the insulin more effective. In addition, the insulin will put the brakes on the liver's production of glucose. Thus your BG levels should go down.

Another approach is simply to exercise *after* your meals instead of before.

Exercise has effects that don't depend on insulin

When you exercise, the muscles can take up glucose even without insulin. No one is sure exactly how this happens, although there is some evidence that nitric oxide (NO) and a molecule called *AMPK* are involved. AMPK levels are also raised with the drug metformin. Somehow, the exercise is able to do the same thing as insulin does: it increases the number of GLUT4 transporters (the little boats that ferry glucose across the cell membrane) in the membrane of the cell. However, the pathways are different, so the effects of insulin and exercise are additive. If you have insulin resistance, the effect of insulin is reduced, but the effect of exercise is still normal.

In addition, the exercise increases your circulation. When you're lounging around in front of the TV watching old sitcom reruns, a lot of your capillaries go on strike. The body figures it's not worth the effort to pump blood through muscles that aren't doing any work, so it shuts off some of the capillaries to those unused muscles. When you exercise, these muscles suddenly need oxygen and glucose and fatty acids, so the capillaries open up. This increases the number of cells that are competing for the glucose in your blood, and even without all the other mechanisms for

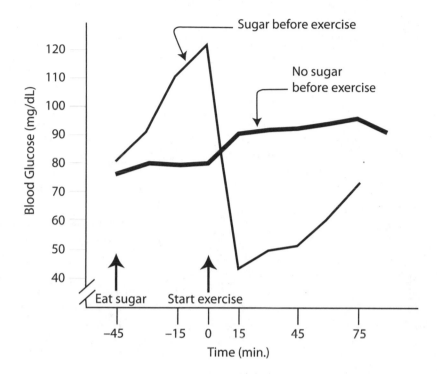

FIGURE 4. The effect of eating carbohydrate before exercise. When a nondiabetic person doesn't eat sugar before exercise, the exercise may cause a small increase in the blood glucose (BG) level (see text). When the same person eats sugar forty-five minutes before the exercise, the sugar triggers an insulin release. When the exercise begins, the insulin becomes more effective and the BG level drops suddenly, in this case down to almost 40 mg/dL, before coming back up to normal levels. In a diabetic person, the exercise-induced increase in BG levels without food, as well as the increase after eating sugar, would be greater.

increasing glucose uptake, your BG uptake would increase and your BG levels would go down.

Strenuous exercise is stressful

I know, I know. For some of us, any kind of exercise at all is stressful. But that's psychological stress. I'm speaking here of physiological stress. You may recall the fight-or-flight reaction to stress that triggers the release of a bundle of counterregulatory hormones (they oppose the action of insulin) that make BG levels go up.

You remember that one reason the body does this is to allow the liver to produce more glucose to ship off to the muscles just in case the body the hormones are living in decides to flee or get involved in a wrestling match.

Well, strenuous exercise is really the same thing as fleeing or wrestling: The muscles need more energy, and they need it fast. So when the body gets a signal that you've started hard exercise, it secretes more stress hormones like adrenaline, growth hormone, and cortisol.

These hormones help the fat cells break down fat into fatty acids, which the muscles can burn for energy. They also tell the liver to crank up its production of glucose, which the muscles can also burn. These signals to the liver are especially strong when the BG levels are not high. If there's already plenty of glucose in the blood when you start to exercise, the liver recognizes that the situation isn't critical yet and doesn't crank up its glucose production so quickly. This is another reason to eat before you start your exercise. The higher BG levels and higher insulin levels will slow down the stress hormone response.

With very strenuous exercise, the liver cranks out glucose, and it may produce more glucose than the muscles are able to take up, even in non-diabetic people. With short bursts of strenuous exercise, the BG levels increase about 20 percent in people without diabetes. Then as soon as the exercise is over, the muscle cells grab the extra glucose to rebuild their glycogen stores and the BG levels return to normal. When you have type 2 diabetes, the BG levels go even higher during exercise and take longer to return to normal.

Prolonged exercise burns glucose

Although short bouts of strenuous exercise may make your BG levels go up, longer bouts of less strenuous exercise may make your BG levels go down. This is because the less strenuous exercise may not be seen by the body as stressful, so you won't get a burst of those counterregulatory hormones that tell the liver to put out glucose.

The less strenuous exercise will also burn a smaller percentage of glycogen. In fact, during low-intensity exercise, as at rest, the muscles actually prefer to burn fatty acids. However, you will burn some glycogen for a longer time. And as your muscles sense that their glycogen stores are going down, they'll do their best to take glucose out of the blood to rebuild them. So you may see your BG levels come down after this kind of exercise.

Many kinds of exercise are somewhere in between these two extremes, so it's often difficult to predict what will happen with your BG levels. You need to test before and after doing the kind of exercise you do the most and see how it affects you.

Anaerobic exercise builds muscle

The kind of exercise that makes you breathe hard, like running or playing tennis, is called *aerobic exercise* because it requires oxygen to produce the energy-currency molecule ATP. Aerobic exercise builds up your heart and the efficiency of your lungs, and it also burns glucose. It's obviously a good thing to do.

But there's another type of exercise called *anaerobic exercise*. This is the kind you *could* do while holding your breath (although you really shouldn't; it's better to breathe while doing anaerobic exercise), for example, weight lifting, push-ups, or climbing a steep hill (see Day 5).

Weight lifting doesn't make you breathe hard while you're doing it, and it won't increase the efficiency of your lungs. But weight lifting will increase the strength and, especially if you're male, size of your muscles. Because the muscles are one of the main organs that take glucose out of the blood, the more muscle you have, the better you'll be able to control your BG levels in the long run.

Muscle also burns calories faster than fat cells do, so as you increase the ratio of muscle to fat, you'll make it easier to lose weight. If you *are* trying to lose weight and you're also lifting weights, remember that muscle weighs more than fat. As you lose fat and gain muscle, you may actually gain a little weight. Don't worry about it. The inches that you're losing will tell you that you're just gaining more muscle.

Exercise causes a virtuous circle

As you can see, there are many kinds of exercise, and they may all affect your BG levels and your type of fitness differently. But they're all beneficial in the long run. Exercise is a virtuous circle. More exercise creates more muscles, which make more exercise easier. Short-term effects are sometimes hard to predict. But long-term effects are clear. In the long term, exercise makes the BG levels go down.

IN A SENTENCE:

■ *In the long run, both aerobic and anaerobic exercise will help keep your blood glucose levels low, but in the short term, the effects of exercise are sometimes difficult to predict.*

living

Tracking
Your Progress

When you started out managing your diabetes, the important thing was to get into the habit of testing your blood glucose (BG) levels. Now you may want to get a little fancier in the way you keep track of your BG levels so you can spot trends and see how different foods and exercise patterns affect your control.

Start with logbooks

You probably already have a few *logbooks* designed for this purpose. Most meters come with logbooks, which include spaces to enter your BG readings at standard times, usually before meals and at bedtime, sometimes more, as well as insulin dosages and comments.

These logbooks are a good place to begin, and maybe they're all you'll ever want. But you may find them limiting and want to document more information; for example, some logbooks don't have space for fasting or postprandial readings. Or you may want the information in a different form.

Even before I was diagnosed with diabetes, I'd written down everything I ate in a little notebook, the kind you can buy at the supermarket, because I thought I might be allergic to wheat. This method continues to work for me. Each day takes up a page, and I can write down what I eat and my BG levels as well as other pertinent information like weight, blood pressure, illness, exercise, or starting or stopping medications.

I also graph some of my results. For instance, when I measure BG levels after trying a new food (see the Learning section), I graph the results in a spiral graph-paper notebook so I don't end up with a mess of sheets I'd probably lose. I also graph my fasting BG levels, which I now measure several times a week instead of daily, unless there's a reason to do so more often, for example, if I'm sick or taking a new drug.

I note on the graphs any different conditions like starting a new drug or not getting exercise because I'm sick or injured, and I find it easier to see patterns this way. Others might find the logbook presentation simpler to analyze.

Everyone has different needs, and as time goes on, you may figure out your own logbook form that tells you what you want to know. Richard H., who had type 1 diabetes, designed his own graph-like BG-tracking forms with a fresh sheet for every day. There were spaces at the top to plot his BG and ketone levels throughout a twenty-four-hour period. He also entered his food intake and his insulin doses. At the bottom, he plotted both his activity level and the way he was feeling, using codes from 0 to 6. For example, activity code 0 was sleeping, 1 was "inactive, boob tube, reading," 3 was "intermittent activity, driving tractor, walking," and 6 was "heavy work, lifting, digging, carrying, shoveling." Feeling code 1 was "quite low [BG level], dull, tense, poor eyesight," 4 was "slightly high, feel safe," 5 was "moderately high, tired, some aches," and 6 was "very high, tired, aches, thirsty, frequent urination." There was also room for comments.

You may not want to devote that much time to documenting daily activities. But if you did it occasionally, you might learn a lot about how various factors do affect you.

Computer programs may help

If you have a computer, much of this documentation and manipulation of data can be done on it. All kinds of computer software are available, from spreadsheet programs with which you can design your own system, to simple free programs that work like logbooks, to fancy Windows- or Macintosh-based graphics programs that let you graph and print your data in myriad ways. Some of these programs can be downloaded from the Internet, sometimes free and sometimes for a fee. In the latter case, you can usually try out an abbreviated form of the program before you buy it.

In most programs, you can enter the data two ways. You can type in your results every day, or you can download your meter directly into the computer. If you think you'll be interested in downloading a meter, you'll obviously need a meter that allows this feature. Ask if the meter has a *data port*. You'll also need a cable that plugs into the meter and into a port on your computer. Sometimes the cable comes with the software, and sometimes it's an additional expense.

Not all software will accept downloads from all meters. So before you buy, make sure the meter you want and the software you want are compatible.

There are more and more diabetes apps for smart phones (one online site said more than a thousand in 2015). Many are free. So if you have a smart phone, look for an app that matches your needs.

Work with your doctor

Sometimes your doctor will want to download your meter at the office. The doctor will then either print out the data and share it with you or use it in a program on the office computer to analyze the results with you. This means you don't need to worry about the technology yourself. But it also means you can't customize the software for your own needs.

If you decide you want to get your own software and print out your results to bring to your doctor, it's a good idea to check first to see what kind of data the doctor wants to see. Some people take fancy graphs and analyses to their doctors and find that the doctors are thrilled. They don't have to deal with difficult handwriting in cramped logbooks, and the graphs and analyses provide additional information.

Other people spend hours printing out fancy graphs and analyses, but their doctors don't want to see all that. They just want to look at the logbook or the A1c. In fact, some doctors don't even want to look at your daily BG numbers; if you have type 2 diabetes, they often only care about the A1c. This can be discouraging if you've gone to a lot of work to manage your data.

Most of the programs produce the same types of information, but they all display it in a slightly different form, and it may be easier for a doctor to spot trends if all the patients present the data in the same way. So if you think a computer program would help you understand what's going on, discuss it ahead of time and see what kinds of information the doctor wants to see and make sure that's included as well as the fancy charts and graphs.

Diabetes programs usually show similar things

Software is constantly changing, so I won't discuss specific programs. Check magazine articles and the Internet for current reviews. Most of them do basically the same thing. They usually have a logbook, which is like the paper versions. Before you buy a program, make sure its logbook works for you. Some of them have only a limited number of spots for entering BG levels, and if you lead a rather unregimented life and eat lunch at 11 A.M. one day and at 3 P.M. the next, or if you don't test for several days and then you test fifteen times the next day, some of the programs' logbooks wouldn't be suitable.

Most of them allow you to input your target levels at various times, and they'll tell you what percentage of the time you were at or above or below your targets. They also usually plot a *modal day*, which is a graph of your BG levels throughout a twenty-four-hour period for a certain length of time, for example for the last week or month or year (usually you can choose the time period). That makes it easy to spot if you're always high in the morning or always low before dinner, so you can take steps to correct the problem.

In some of the programs you can also sort the data by the day of the week, so you can find additional factors. For example, if you find you're off target every Wednesday, you could look at what you do on Tuesdays and Wednesdays that might cause the problem. Is there an office treat every Wednesday morning? A stressful staff meeting? Do you play poker late into the night on Tuesdays?

In various programs you can also sort by events or by the time of day and so forth and view and print line graphs or bar graphs or fancy pie graphs in many colors.

Nutritional programs are useful

Some of the commercial programs also include nutritional analyses, in which you can type in what you eat and the program will tell you how many calories and the amount and percentages of selected nutrients you've eaten so far. Some will even warn you when you've reached your daily limit. If the nutritional analysis is *all* you're interested in, there are handheld nutritional tracking gizmos that are small enough that you can take them with you to work or to restaurants. You punch in what you eat, and they give you daily totals and percentages. Smart-phone apps serve the same function.

Before you invest a lot of money in any of these programs, make sure the program matches your needs. Sometimes too much data is worse than not enough. If you think you'll get swamped with too much information, start out with one of the simpler free programs. If you find it useful, you can upgrade later to one of the fancier ones.

Internet sites will analyze your data

There are also sites on the Internet where you can type in your results or download your meter, and their software will analyze it for you. This raises questions of security, whether you care if your BG data is out in cyberspace somewhere, presumably secure, but not really under your control. Also, the sites might go paws up, and then your data would no longer be available. These sites are also not free.

There is also software that allows you to download your data to your doctor's office through the Internet. Of course this requires that both you and the doctor's office have the same type of software, which is especially designed for this purpose. If you think this might be useful for you, ask at the doctor's office if they're doing this or if they'd be interested in trying it.

The more data you have, the better idea you'll have of what you can do to improve your control. The trick is to not become so overwhelmed with data that you don't know what to do with it. Maybe just writing down the daily BG levels and foods eaten in a logbook would be just fine. That alone is a tremendous advance from the old days in which people with type 2 diabetes had their fasting levels checked at a doctor's office every six months or so. No wonder they often got complications.

But if you enjoy playing around with numbers and charts and graphs, go for it. The software is probably out there. Find what fits the bill and use it. If you can't find what you want, a customized spreadsheet program might work for you. If you're familiar with computer programming, design your own program and then share it with others. Several people with diabetes have done that and offered the programs free via the Internet.

The important thing is not how you keep track of your progress, but the fact that you do. Thinking you're now fine and you don't need to test and keep track anymore often leads to gradually rising BG averages, which may lead to complications. Keeping track keeps you on the track to complication-free years in the future.

IN A SENTENCE:

■ *Keeping track of your blood glucose levels—whether in a logbook or on a computer—helps you maintain good control.*

Estimating Your Personal Glycemic Index Values

By now, you should be comfortable measuring your blood glucose (BG) levels regularly. If so, you're probably controlling better than most people with type 2 diabetes. Simply accepting that you have the disease and being willing to invest the little time it takes to do BG tests is a giant step toward good control. But you can do even more with your meter than just test your BG levels at various times of the day.

Although these little home meters aren't as accurate as expensive clinical lab equipment, they can provide sophisticated information. You can even measure your own *glycemic index* values, which estimate how much a particular food will raise your BG levels.

A first step in understanding how food affects your control is to measure your BG levels immediately before and two hours after you eat. That gives you a general idea. But it doesn't tell the whole story. Different foods raise BG levels at different speeds.

The BG level after eating glucose or another simple sugar usually peaks at about thirty minutes, and the level after eating white bread peaks a little later, at about sixty minutes. But if both foods contained the same amount of carbohydrate, the overall increase in the BG level would be about the same with

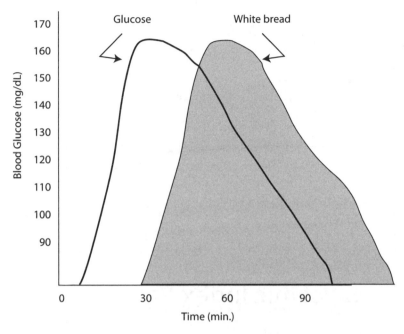

FIGURE 5. Different blood glucose responses to different carbohydrates. Glucose tablets (left) usually peak in about thirty minutes. Starch (white bread) peaks at about sixty minutes.

both foods. This is shown in Figure 5. If you measured only at thirty minutes, you would conclude that glucose causes a much greater increase in BG levels than bread. But if you measured at ninety minutes, you would conclude that bread causes a much greater increase in BG levels than glucose (see Figure 5). This illustrates the problems when your certified diabetes educator (CDE) says to keep your BG levels under 140 mg/dL (milligrams per deciliter) after meals. You might have a different definition of "after meals" than the CDE.

Testing more often. The way to overcome this problem is to test more often after eating a particular food, enough to produce a real *BG curve*, meaning you can see when the BG level goes up, when it peaks, and when it comes down to baseline again, as shown in Figure 5. Of course this takes more test strips than simply testing once or twice a day. If money is no problem, you can buy extra strips for this purpose. Otherwise, if your control has been pretty steady, you can test fewer times for a few days, or even every other day, for a while, save up the strips, and then do a good curve on a new food.

When measuring BG curves, first you need to decide what time of day you're going to do the tests. The effect of a particular food can sometimes depend on what you ate at the previous meal. For example, a soluble-fiber-filled meal for breakfast may result in lower BG level increases after lunch. A BG curve can also depend on how much exercise you had before the test. If you're one of those people who always has the same breakfast and the same lunch and pretty much the same dinner and always exercises at the same time of day for the same length of time, then it won't matter much when you decide to do your tests as long as it's always the same time.

If your daily schedule differs a lot, however, it's probably safer to do your tests in the morning, before you eat. The problem here is the *dawn effect* (see Day 6). If your BG level increases before you get up in the morning and then stays the same until you eat, this won't be a problem. But if your BG level starts increasing when you get out of bed and increases different amounts on different days, then you might want to postpone your testing until the level becomes steady.

This kind of testing requires more than one reading

Let's assume you've decided to test the effect of eating a slice of bread, and you want to start first thing in the morning. What do you do? First, of course, you measure your BG level at time zero. Then you eat a slice of bread as quickly as you can. Five minutes to eat a test food won't matter, but it's obviously not a good idea to savor it for a half an hour or so. If you know that coffee or tea (with no milk or cream and obviously with no sugar—not even sugar substitutes that contain bulking agents) or soda won't affect your BG level, you can drink them. Otherwise drink water.

Then you start measuring. As a general rule, a reasonable amount of glucose tablets will peak in about 30 minutes. Processed carbohydrate like bread will peak in about 60 minutes. A slower carbohydrate, or starch with fat added, will peak even later, at about 90 minutes. Some very slow carbohydrates won't increase BG levels much until about 4 or 5 hours, the same as protein foods.

If you're measuring a simple sugar like glucose, you'll probably want to do the first test at 15 minutes. When you're testing something that you expect to peak at 60 minutes, you can wait until 30 minutes to do your first test.

How often should you test? Again, that depends on how many strips you can afford to use and how many finger sticks you can stand to endure. I usually measure at 30 minutes, 1, 1.5, 2, and 3 hours, or until the numbers return to baseline. If for some reason I really want to know exactly where the peak is, I might measure at 30 and 45 minutes, 1, 1.25, 1.5 hours, and so forth, assuming the peak is around 1 hour. The more points you measure, the more accurate the curve. The more tests you do, the better sense you get of what times you should test. If you plot your results on graph paper as you go along, you'll see what's happening, and if one point seems unreasonable, you can take a second reading.

Figure 6 is an example of what you can learn by doing this type of test. In this test, I ate a piece of French bread with sugar-free jam and then took a thirty-minute walk up and down a steep hill. When the BG level had returned to baseline, I ate another piece of bread and jam and worked at my computer. You can see from the figure that without the exercise, my BG level went about twice as high. And because I started 20 mg/dL lower, the increase without exercise was almost three times as much (up 115 compared with up 40 mg/dL).

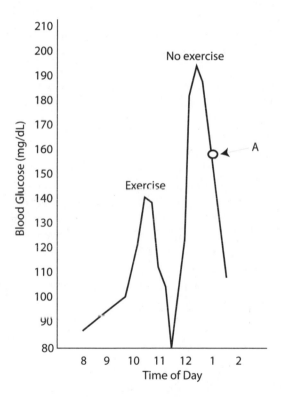

FIGURE 6. Effect of exercise. When exactly the same food was eaten (French bread and sugar-free jam), the blood glucose level rose almost three times as much when I sat at my computer as when I hiked up a steep hill immediately after eating the bread and jam. The food was eaten at 9:45 and 11:30 A.M. Between 8 and 9:45 A.M., the slight rise from 85 to about 100 mg/dL is due to the dawn effect. The point marked A is where I started feeling ravenously hungry.

You can do your own mini glucose tolerance test

This method can even be used to do what I call a *mini glucose tolerance test (mini GTT)*, using glucose tablets. A real GTT (see Day 5) done in a lab to diagnose diabetes usually uses a whopping 75 grams of glucose. I don't like to subject my system to such huge doses, so I use 12 grams, which means quickly eating three of the 4-gram glucose tablets washed down with water. Bread and jam taste a lot better, but manufacturers often change their recipes or suppliers. Glucose tablets tend to be more uniform. I stick with one brand when I can.

Then when you have a baseline glucose curve, you can try different things to see how they affect it. For example, Figure 7 shows the effect of fat. Fat delays the emptying of the stomach, and if you have some insulin production, as you usually do with type 2 diabetes, sometimes your beta cells are able to cope better when little spurts of carbohydrate come out of the stomach instead of a huge carbohydrate dump all at once.

To test this idea on myself, first I measured a curve after eating 12 grams of glucose. Then I ground up the glucose tablets and mixed them into whipped cream (no sacrifice too great in the name of science; this was really good). You can see that in my case, the fat actually reduced the BG level. Then, just to make sure the second curve wasn't lower because of some residual effect from the first curve (for example, maybe the first dose of glucose had induced enough insulin to carry over into the second curve), I did another 12-gram glucose curve without any fat. This was very similar to the first curve, suggesting that the effect of the fat was real. In order to prove it, I'd have to do a lot more tests. But this suggested that for me a little fat will reduce my BG levels, at least in the short run.

But YMMV (Your Mileage May Vary). Some people say fat *increases* their BG levels after a meal. It's possible that fat would decrease the BG level in the short term and increase it in the long term. Several people with type 1 diabetes have remarked that when they eat a lot of fat, their insulin requirements go up later, from six hours to several days after eating the fat.

One interesting thing I've discovered when doing these mini-GTT curves is that I often get ravenously hungry shortly after the BG peak, when the BG level is falling rapidly, as shown in point A in Figure 6. I don't know if this is a universal phenomenon or not, but others have said they've found similar things. "Most of my food cravings occur when my blood sugar changes, either up or down. If I can hold it constant, or near constant, I eat less and feel better," said Jim D. This is one reason to avoid a diet that will cause postprandial BG spikes. If you're trying to lose weight, ravenous hunger is not something you want.

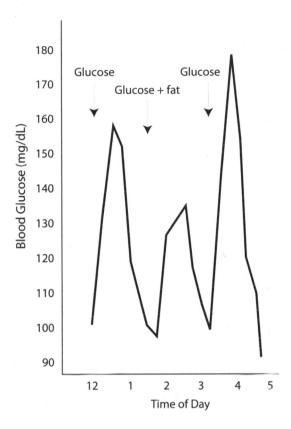

FIGURE 7. Effect of fat. When I eat fat, the blood glucose (BG) peaks are smaller. In this case I first ate glucose tablets (curve on left), then glucose tablets mixed into whipped cream (center curve), and then pure glucose tablets again (right curve). In each case the pure glucose caused a greater BG-level increase than the glucose mixed with fat. Note that some people find that fat *increases* their BG levels.

I also discovered that no-sugar-added ice cream raised my BG level just as much as the same amount of regular ice cream (same brand). The real stuff also tasted better.

The area under the curve gives you a number

Now that you know how to measure a BG curve, you might like to get a number that would let you compare the results of eating one food or trying one exercise with the results of another. How do you do that? You measure the *area under the curve*, often called just the *AUC*. This means the area on the graph that has increased as a result of trying a particular food or exercise, as shown by the shaded area in Figure 5. If the food didn't make the BG level go up at all, then the AUC would be zero.

If you happen to have a computer with sophisticated graphing software, you're in luck. Otherwise you'll have to use approximations of the AUC. One way is simply to look at two curves and get an idea of which food causes a greater increase. When the curves are the same shape, this is pretty simple. But sometimes if one food causes a high peak that comes down quickly and another one causes a lower peak that extends for a longer time (Figure 8), it's more difficult to compare them.

One method of doing a rough estimate is simply to count the number of squares under the curve on a sheet of graph paper. This gives you a numerical estimate, but it's rather tedious. If you are mathematical or have a mathematical friend and a computer, you can set up a spreadsheet to calculate the AUC for you.

The A1c depends on the cumulative AUCs throughout the day. As shown in Figure 8, you could have two different foods with the same AUC, one that gave you a high peak that quickly returned to baseline and the other that gave you a low, long-lasting peak. Which would be more damaging? Not everyone agrees on the answer to this question. Some people say that short peaks, even high ones, are no problem as long as they don't last very long, that the only important factor is the AUC. Others think high peaks can be damaging, even if brief. Recent research tends to support the latter view.

The glycemic index measures blood glucose increases

This approach (using sophisticated computer integrations) can be used to get the AUC of various foods, and this is what researchers do when they measure the *glycemic index* of food. They give both diabetic and nondiabetic people an amount of food that contains 50 grams of carbohydrate. Then they test the BG level every fifteen minutes for the first hour and every thirty minutes for two hours in nondiabetic volunteers and an additional third hour in diabetic volunteers, and from this they calculate the AUC. They test each food two or three times with each person and then average the results from eight to ten people to get an official glycemic index number, which describes how much a particular food will raise the BG level relative to glucose or white bread. Glycemic index results compared with glucose are always a little lower than the glycemic index results compared with white bread.

Researchers have found that although the BG levels rise different amounts in different people after eating the same food, the *relative*

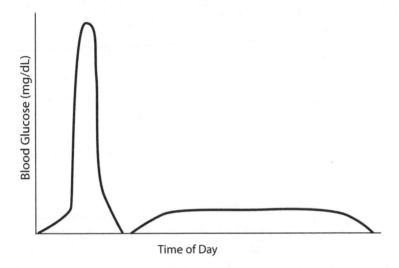

FIGURE 8. Areas under the curve (AUCs). The hypothetical curve at the left shows a high peak but a short duration. The hypothetical curve at the right has a low peak but a long duration. The AUCs are approximately the same. The hemoglobin A1c values are thought to reflect the AUCs. If so, it wouldn't matter if you ate a food that caused a high, short spike or one that caused a lower peak if that lower increase persisted for many hours.

amounts are usually the same. In other words, Dennis's BG level might go up 100 points with rice cakes and 40 points with a pear, and Chanelda's BG level might go up only 30 points with rice cakes and 15 points with a pear. The effects of the carbohydrates are quite different in these two different people, but in both cases the rice cakes raised the BG level a lot more than the pear.

Foods with a large particle size, high fiber and fat content, and high acidity have lower glycemic index values than highly processed foods with very little bound-up fiber and small particle sizes. Raw foods have lower glycemic index values than cooked.

Substance glycemic index includes noncarbohydrate foods

Researchers working with the glycemic index have measured only foods containing carbohydrates, and the glycemic index gives you a good idea of how much two different high-carbohydrate foods will raise your BG level, for example, white bread compared with whole-grain bread. But there are no glycemic index values for low-carbohydrate foods like steak or cheese.

Furthermore, the glycemic index researchers have tried to standardize the foods relative to the same amount of carbohydrate in each food. The glycemic index values tell you only that 50 grams of digestible carbohydrate in carrots will raise your BG level more than 50 grams of digestible carbohydrate in chickpeas. But carrots contain a lot of fiber; a half cup of raw carrots contains only about 3 or 4 grams of nonfiber carbohydrate, and you'd have to eat 6 or 8 cups of carrots to get those 50 grams of carbohydrate. Chickpeas contain about 15 grams of nonfiber carbohydrate per half cup, so you'd have to eat only 1.7 cups of chickpeas to get the same amount of carbohydrate.

Thus although the glycemic index provides a lot of useful information, it can sometimes be misleading. For this reason, Derek Paice, an engineer with type 2 diabetes, came up with a concept he calls the *substance glycemic index*, or *SGI*. This is similar to the glycemic index except that instead of comparing foods with the same amount of carbohydrate, he compares foods with the same total weight.

This means he can get SGI numbers for noncarbohydrate as well as carbohydrate foods. He's also comparing weights of foods one might actually eat (60 grams are about two ounces) instead of amounts that contain 50 grams of carbohydrate, which can be enormous with foods that don't have a lot of carbohydrate. As his standard he uses 60 grams of whole wheat bread, and he expresses the numbers as a percentage of the AUC for a similar weight of whole wheat bread.

For example, with his sample size of one person (himself) and using a home BG meter, he finds that if whole wheat bread has an SGI of 100, some sausage rolls made with wheat flour have an SGI of 56, steak has an SGI of 17, and a cheese omelet has an SGI of 6.

Your results can provide useful information

Doing tests like this can be quite tedious and time consuming. Some people just measure the AUC for the first two or three hours, as the glycemic index researchers do. I don't like to test a substance without doing a complete test, waiting until the BG level returns to baseline. In some cases, this can take hours. For example, some foods containing protein or slowly digested carbohydrate that acts almost like protein cause very little BG increase until five or six hours after you eat them. Pasta, for example, has a second peak that would be missed if you stopped testing at two or three hours.

Because exercise can affect the results, I also like to avoid any kind of exertion when I'm testing, and of course I can't eat anything else when I'm doing a test. This means every test curve requires a real investment of hunger and effort, not to mention holes in the fingers. Some of you may not want to invest this much time and energy in getting AUC numbers for all your foods.

If not, doing just a few curves so you'll understand more about when the various foods you eat will peak might make sense. Then you could always measure at those times. Even just always measuring one or two hours after a meal or a new food will give you a rough estimate. As shown in Figure 5, it can give some erroneous results, but it's better than not testing at all. The continuous monitors are a godsend for this type of testing, except for their high prices.

Even the AUC method can give inconsistent results. Type 2 diabetes is complicated, and many different things can affect how much your BG level will go up after a meal. For example, an unknown infection, a telephone call saying a close friend or relative is sick, having to get a cat out of a tree, or other stressful events could affect the results of a test. This doesn't mean they're not worth doing.

Figure 9 shows some of the variations that can affect an AUC test. I was trying to find out if I could eat some of the supersweet local cantaloupe being sold at a local farm stand. So first I ate six ounces of melon first thing in the morning, which is when I do AUC tests. As you can see, my BG level went quite high, too high for me. Then I wondered if I could tolerate slightly less cantaloupe with other food, so I had a lunch of beef, broccoli, pepper, and four ounces of melon. This time, my BG level hardly moved.

Then, to see if the lower BG rise had to do with the food I ate with the melon or to other factors, I had another seven ounces of melon with no other food. You can see that the BG level didn't rise nearly as much as it had in the early-morning test, even though I ate more melon. This lower rise with more melon could have been caused by several factors. (1) Most people are more sensitive to carbohydrates in the morning. Maybe the large rise early in the day was just part of the dawn effect. (2) I had other food before the seven ounces of melon. Even though the BG level had returned to normal, some food might have remained in my stomach and could have slowed down the digestion of the melon. (3) Some people show what is called a *priming effect*. This means that if you eat a lot of carbohydrate at one meal, you produce more insulin the next time you eat carbohydrate (see Figure 3 in Month 7). This seems to be true for me. A second mini GTT usually shows a lower BG peak than the first one.

So it's difficult to know what caused the difference. But it does suggest that if I want to eat a little bit of fruit, I'm much better off eating it along with some protein and fiber-rich vegetable, especially later in the day.

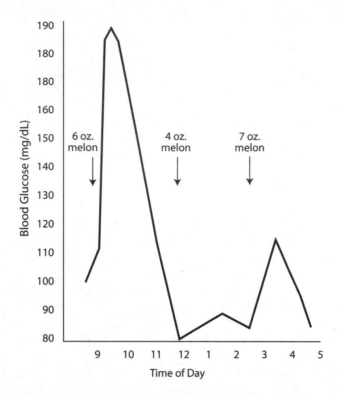

FIGURE 9. So many variables, so little time. When you're trying to figure out how a particular food affects your blood glucose (BG) levels, you have to remember that many factors can be involved. This shows how my BG levels responded to three different meals containing cantaloupe. In the curve at the left, I ate six ounces of melon with no other food, and my BG level went quite high. Then I had four ounces of melon along with meat and vegetable (beef, broccoli, and pepper), and my BG level hardly increased at all. Finally, I had seven ounces of melon with no other food, and the BG level increased just a little. Measuring after only one melon-containing meal might have led to an erroneous conclusion. The time of day, accompanying food, and previous meals, as well as exercise and stress, can all affect the response.

What's true for me might not be true for you. The graphs of my results shown in this book are what are called *n = 1 experiments*, meaning the number of people tested was only one. With only one person, the results are only suggestive. If your results don't match my results, don't worry.

You may have a different type of diabetes, or just a different metabolism than I do. Trust your own results. If you do have the time and energy to invest, testing this way and getting AUC numbers for your favorite foods will give you a much, much better idea of which foods and activities you can choose for maximal control.

IN A SENTENCE:

■ *With a little extra work, you can use your home glucose meter to get approximate values for your own personal glycemic index values.*

living

Complications

I hope that by keeping your blood glucose (BG) levels close to normal, you will avoid ever developing any diabetic complications. As discussed in Day 6, there is now real evidence that the lower your average BG level is, the smaller the risk of complications, especially the *microvascular* ones.

Unfortunately, however, because you may have had diabetes for many years before being diagnosed, you may already have had early signs of complications when you were diagnosed. If not, you should at least be aware of what kinds of complications can occur so you can be alert for their early signs and insist that your periodic health examinations test you for their presence.

Microvascular complications are serious

Microvascular complications are the ones caused by problems in your small blood vessels and include *retinopathy* (eye problems), *nephropathy* (kidney problems), and *neuropathy* (nerve problems): the Three O'Pathy Sisters. They are more common in people with long-standing type 1 diabetes, but people with type 2 diabetes are not immune. Microvascular complications usually occur only after about ten years of high BG levels.

Eye problems can be detected with regular eye examinations

Glaucoma and cataracts are not limited to people with diabetes, but if you have diabetes, your chances of getting glaucoma and cataracts are increased.

Glaucoma. *Glaucoma* means the pressure in your eyes is greater than normal. This pressure can damage the optic nerve, the one that sends messages from your eyes to your brain. Uncontrolled, glaucoma can cause blindness, usually starting with a loss of peripheral vision. When caught early, however, glaucoma can be controlled with eyedrops, and your chances of losing sight are small. Make sure your *intraocular pressure* is measured when you have your regular eye examinations. Ask your ophthalmologist about the symptoms of acute glaucoma, which include pain, nausea, and halos around lights, and seek medical attention immediately if they occur.

Cataracts. *Cataracts* result from clouding of the lens of the eye and are common in elderly people. If you have diabetes, you're more likely to have cataracts and to get them at a younger age. These days, the lens can be removed and replaced with an artificial lens in a fairly routine outpatient procedure, and some people report that their vision is much better after this operation than it ever was before.

Retinopathy. *Retinopathy* is an eye condition that is limited to people with diabetes, and it's been shown that lowering BG levels slows the onset or progression of the condition. When BG levels have been elevated for ten or twenty years, most people show signs of early retinopathy. About 20 percent of people diagnosed with type 2 diabetes show such signs when they're diagnosed.

This early stage of retinopathy is called *nonproliferative* or *background retinopathy*, and it doesn't usually cause any loss of vision. For some reason that is not completely understood, when BG levels are elevated, the capillaries become more fragile and leaky. Some of the capillaries in the eyes form *aneurysms*, or outpouchings, that can be seen when a doctor examines the *retinas* of your eyes, the part of the back of the eye that is responsible for detecting light and converting it into nervous signals that are sent to the brain. Sometimes the capillaries also leak fluid, and fats from the fluid can condense and form what are called *hard exudates* because their borders look sharp.

As long as the retinopathy doesn't proceed any further, your vision should remain normal, unless some of the fluid leaks into the *macular* area of the retina and causes swelling, called *macular edema*. The macula is the part of your eyes responsible for central, detailed vision, so when this area is swollen, your vision may be reduced. The glitazone drugs occasionally produce macular edema.

If BG levels aren't controlled, retinopathy can proceed through several other stages to *proliferative retinopathy*, which can cause loss of vision. As in the rest of the body, when circulation through the capillaries is slowed down or stopped, the body tries to fix the problem by making new capillaries. If this happens in your heart, it's a good thing. When it happens in your retina, it's not.

The new blood vessels can obstruct your vision or, worse, because they are even more fragile than normal, they can leak blood into the clear fluid in your eyeball (called the *vitreous humor*), causing clouding of your vision. If they bleed and then clot, the clot can contract and pull the retina away from its attachments. This is called *retinal detachment* and is a serious condition that can lead to blindness.

These days, laser surgery can be used to seal the leaky capillaries before serious damage occurs. The procedure does hurt; most books say a little, some patients say a heck of a lot. But it works. Studies have shown significant reduction in serious vision loss when laser surgery is used this way.

A better way to save your sight is to keep your BG levels down so you'll never need the surgery. Early retinopathy has no symptoms, so it's important to get an annual eye examination (see Week 2) to detect retinal changes early, before they've done any damage. It's also important to keep your blood pressure down, as high blood pressure increases the chances of bleeding throughout the body.

Nephropathy can be detected with lab tests

Diabetic nephropathy, or damage to the kidneys, usually goes along with retinopathy. So if there are no signs of damage to your eyes, your kidneys are probably OK. Conversely, if you have signs of early retinal problems, you probably have early kidney problems as well, so make sure your doctor checks you carefully for this (see Day 5) and continues to do so in the future.

Early nephropathy can be reversed by maintaining BG levels at near-normal levels, but if you wait until there is a lot of protein in the urine, the damage probably can't be undone. If you keep your BG levels in the normal range, or close to that, you probably won't get either kidney or retinal damage in the first place. However, the risks of both problems are partly genetic, and if you're Native American, Hispanic American, or African American, the risks of these complications are greater even with good control.

How kidneys work. The kidneys are the body's garbage collectors, including an efficient recycling center. They basically filter metabolic waste products, toxins, some drugs, and extra fluids out of the blood, producing urine, while retaining proteins and anything else that the body can reuse.

Here's how they work. The kidneys have a lot of structures called *nephrons*, each of which consists of a pompon-like tuft of capillaries (called a *glomerulus*) inside a balloon-like pouch. When healthy, these capillaries have small pores in them, and they are surrounded by a mesh of material called *basement membrane* that also acts like a filter. Both the pores and the basement membrane have a negative charge.

Blood flows through the capillaries, and much of the liquid and small molecules like glucose and sodium chloride can go through the pores and the basement membrane and are secreted into the pouch and then down a series of tubes into the bladder. Large molecules like proteins usually can't fit through the holes. Even when the proteins are small enough, the negative charge on the pores and basement membrane tends to keep them out.

On the way to the bladder, through a complicated series of steps, many of the beneficial small molecules are reabsorbed into the blood and recycled by the body, so only the stuff the body really doesn't want ends up in the urine.

How damage occurs. Even when BG levels are normal, some nephrons become damaged with age; after age forty, we lose about 10 percent of our nephrons every ten years. But that doesn't make much difference because we have a lot more nephrons than we really need, so the damage is often not apparent until 80 percent of the nephrons have been damaged.

When BG levels remain high for a long time, this degeneration is much faster than normal. It is thought that **AGEs** (*advanced glycation end products*) contribute to the changes (see later in this chapter). The basement membrane gets thicker. The negative charges are lost. Just as happens in the retina of the eye, the capillaries become leaky, and they start letting proteins escape into the urine. When tiny amounts of the protein albumin can be detected in the urine, a state called *microalbuminuria* (meaning "tiny amounts of albumin in the urine"), this is a sign that the nephrons are showing damage.

Cells between the capillaries called *mesangial cells* begin to proliferate until they squeeze the capillaries and increase the capillary blood pressure. Eventually, the capillaries become completely blocked and can't do their job at all. Essentially, what was formerly an exquisitely engineered waste-processing plant has been turned into a mass of scar tissue.

High blood pressure makes the damage to the nephrons worse, so controlling blood pressure, especially with drugs called **ACE** (*angiotensin-converting enzyme*) **inhibitors** or the related **ARBs** (*angiotensin receptor blockers*), is a good way to reduce the probability that you'll ever develop nephropathy and a good way to minimize the damage if it's already begun. High cholesterol levels and smoking also increase the damage. The other important thing to do is to bring your BG levels to normal levels as soon as the microalbuminuria is detected.

Neuropathy can be painful

Neuropathy means damage to the nerves. Like damage to the kidneys and eyes, neuropathy is much more likely to occur when your BG levels have been high for many years. However, about 20 percent of people with type 2 diabetes already have signs of early neuropathy when they're diagnosed, and sometimes the neuropathy is what brings them to the doctor in the first place.

Peripheral neuropathy. No one is sure exactly how the nerve damage occurs. It may be from direct damage to the nerves or from damage to the blood vessels supplying the nerves, or both. What is called **peripheral neuropathy** is the most common form and involves damage to the nerves of the hands and feet, especially the feet. You may feel tingling, burning, or prickling in your feet, especially at night and in the winter. Drinking alcohol can make the pain worse. Sometimes the feet are so sensitive that even the pressure from blankets causes pain.

Luckily, this early stage of neuropathy can usually be reversed by bringing your BG levels back to near-normal levels. As you improve your control, the pain in your feet may get worse at first. Don't worry about this. It just means the nerves are healing and are better able to feel pain. This increased pain should be temporary.

If you don't improve your control, the neuropathy will progress, the pain will eventually subside, and your feet will become numb, unable to feel pain at all. At this point, the nerves are probably dead, and bringing your BG levels back to normal probably won't make the feeling return. You might think this would be a relief, but actually it's a great danger. Without feeling in your feet, things like splinters or calluses can go unnoticed and turn into ulcers that are difficult to heal.

Note that if you do have neuropathy and the pain is so bad that you need medication, the doctor may prescribe a type of antidepressant. Don't worry. The doctor isn't implying that your pain is psychological. Some antidepressants reduce the pain of neuropathy by a mechanism unrelated to their antidepressant effect.

Having diabetes makes all your nerves more sensitive to damage from other causes. For example, people with diabetes are twice as likely to have *carpal tunnel syndrome*, which is caused by pressure on the nerves going into the hand, often by repetitive actions. People without diabetes also get carpal tunnel syndrome, but not as easily.

Motor neuropathy. The damage I've mentioned so far is damage to *sensory nerves*, the nerves that allow you to feel sensations of hot, cold, pain, and so forth. The *motor nerves*, which make your muscles move, can also be damaged, although this is less common.

Autonomic neuropathy. High BG levels can also damage what are called *autonomic nerves*, the nerves responsible for all the actions that the body carries out automatically, without conscious effort, for example, breathing, beating of the heart, and digestion. This is called (surprise) *autonomic neuropathy*. It can cause problems with bladder emptying, sexual functions, digestion, sweating, and control of the heartbeat. Autonomic neuropathy usually occurs after sensory neuropathy, but if you have a lot of neuropathy in your extremities, you may have some autonomic neuropathy as well. The HRV test (see Week 2) can test for autonomic neuropathy.

When autonomic neuropathy affects the heart, it may not speed up or slow down properly, or the rhythm may be out of whack. Sometimes the typical symptoms of heart attack are absent, so you might think a heart attack was something else.

Gastroparesis. A common result of autonomic neuropathy to the *vagus nerve* is *gastroparesis*, or slow emptying of the stomach. This is especially dangerous if you're taking sulfonylureas or injecting insulin, as you take a certain amount based on when you expect the food to be digested. If the food doesn't leave the stomach on time, the drugs will make you go low. If then the food is suddenly dumped, you'll go too high.

Even if you're not using insulin, gastroparesis can cause what appear to be random fluctuations in your BG levels that you can't explain. If you also feel full after eating very small meals and have a lot of indigestion, nausea, and maybe constipation or diarrhea that you can't explain, ask your doctor about the possibility of gastroparesis. There are drugs that help with this, as does eating small meals with very little fat or fiber.

If you have neuropathy in your extremities, there's a good chance you have some early signs of gastroparesis, so be alert for them.

Other neuropathies. Autonomic neuropathy can also cause changes in the way you sweat, with very dry feet that tend to crack and increased sweating in the face.

Unfortunately, another possible type of neuropathy in men is impotence. Because there are many other possible causes of impotence, including psychological ones, you can't assume that it stems from neuropathy without excluding those other causes. Again, high BG levels increase the probability of impotence, so do what you can to keep them in the normal ranges. In women, autonomic neuropathy can cause a decrease in lubrication.

Some complications are not unique to people with diabetes

Some conditions are not unique to people with diabetes, but they are more common. These include yeast and other fungal infections; thickened skin; Dupuytren's contracture, a thickening of tendons in the hand that causes a finger to refuse to straighten out; and frozen shoulder. Some skin conditions include a flushed face that returns to normal when BG levels are controlled and yellowish skin that may result from AGE formation.

Macrovascular complications can be lethal

Macrovascular complications are those related to the larger blood vessels and include heart attacks, strokes, and *peripheral vascular disease*, which can be lumped together as *cardiovascular disease*. Most people with type 2 diabetes will eventually die from cardiovascular disease. If this sounds grim, remember that most people will eventually die from something or other; your high risk factors for cardiovascular disease are like an early warning system, letting you know where you should focus your preventive actions.

Macrovascular complications can be reduced by keeping your BG levels close to normal, but not as much as microvascular ones. One reason may be that much of the damage from the insulin resistance (IR) that is usually the cause of type 2 diabetes has already occurred by the time you are diagnosed and can't be easily reversed.

Cardiovascular disease is not limited to people with diabetes. When you have all the symptoms associated with type 2 diabetes except high BG levels (IR, an apple shape, high blood pressure, high levels of triglycerides, low levels of HDL, normal or only slightly elevated levels of LDL), this is called *metabolic syndrome*, *Syndrome X*, or *insulin-resistance syndrome*, and I discussed the details in Month 6. Treatment for cardiovascular risk factors is similar in diabetic and nondiabetic people. However, because of the increased risks, it's a good idea to try to keep your cholesterol levels and blood pressure a little lower than you would if you didn't have those additional risks.

Plan ahead for pregnancy

Pregnancy isn't really a complication of diabetes, unless you happen to meet your sweetie at a diabetes support group. But it can complicate your control.

Because type 2 diabetes is usually diagnosed in older people, most of you probably won't have to deal with this complication. But more and more young people are being diagnosed with the disease and need to know of the potential problems.

The important thing to know is that high BG levels or high ketone levels *early in pregnancy* can cause birth defects, so it's essential to plan your pregnancy ahead of time and make sure you're in excellent control before conception and in the early months. This would be a good time to see an endocrinologist if you haven't already done so, or an obstetrician who is experienced treating people with diabetes.

The other important thing to keep in mind is that many drugs can harm the fetus, so if you're taking oral diabetes drugs, you need to switch to insulin before you become pregnant. IR goes up two or three times in late pregnancy, so you may need insulin at that time even if you were controlling with diet and exercise alone before you became pregnant. Once the baby is born, the IR returns to prepregnancy levels.

Some other drugs such as ACE inhibitors for kidney problems may also damage the fetus, and other drugs should be substituted. Again, plan ahead and stop taking any potentially damaging drugs *before* you get pregnant. This includes caffeine and alcohol.

If you already have any eye or kidney damage, it may become worse during the pregnancy but usually returns to former levels after the baby is born.

With planning and normal BG levels, you should have just about the same chances of having a normal baby as someone without diabetes. If you're male, your diabetes shouldn't affect the outcome of the pregnancy. Type 2 diabetes has a strong genetic component, so your children will be at increased risk. However, knowing that ahead of time should help them keep their diabetes genes under control by exercising regularly and moderating their consumption of processed carbohydrates and saturated fat.

There may be several causes of complications

No one is sure exactly what causes diabetic complications. However, it's quite clear that high BG levels are a major factor. As mentioned in Day 6, several long-term studies of people with both type 1 and type 2 diabetes proved without a doubt that keeping your BG levels down will reduce the statistical probability that you will develop diabetic complications.

Table 2 in Day 6 shows the relationship between BG levels and retinopathy. Risks of other complications are reduced in a similar way. It's quite clear that keeping your BG levels down gives you just about the same risk of developing complications as someone who doesn't have diabetes. Letting your BG levels stay high almost ensures that you will eventually have problems. And remember that type 2 diabetes develops slowly, so you may already have had high BG levels for several years, or even more, before you were diagnosed.

It's not very surprising that scientists haven't figured out the exact mechanisms of diabetes complications yet even though so many people develop them. They haven't figured out the exact mechanisms of aging yet either, and 100 percent of people age, if they live long enough. In some ways, diabetes simply accelerates the normal aging process.

One way high BG levels are thought to cause complications is by means of AGEs. Everyone's blood contains some glucose. If you heat glucose with proteins at a very high temperature, you get what scientists call the *Maillard reaction*; others call it *browning*. That's what happens when you brown beef in a frying pan. Even at normal BG concentrations and normal temperatures, glucose reacts slowly with many of the proteins in your body in a similar reaction, forming AGEs. When your BG levels are high, more AGEs are formed.

Smoking can cause the formation of AGEs. And you can also get AGEs from your food. Some research has suggested that even these ingested AGEs can cause problems.

Cooks often treat food in ways that encourage browning, such as frying or roasting at high temperatures to encourage browning of the outer layers of meat. Broiling also results in browning, and broiled poultry skin is especially high in AGEs (more than a hundredfold higher than when uncooked).

Adding a sugary sauce, for example, barbecue sauce, to meat before cooking causes even more browning. Even bread crusts include some AGEs, as does roasted coffee. On the other hand, moisture discourages the formation of AGEs, so boiled foods don't contain very many. But microwaving food produces AGEs even when the foods don't turn brown. Warming milk in the microwave, for example, increases the AGE level by two or three times.

Browning reactions tend to improve the flavor of food, and not only good cooks but Western food manufacturers have taken advantage of this fact to increase the appeal of food by encouraging browning, for example, by adding sugar to crusts and sauces so they'll brown more.

Studies have shown that when you feed human volunteers foods that are high in AGEs, the levels of AGEs in their blood increase dramatically. In people with normal kidney function, many of the AGEs are excreted in the urine, but some remain. There are receptors for AGEs called *RAGE* that bind the AGEs and cause oxidative stress. Other receptors called *AGE-R1* bind the AGEs and help to detoxify and eliminate them. The balance between receptor types is important, and when there are too many AGEs, the balance in this complex system can be disrupted.

When researchers fed diabetes-prone mice a low-AGE diet, 60 percent of the mice were diabetes-free after fourteen months. But when they fed another group of mice regular feed that included ten times more AGEs, more than 90 percent of the mice developed diabetes within three months. Another study showed that a low-AGE diet resulted in a decrease in IR.

AGEs may be one cause of aging, and thus when your BG levels are high, you're causing accelerated aging.

In diabetic cataracts, it is believed that high glucose levels inside the lens of the eye cause the formation of the sugar alcohol *sorbitol*. This reaction is catalyzed by an enzyme called **aldose reductase**. The sorbitol can't get out of the lens again and draws in water, so the lens swells. Note that eating sorbitol isn't apt to cause cataracts. When you eat sorbitol, it is converted to fructose in the liver.

There is some evidence that sorbitol in nerve tissue contributes to nerve damage, but not primarily by causing swelling. In this case, the sorbitol may somehow keep a compound called *myo-inositol*, which is important for membrane function, from entering the nerve cell, which doesn't conduct current as well as a result.

Aldose reductase inhibitors have been able to improve some complications including nerve function and cataracts, but serious side effects have been reported, and at the time of this writing none have been approved by the Food and Drug Administration.

Free radicals may contribute to diabetic complications. Other mechanisms may cause complications, but they are not well understood. One seems to involve a particular form of a protein called *protein kinase C*. Another pathway thought to be involved with complications is the *hexosamine pathway*. Unless you're a biochemist, you needn't worry about what all these pathways involve, just that there are thought to be several ways in which diabetes can cause complications.

One compound, *benfotiamine*, which is a fat-soluble derivative of the vitamin thiamine, has been shown to inhibit four of the major pathways thought to cause complications in model systems (rodents and cell cultures). Like alpha-lipoic acid, benfotiamine has been used for some years in Germany to treat neuropathy. However, it is not yet in general use to prevent diabetic complications in humans. And because it's fat soluble, it could be harmful in excess, like the fat-soluble vitamins A and E.

Other compounds seem to reduce the formation of AGEs, and some can even break down the AGEs after they've been formed. These include *pyridoxamine*, which is a form of vitamin B$_6$; *aminoguanidine*; and *ALT-711*. These have been studied in model systems, where they seemed to show benefits. However, studies in humans are preliminary, and the drugs could prove to be toxic with regular use. Several companies that were researching such drugs have abandoned the projects. The diabetes drug *metformin*, the *ACE inhibitors* and the related *ARBs*, *carnosine*, *D-penicillamine*, and *vitamins C, E,* and *A* have also been reported to reduce the formation of AGEs.

No one understands why some people get complications and others do not. Some people can have high A1c results for years and never have serious complications, whereas others have much lower A1c's and still develop complications. Some ethnic groups like Native Americans, Hispanic Americans, and African Americans seem to be more prone to developing microvascular complications.

Be in charge

When discussing complications and testing for early signs, many books on diabetes say things like, "Your doctor will check you for this regularly." But in fact, many doctors *won't* check you regularly, especially when you belong to a health maintenance organization that is concerned with keeping costs down.

So it's up to you to understand which complications you think you're at most risk for and to make sure your doctor orders the appropriate tests.

It's also up to you to make sure you keep your BG levels close to normal so the risks will be low or, if you already had some complications when you were diagnosed, the complications can be reversed as much as possible.

IN A SENTENCE:

■ *High blood glucose levels can cause diabetic complications, but microvascular complications can usually be controlled or even reversed if you are alert for their symptoms and seek early treatment.*

Diet Wars:
Getting Beyond the Hype

Diet and exercise are the cornerstones of treatment of type 2 diabetes, even if you are also using oral drugs or insulin. Everyone agrees that if you have type 2 diabetes you should "eat healthy." The problem is, no one can agree on what healthy eating is. No topic raises more passion than a discussion of dietary prescriptions for people with diabetes—or, for that matter, without.

Diet gurus push their agendas

Some of the popular diet books would have you believe that if you follow their diet, you'll cure everything that ails you. The authors tend to cite all the evidence that supports their point of view and ignore all the evidence that doesn't.

For example, it has been found that many groups of people who switch from a traditional way of life that includes a lot of hard work and an adequate but not excessive diet develop diabetes when they move to the city and adopt a so-called civilized way of life. This usually includes a lot less physical labor and a varied diet that includes a lot more calories, including both more fat and more processed carbohydrate.

Proponents of low-fat diets cite people like the Bantu, who traditionally had a low-fat, high-carbohydrate diet and say, "See, these people didn't eat a lot of fat until they moved to the city and adopted Western high-fat diets and got diabetes. Therefore, fat causes diabetes."

Proponents of low-carbohydrate diets cite people like the Eskimos or Yemenite Jews, who traditionally had a high-protein, low-carbohydrate diet, and say, "See, these people didn't eat a lot of carbohydrates until they adopted Western high-carbohydrate diets and got diabetes. Therefore, carbohydrates cause diabetes."

Like politicians, various popular diet authors sometimes seem so busy pushing their own agendas that they don't have time to listen to each other or cooperate in trying to reach the truth. For example, in February 2000 the US Department of Agriculture sponsored what was called "The Great Nutrition Debate," at which authors of the leading diet books and representatives from government agencies were given a few minutes to present their cases. Reading a transcript of the debate, I got the feeling they were all wearing earplugs when the other people were speaking.

Dietary prescriptions seem to yo-yo from low carbohydrate to high carbohydrate back to low carb. In 2015, the trend is more and more toward low-carbohydrate diets for people with diabetes. But we still have no long-term studies of the success of *any* dietary approach.

As always, the diet that has the most popular support may not be the best diet for you. A good approach is to start with a low-carbohydrate diet and test its effects on your weight, your hunger levels, your BG levels, and your budget. If it works, that's wonderful; stick with it. If not, try tweaking it in one way or another until you find a diet that controls your diabetes and also allows you to enjoy life.

Just remember to give a new dietary approach time before you conclude that it doesn't work. When I first gave up bread, I really missed it. Now I don't give a hoot about baked goods and can walk into a bakery without being tempted in the slightest.

Never rely on just one author's interpretation of the limited studies that have been done so far. The important thing is how any diet affects you.

Evaluate blood glucose and lipid control as well as weight loss

When you read about various types of diets, keep in mind that when the writers in the popular press discuss a *diet*, what they usually mean is a *weight-loss diet*. When they evaluate a diet, they are evaluating how well it works to make you lose weight. They are not evaluating how well it controls diabetes.

One standard criticism of the more extreme diets, for example, very low fat or low-carbohydrate diets, is that "no one could stick to a diet like this for more than a month or so." Although that might be true for someone dieting simply to get into a smaller size of jeans by the next high school reunion, for anyone with serious health problems, those criticisms are no more valid than saying a person with high blood pressure wouldn't be able to give up salt for more than a month or so. Giving up butter or giving up bread is better than giving up your eyesight and your feet. In the old days, people with diabetes had to weigh their food, and they followed such rigid regimes for years.

Weight loss usually does reduce insulin resistance (IR). However, you should never forget that controlling your blood glucose (BG) levels is more important than losing weight. If you found some nutso diet that made you lose weight but also made your BG levels stay around 300 mg/dL (milligrams per deciliter) all day, this would not be a good diet for you. The reduction in IR from the weight loss would not balance the damage you'd have from the high BG levels.

Because you are at increased risk for heart disease, you also need to evaluate the effects of any diet on various lipid levels, including LDL, HDL, and triglycerides. As tests for new heart-disease risk factors become common, you must evaluate the effects of the various diets on these factors as well.

So if you want to try a new dietary approach, keep testing your BG levels before and after meals and keep track of your A1c and blood lipid levels before you settle on a particular diet for life.

Don't rely on the popular press.

Keep in mind amounts versus percentages

Most diets are described in terms of the percentages of carbohydrate, fat, and protein (see Day 3) that they allow, and they are often labeled according to these percentages as "high this" or "low that."

But percentages aren't the same as amounts. For example, the American Heart Association (AHA) recommends a diet that contains 30 percent fat or less. You've probably always been a big eater, and let's say that before your diagnosis you were eating 3,000 calories a day. That means you could have been eating a "perfect" AHA diet and guzzling 900 calories (100 grams) of fat a day.

Now let's say you go on a strict diet and eat only 1,500 calories a day, limiting your fat intake to 675 calories (75 grams) a day. In this case, you'd be eating less fat, but it would represent 45 percent of your total caloric intake. So even though you'd now be eating less fat than before, some people would castigate you for your "increased" fat intake.

The same is true of protein. When people are limiting calories, some so-called **high-protein diets** actually contain smaller *amounts* of protein than the average American eats, yet because the *percentage* of protein is higher, the diets continue to be criticized on the theory that eating a lot of protein could damage the kidneys (see later).

This is also true of carbohydrate foods. If you're not eating a lot of calories, even though the carbohydrate percentages may be high, on a "high-carbohydrate" diet, the amounts may be relatively low compared with what you were eating before. This is particularly true if you're eating low-glycemic-index foods that are rich in fiber.

Don't be swayed by popular labels such as "high-carbohydrate diet" or "high-protein diet."

All the diets make you eat less

I described various diet approaches on Day 4. Despite claims about their miraculous properties, most weight-loss diets work by tricking you into eating fewer calories, and some studies have shown that people lose weight at about the same rate no matter which approach they take. Let's look at how this works.

Exchange diets. The *exchange diets* are the most obvious. You are given a certain number of exchanges that total a certain number of calories, depending on your size and goal weight. As long as you stick to the prescribed exchanges, your calories will be controlled.

Low-fat diets. With the *low-fat, high-carbohydrate diet*, sometimes you don't need to count calories, but because carbohydrates have only four calories per gram and fats have nine calories per gram, when you eat a lot of carbohydrate, you're eating fewer calories with an equal amount of food. You feel full sooner and tend to eat less.

Low-glycemic-index diets. Low-glycemic-index foods are usually high in indigestible fiber. Most *low-glycemic-index diets* also emphasize substituting the low-glycemic carbohydrates for fats, and the low-glycemic-index foods have even greater bulk for the number of calories they contain and fill you up even sooner. Again, the net result is eating fewer calories.

Low-carbohydrate diets. *Low-carbohydrate diets* work another way. Eating a lot of fat makes many people slightly nauseous. Most people can imagine downing stacks of pancakes or bagels, but the thought of eating several sticks of butter or drinking a cup of olive oil doesn't have the same appeal. So when you're allowed to eat all the fatty meat and cheese you want, most people automatically limit the amount they eat, especially after a few days. In addition, low-carbohydrate diets cause *ketosis*, and ketones in the blood also cause people to lose their appetite. The mild ketosis caused by eating very few carbohydrates or burning a lot of fat occurs when BG levels are normal and is not the same as *ketoacidosis* (see Month 2), which is a serious condition that occurs when BG levels are high. As long as your pancreas is able to produce some insulin, the insulin will slow down the production of ketones before they cause acidosis.

Note that the appetite-reducing effect of low-carbohydrate diets lasts longer than the full-stomach appetite control of high-bulk diets. With the latter, you may feel full right after eating, but without fat to slow the emptying of the stomach, you may be ravenous three or so hours later.

Food-combining diets. Weight-loss diets that prohibit combining certain foods also result in eating fewer calories. For instance, one such diet says not to eat protein and starch at the same meal. So instead of eating meat and potatoes for lunch and dinner, you eat meat and green vegetables for lunch, and potatoes and green vegetables for dinner. Net result: you've substituted low-calorie green vegetables for high-calorie potatoes and meat.

One-food diets. Real fad diets such as those that limit your intake to one or two foods make you eat less because you quickly become bored with those foods. It's having a variety of foods available that makes most people eat too much. You probably remember trying to explain to your mother when you were a child why you were too full to finish your spinach, but your appetite miraculously reappeared as soon as she brought out the chocolate cake. One man told his mother he had a separate stomach for dessert.

Apparently rodents have the same problem. Some studies have shown that mice that are genetically engineered to gain weight easily do so only when offered "cafeteria diets," meaning foods with different tastes. When offered nothing but ordinary mouse chow, they don't eat as much and remain normal weight. This is a good example of the fact that like type 2 diabetes, obesity often has both a genetic and an environmental component. In order to be overweight you usually need both the genes that predispose you to easy weight gain and an environment in which there is a bountiful, varied food supply.

Complex theories. Diet books may cite complicated theories of why their diets allow weight loss with no effort on your part, but in general they simply get you to eat less food. Eating less food is a good thing. As I discussed in Month 8, often simply reducing your caloric intake will help reduce your BG levels, even if you don't lose weight. So if one of the popular approaches works for you *and doesn't result in an increase in your BG levels,* that's the way for you.

Don't be influenced by complex theories of how a particular diet will let you lose weight while eating all you want.

Dietary misunderstandings are common

Many things you'll read in diet books are based on truth. But sometimes they're only half-truths that have become garbled with time. Following are a few examples of this.

If a carbohydrate isn't a sugar, it's "complex." For many years, doctors and dieticians urged people with diabetes to eat a lot of so-called complex carbohydrates (meaning *polysaccharides*; see Day 3). They explained that "simple sugars" like sucrose were quickly broken down by the body and raised the BG level quickly. Instead they told people to eat a lot of complex carbohydrates like potatoes and rice, because the big molecules were supposed to be broken down slowly and raise the BG levels slowly.

Why no one thought to test this idea is beyond me, but they didn't. Then someone realized that in fact starch is digested so quickly that it raises the BG level as fast as sucrose (table sugar)—in fact a little faster, because starch is all glucose, and sucrose is only half glucose, the other half consisting of the sugar fructose, which doesn't raise BG levels as fast.

Nevertheless, many health-care people continued to urge people to eat more complex carbohydrates, and a few still do. Some dealt with this situation by redefining complex carbohydrate to mean slowly digested (low-glycemic-index) carbohydrates, such as those bound up with a lot of fiber, and not high-glycemic-index carbohydrates, such as the starch found in potato or white bread. Others urge that we dump the term *complex carbohydrate* altogether and refer to dietary carbohydrates by their formal names: *monosaccharides* and *disaccharides* (which can both be called *sugars*) and *polysaccharides* (or, more specifically, *starch* and *fiber*, depending on whether or not it can be digested by humans).

Protein is bad for kidneys. Another oft-cited half-truth concerns the effect of low-carbohydrate diets on kidneys. Many dieticians frown on low-carbohydrate diets because they say high-protein diets (meaning high *percentages*) are damaging to kidneys.

Most everyone agrees that a high-protein diet is not good for kidneys that show some signs of damage. But in those without kidney damage, there is no published evidence that a high-protein diet causes damage. Body builders eat large amounts of proteins, and there is no evidence that doing so harms their kidneys.

A low-fat diet gives you license to eat all the carbohydrate you want. Another misconception concerns low-fat diets like the famous US Department of Agriculture's **food pyramid**, which many of you learned about in school. The pyramid has morphed into MyPlate, with slightly less emphasis on carbohydrate. But it continues to prescribe lean meat and low-fat dairy and advises limiting fats. Some people think, "If I don't eat fat, I can eat all the carbohydrate I want." In fact, MyPlate, like the old food pyramid, limits carbohydrate, the recommended amount depending om your age, activity level, and sex. So MyPlate is really a calorie-restricted exchange-type diet. If you follow it, you'll probably lose weight because you're eating fewer total calories, not because you're eating a lot of carbohydrate.

A low-carbohydrate diet gives you license to eat all the fat you want. If you are large and need a lot of calories to maintain your weight, you may be able to eat all you want on a low-carbohydrate diet and still lose weight, because you may lose your appetite after eating a lot of fatty foods. But if you're small and your caloric needs are also small, you may have to pay attention to how much you eat on this kind of diet if you want to lose weight as well as keep your BG levels down. One of the popular low-carbohydrate diets (*Protein Power*) even mentions this, but they do so in a footnote, in tiny type, so some readers may not notice.

Carbohydrate is good for diabetes. Some dieticians still prescribe a "heart-healthy" low-fat diet with about 60 percent of the calories coming from carbohydrate, although recommended carbohydrate amounts seem to be decreasing. You may recall the rationale for this diet. Having diabetes, you are already at increased risk of heart disease. The standard American diet, which tends to contain a lot of fat, is associated with a higher risk of heart disease.

Hence the real reason for promoting this diet is to **reduce your fat intake, not increase your carbohydrate intake.** The carbohydrate content is high because you have to replace the fat calories with something, and many dieticians are taught that too much protein is bad. The only thing left is carbohydrate. The carbohydrate does increase your *postprandial* BG levels, but people endorsing this diet think that's not as important as eating less fat.

Unfortunately, the basic message is sometimes garbled. Instead of telling you to eat less fat, some dieticians may tell you to eat more carbohydrate. Some people say they go to their dietician complaining that their BG levels are too high, and the dietician tells them to add more carbohydrate to the diet. After getting this type of advice, Bobbie K. used to eat the same dinner she'd always eaten and then *add* extra bread or potato. "Gotta get my carbs."

Current recommendations *do* distinguish between "fast," or high-glycemic-index carbohydrates like white bread and white flour and low-glycemic-index carbohydrates like whole grains or broccoli and recommend eating more of the latter. Early studies that showed that low-fat, high-carbohydrate diets could reduce IR in people with diabetes used low-glycemic-index, high-fiber carbohydrates. Somehow the message that "carbohydrates are good" got through, and the message that "they should be unprocessed and high in fiber" got lost and is now being rediscovered.

If it's popular, it's a fad diet. After years of being told to avoid fat like the plague, many people are now going to the other extreme and avoiding carbohydrates in order to lose weight. These diets are now very popular, and in that sense they are fad diets.

Critics say things like, "The only reason people try these diets is because they give them an excuse to eat the fatty foods they love, like roast beef and whipped cream." This makes as much sense as saying, "The only reason people go on low-fat diets is to give them an excuse to eat the starchy foods they love, like spaghetti and freshly baked bread."

When you have diabetes, you need to choose the diet that will do the best job of keeping your BG and lipid levels close to normal. If a low-fat or a low-carbohydrate diet or some mixture of the two does this for you, it's a medically necessary diet for you. It's not a fad diet. Don't let the knee-jerk critics influence your choice.

Low-carbohydrate diets lack nutrients. Critics of low-carbohydrate diets for weight loss often say they are devoid of the important nutrients you get in fresh fruits and vegetables. The media often describe these diets as consisting of nothing but fatty meat, cheese, and whipped cream.

Those using such diets simply to lose weight might, in fact, take them to these extremes. If you have diabetes, you are in this for the long run and should be more interested in nutrition and variety than in superquick weight loss.

Such diets do not usually prohibit fruits and vegetables, just those that are high in sugar and starch. You can eat nutritious green leafy vegetables and reasonable amounts of high-fiber vegetables such as broccoli and cauliflower and even small amounts of fiber-rich fruits such as berries. In fact, the produce eaten on such diets is often more dense in nutrients than the starch-filled ones prescribed in low-fat diets.

Learn to analyze the claims

When you have diabetes, you need to understand diet and nutrition better than most people, even some experts. With experience, you can evaluate the effect of a particular diet on your own particular physiology better than any diet analysts.

IN A SENTENCE:

■ *Diet book authors don't agree on what is the best diet for people with diabetes, so you'll have to learn to find the truth beyond the hype.*

MONTH **11**

Burnout

Many people work through a period of depression after their diagnosis (see Week 4) and then move on, focusing on the positive things in their lives.

Unfortunately, however, this does not mean that depression has gone from your life forever. After many months, or years, of dealing with diabetes, many people suffer a bout of secondary depression, or "diabetes burnout." You probably won't reach this point in your first year, but you should know that it may lie ahead and not be surprised if it occurs.

You can't sell out

One problem with diabetes is that it's relentless. Like the farmer who has to milk the cows twice a day 365 days a year whether healthy or sick, whether holiday or none, you never get any time off. You have to deal with controlling blood glucos (BG) levels twenty-four hours a day, seven days a week. It never stops. And unlike the farmer, you have no choice. You can't sell your diabetes at an auction.

Some people quickly accept the diagnosis and the challenge ahead and work incredibly hard to control their BG levels. They go on a strict diet and lose a lot of weight. They start exercising and develop muscles they hadn't used in years. Their A1c levels drop into normal levels. They are enthusiastic and preach the rewards of taking charge to the newly diagnosed.

Then one day after several years of this good control, they just get tired of it all: the constant testing, the constant deprivation, the tantalizing treats they can't have, all those medical appointments, the extra expenses of it all, and, most of all, the fact that there are no vacations from this rigid routine.

"Mostly I'm just kind of, for lack of a better word, *disenchanted* with the whole thing," said Fran R. "For all practical purposes I'd have to honestly say I've back-burnered the diabetes and lost the desire to test, and exercise has gone by the wayside in my busy life with work, kids, dog, etc. I keep thinking I'll 'snap out of it,' but I think I felt really discouraged with the months of 180-something morning highs and that kind of thing. I *know* all about the horrendous complications that can happen, and it just seems getting the routine of exercise and trying to lose weight have been, well . . . so damned hard."

Remember the second fantasy in Day 2, that your diabetes would suddenly disappear. Many people carry this fantasy for years. Unfortunately, this tendency is encouraged by some members of the medical profession, who tell you that if you would just lose a little weight, your diabetes might go away. "Sometimes just five or ten pounds will make a difference."

As described in Month 8, weight loss can normalize BG levels, especially if the diabetes is diagnosed in the very early stages. But that's not universal, because most people aren't diagnosed until their BG levels are fairly high. Weight loss can help with insulin resistance (IR), but usually once your BG levels get high enough for you to be diagnosed, about 50 to 80 percent of your pancreas has been destroyed, and no matter how much weight you lose you'll always have trouble with BG control. Feeling betrayed, promised something that didn't happen after you worked so hard to do what they said would help, can contribute to burnout.

Diabetes doesn't show

Always feeling different, always having to explain can also cause you to suffer burnout. Diabetes doesn't show. It's not like you are in a wheelchair or have a cast on your arm. If you've lost weight and gotten a lot of exercise, you probably look a lot healthier than before you were diagnosed. It's difficult for people to remember that you have a disease.

"I just got some delicious cheesecake from a friend in New York. Why don't you come over and share it with me?" or "Would you like a cookie? I baked them myself." Even your best friends may make offers like this, and once again you have to explain that you can't (or won't) have those things. "Oh yes, I forgot."

Each time a friend describes in tantalizing detail the extra-rich chocolate pie someone made for a birthday, you are reminded once more that you are different. You can't eat that stuff. You know they don't do it on purpose. Diabetes doesn't show, so they forget you're sick.

"We don't look or most of the time act as though anything is wrong with us," said Barbara F. "Plus, most of the time we don't even notice what other people are eating, and they don't notice what we're eating. Just once in a while it hits. Chet invariably comes to wherever I am to eat his afternoon snack. Most of the time I don't notice or it doesn't bother me. But once in a while it really gets to me. This afternoon he was eating a brownie, which he consumed in about three bites, hardly tasting it. I had to get up and walk away. I really wanted just a bite, and I'd have let it roll around in my mouth just to enjoy the flavor. At the moment it seemed to me he was doing it on purpose just to make me suffer. I know that's not true. If he knew how it made me feel, he'd never do it again. The next time he eats a brownie, I won't even notice he's eating it."

Even those who remember that you have diabetes often don't understand the realities of the disease. Well-meaning friends or relatives may suggest that if you'd just take the right vitamins or supplements, "your little sugar problem" would go away. Or they'll say, "I saw on the news last night that eating fiber prevents diabetes," not realizing that what might statistically reduce the chances of getting diabetes is not going to cure it once most of your pancreas has been destroyed.

Others won't understand the reality of being on a restrictive diet for the rest of your life. "I did Weight Watchers for six months, and it wasn't so bad," someone might say when you are feeling down about having to yet again miss out on an exotic Asian rice dish at a potluck supper. Of course diets are never fun, but most people dieting for weight loss expect to see light at the end of the tunnel. Your diet will never end.

Sometimes it all seems overwhelming

Sometimes all these little things seem to happen all at once, and suddenly the depression that you overcame after the diagnosis returns. It all just seems overwhelming. You want the diabetes to go away.

Again, the solution is time, getting in touch with people who understand, and venting your frustrations. I tend to be like Mary Mary, Quite Contrary. If someone tries to tell me diabetes is no big deal, it's better than having brain cancer, I'll feel they don't understand, get grumpy, and go home and whine a lot. But if they do something thoughtful, like making sure there's something I can eat at their party, then I'm so touched by their caring that I realize diabetes really isn't that much of an extra burden and many of my friends are dealing with things that are much worse. Then I can get on with my life.

As with so many other aspects of life, you want to be understood. If your friends and relatives take the time to listen and understand, you may be able to minimize the number of times you are blue. If they won't, try to find people who do understand and share with them. "Maybe I just need to whine and vent now and then, then turn around and just get on with it, eh?" Bexie G. concluded after venting on an email list.

Set an example

If things suddenly seem like too much and you can't get motivated to keep good control even though you know it will make you feel better, think of the others in your life. Taking care of your diabetes will set a good example in case they ever develop the disease. We all know someone who had a diabetic Uncle Denial who refused to change his diet or drinking habits and lost both his legs and went blind and sat in a wheelchair listening to the radio until kidney failure did him in. The fear that you'll end up like Uncle Den may be one reason for denying your diagnosis at first or feeling it's not worth the effort to control your diabetes because his fate is inevitable.

Now you have a chance to change that image for your children and your grandchildren and all your friends as well. Imagine that one of your nephews is diagnosed with diabetes in twenty years. Maybe instead of feeling that things are hopeless, he'll think of Uncle Moderation, who took good care of his diabetes and had no side effects and kept active and healthy for a long time—and still is. Instead of denying his disease, he might come to you for advice, ask how it is that you are managing to control so well and to lead such a normal, active life.

Others often aren't interested

When you find out what a bother it is to have diabetes, you most likely want to do what you can to prevent the disease in other people, especially close friends and relatives. You may often think, "If only I'd known then what I know now about the dangers of 'slightly elevated' BG levels and diets high in processed carbohydrate and fat, I could have done something to prevent this thing from ever progressing so far." You'd like to educate others, to warn them.

Unfortunately, in most cases, you'll find they're not interested. In teenagers, this is no surprise. Teenagers almost always think they're immortal, that nothing bad will ever happen to them. But you'll probably find pretty much the same reaction in others you try to warn. Diabetes is your problem. It won't happen to them. If you keep preaching and talking about it, they'll get bored with the topic and tell you to get a life.

Whatever you do, don't nag. If you tell young people that if they eat too many sweets they'll get fat and get diabetes when they're older, then if they do get diabetes when they're older, they'll always feel guilty about it. They'll feel that it's all their fault, even though they know it's partly genetic and eating sugar doesn't cause the disease.

That happened to Natalie S. "I was raised with the admonishment (from *all* of the older generations) 'Don't eat that, you'll get fat and you'll get diabetes!' I remember thinking, as a teenager and young adult, 'The hell you say!!' And when I was indeed diagnosed with diabetes, I could hear all those voices saying, 'I told you so!!!!!' I spent my whole first visit with a CDE and dietitian bawling my eyes out. The ironic thing is that, in my family, diabetes is *not* associated with obesity. But the voices had done their dirty work, and I still struggle with feelings of guilt and self-blame. The media certainly tries to reinforce the guilt trip too, implying that by keeping your weight down, or losing weight, you can prevent diabetes."

The only thing you can really do to help is to be there if they do ask and to stick to your diet and your exercise plans even when you're feeling blue. Who knows. Maybe if they notice that you're losing weight and feeling more energetic when you eat more vegetables and less pizza, they'll be tempted to try it themselves.

Don't stop testing

Another form of burnout is simply getting tired of pricking your fingers all the time. If you've done a lot of testing and you have a good idea of which foods keep your BG levels at near-normal levels and which kinds of exercise help you the most, and if your BG tests are usually where you'd expect them to be, you may decide it's not worth the trouble to test.

Then there's the trick of having something you know isn't good for you and "forgetting" to test afterward because you really don't want to know how much it made your BG level go up. This is human nature. Everyone does it. "I had a piece of chocolate and as far as I know, my blood sugar didn't go up at all—of course that could be because I didn't test."

As long as you do occasional spot checks at different times of the day, not testing as often after you've learned how different foods affect your control is usually OK. It's avoiding the spot checks too that can be dangerous.

Sometimes, without realizing it, you'll start eating just a little more of "problem foods," and then a little more, and a little more, until you've returned to your former eating patterns.

"I've gone through a couple periods of no testing," said Alex E. "I thought I might save some money by not testing every day. I was doing OK, so I skipped a day here, a day there. Then a few days at a time, and then all of a sudden, I'd gone three months without testing. And sure enough, my BGs had drifted back up. Once wasn't enough. I had to go through that twice."

Just be alert for this and try to do spot checks now and then. It's always easier to get back on the wagon when it isn't moving too fast.

Don't despair

Diabetes burnout and having the blues is, unfortunately, probably going to be an occasional companion as you learn to deal with this new way of life. Just understand that some initial mourning is normal, and burnout may crop up occasionally in the future. Don't despair. This is also normal. Take time out. Reevaluate. Spoil yourself. Connect with fellow travelers. This mood should pass, and you should soon be back in the saddle of diabetes control. Once you get control, it's really not as bad as it seemed at first. Life goes on. Enjoy it.

IN A SENTENCE:

■ *You may occasionally have to deal with diabetes burnout, but don't despair, the mood should pass.*

Diet Wars: Finding What Works for You

In the last Learning section I discussed how you can learn to get beyond the hype in the diet books. Now you need to learn how you can evaluate any particular diet's effect on your diabetes and weight loss.

Evaluate both short-term and long-term hunger

The high-carbohydrate diet supporters say that carbohydrate will fill you up sooner, and indeed, studies have shown that a boiled potato makes you feel full sooner than an equivalent number of calories eaten as fat. Some people have even worked out a *satiety index* that classifies foods according to how fast they fill you up, and carbohydrate foods lead the list. *Low-glycemic-index* carbohydrates tend to fill you up even more than other carbohydrates because they have more bulk and take longer to digest.

When you're taking hunger into consideration in choosing a diet, remember to consider how long that feeling of fullness will last. Some people find that high-carbohydrate diets (especially those with high-glycemic-index *processed carbohydrates*) make them feel stuffed for an hour or so, but then they get ravenously hungry. This may be especially true of people who have fluctuating blood glucose (BG) levels, that is, people with diabetes. Rapidly rising and falling levels of glucose or insulin or both may trigger hunger pangs as well as surges of *adrenaline*, which also stimulates hunger.

In Jennifer L.'s experience: "I could eat a pound of pasta (with the 'regulation' fat-free sauce) and an hour later be standing in the kitchen in front of the fridge, starving. Needing to eat something, anything. Unable to stop thinking about food. Feeling very, very, very hungry, even though my stomach was full."

Protein and fat leave the stomach more slowly and may keep the hunger pangs away for a longer period of time than carbohydrate, even if they don't fill you up quite as quickly. The same is true of low-glycemic-index carbohydrates such as lentils, high-fiber vegetables, and some beans. They are digested slowly and may keep your BG levels on an even keel.

"I chose to follow a lower-carb plan to control my BG," said Jennifer. "It worked. But more amazing to me was that those almost daily crave attacks disappeared completely. Entirely. At least for the last year and a half. I have had *none*. It is the first time in my forty years that I have not had these cravings. And for a person that had them daily, it's amazing."

Also try to figure out if your main problem is starting to eat (eating more often than usual because you're hungry all the time) or stopping eating (eating only at the normal times but eating a lot because you don't feel full). A diet that fixed one of these problems might not be as good for the other.

Pay attention to other short-term versus long-term effects

Sometimes when you try a new type of diet, you'll find that your BG or lipid levels change. If so, don't make any decisions right away. Sometimes it can take days, weeks, or even months for your body to adapt to a new way of eating.

For instance, some people find that when they start on a low-carbohydrate diet, their lipid levels go down at first. But after six months, they may go back up again. Others may find the exact opposite. Still others find their lipid levels go in one direction and stay there.

Some people report extreme fatigue when they suddenly switch from one type of diet to another. One reason for this is that the body is a very adaptable, efficient machine and doesn't waste energy producing enzymes it doesn't need. So if you've been living on a low-fat, high-carbohydrate diet for a long time, your body has been producing the enzymes it needs to process carbohydrates, but not many of the enzymes that are needed to process fat. If you switch suddenly, it doesn't have the "machinery" it needs to get energy from fat and ketones, and you may feel tired for a while until the body has time to "manufacture" enough of the enzymes needed to process the new type of diet.

The same is true if you go the other way. If you've been living on a low-carbohydrate, high-fat diet, your body hasn't been producing many of the enzymes it needs to process carbohydrate. If you suddenly eat a lot of carbohydrate, your BG levels will go very high. In fact, people who have been on low-carbohydrate diets or who have been starving (the ultimate low-carbohydrate diet) will test diabetic even when they're not. This is called *starvation diabetes*, and it's the reason you're usually asked to eat 150 to 300 grams of carbohydrate a day for several days before taking a glucose tolerance test.

These enzymes that are only produced in the presence of the substances that they process are called *inducible enzymes*.

This means that you should never make any decisions on a new way of eating after just a day or so. Try it for at least a week. In terms of lipid levels, a few months is better. Then keep testing every six months or every year to make sure.

Low-carbohydrate diets make you more sensitive to carbohydrate

When you go on a low-carbohydrate diet, you may find that as long as you avoid carbohydrates, your BG levels will stay fairly low. But if you give in to temptation and eat more carbohydrate, your BG levels will go higher than they used to.

This is because, as explained in the previous section, your body stopped producing a lot of the inducible enzymes that process carbohydrate. What this means is that if you don't think you'll be able to stick to a low-carbohydrate diet most of the time, you might be better off with one of the other diet approaches. An occasional spike when temptation is overwhelming probably won't hurt you, but high BG levels on a regular basis could.

Let's look at how some of these diet changes might work. Assume you're starting from a standard American diet with plenty of calories, fat, and carbohydrate. Just reducing calories, as on an exchange diet, usually brings your BG levels down. You're eating less food, so even when BG levels rise after eating, they don't rise as far.

Now let's say you decide to try the high-fiber, high-carbohydrate, low-fat diet instead. Let's say on the exchange diet, after eating 57 grams of carbohydrate (two starch exchanges, one fruit exchange, and one milk exchange), your BG level went up to 200 mg/dL (milligrams per deciliter). On a high-fiber, low-fat diet, you might be eating even more carbohydrate than that, say 70 grams per meal. When you began such a diet your BG level might go even higher than 200 mg/dL, maybe to 250 mg/dL.

But after a few days, your body would adapt, and you might find that even when eating 70 grams of high-fiber carbohydrate, your BG level wouldn't go over 180 mg/dL. Your glucose tolerance would have improved, because both the machinery needed to process carbohydrates was stimulated and your insulin resistance (IR) was reduced.

Now let's see what would happen on a low-carbohydrate diet. In this case you'd be eating only about 6 to 20 grams of carbohydrate per meal, preferably "slow" low-glycemic-index carbohydrates, along with more protein and fat. In this case, your BG level might not go above 120 mg/dL because you simply weren't eating a lot of carbohydrates and the increased fat meant that your stomach emptied more slowly. As long as you stuck to this diet, your BG levels would remain low.

The trade-off would be that if one day you gave in to temptation and ate the same 57 grams of carbohydrate that sent you up to 200 mg/dL on the exchange diet, you might go even higher, maybe 300 mg/dL now, because your body would no longer be accustomed to processing carbohydrates and your IR might have increased if you were eating a lot of saturated fat.

So again, consider which diet you think you could maintain in the long haul, and wait a few weeks before evaluating its effects.

The effects of different diets on your postprandial lipid levels are not so easy for you to see as the effects on postprandial BG levels, because cholesterol levels don't change as quickly as BG levels. So you're probably relying on fasting lipid panels to see how these various diets affect your lipids.

An experiment

You can buy home meters that measure your levels of lipids. One meter measures total cholesterol, HDL, and triglycerides as well as glucose and ketones. Using the results, you can calculate your LDL levels: LDL = Total cholesterol − HDL − (triglycerides/5). However, the strips are more expensive than those for BG meters, and insurance won't pay for them.

I have such a meter, and several years ago I received a windfall of triglyceride strips that would expire in a week or so. I hated to waste them, so I decided to use them to test my triglyceride and BG responses to two different diets: low carb and low fat.

The first day I followed a low-fat diet. For breakfast I ate a lot of carbohydrate, including one ounce of spaghetti cooked al dente and three-quarter cup of white rice (about 60 grams of carbohydrate, or four starch exchanges). For the rest of the day, I ate less carbohydrate but continued to eat low fat.

The second day I followed a low-carbohydrate diet. For breakfast I ate a lot of fat, including a sausage, mushrooms fried in butter, two slices of bacon, and one-quarter cup of the creamy topping of whole-milk yogurt. Unfortunately, I didn't keep a record of the type of sausage, and the fat content on the top of the yogurt is difficult to estimate. But picking a sausage from a nutritional program and assuming the creamy part of the yogurt was the equivalent of half-and-half cream, I calculate about 50 grams of fat, or ten fat exchanges. For the rest of the day, I ate less fat, especially less saturated fat, but continued to eat low carb.

Both days I measured both BG and triglyceride levels every hour or so until I went to bed. On the low-carbohydrate day, I had three meals and one small snack. On the low-fat day, I was constantly hungry, had four meals, and kept snacking.

You can see the results in Figure 10. After a "healthy" low-fat breakfast, my BG levels shot up to more than 200 mg/dL and took more than six hours to come down.

My triglycerides, however, remained low for a while, and at first I thought perhaps the low-fat diet might be better overall. However, after about six hours, the triglyceride levels started to increase steadily, and by the next morning, they were higher than they had been the day before.

On the low-carbohydrate diet, my BG levels stayed low all day. However, after the very high saturated fat breakfast, the triglyceride levels skyrocketed. The second, smaller triglyceride peak was after about three ounces of farmed salmon (7 to 10 grams of fat) for supper. Then they started coming down, and by the next morning *they were lower than they had been the day before.*

As I interpret these results, the high triglyceride levels after eating the high-fat meals represent *chylomicrons*, the lipoproteins that transport fat from your meals to the cells of your body. The high triglyceride levels after eating the low-fat meals represent *very low density lipoprotein*, which takes fat from the liver—including the fat your liver synthesizes when your intake of dietary fat is low—and distributes it to cells that need it, or again, to the fat for storage. Note that the fat synthesized by the liver tends to be saturated fat.

There are several interesting factors to consider here. First, when you have a lipid test done at the lab, it's usually done fasting, which means first thing in the morning after not eating for six to fourteen hours. It tells you nothing about what your triglyceride levels were all day.

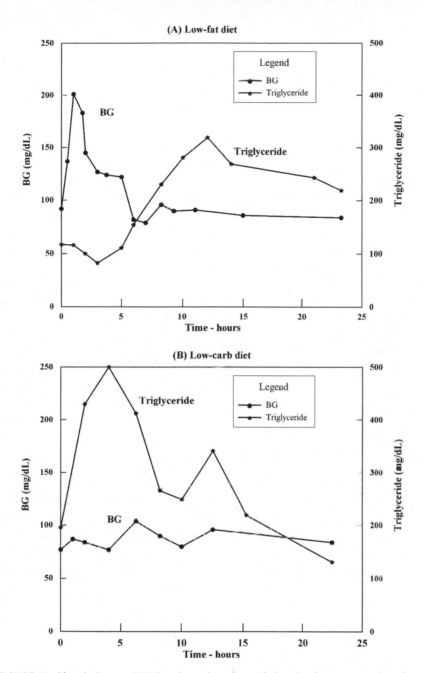

FIGURE 10. Blood glucose (BG) levels and triglyceride levels after eating a low-fat diet and a low-carbohydrate diet. On the low-fat day (A), meals were eaten at time zero, 3.5, 7, and 9.25 hours. On the low-carbohydrate day (B), meals were eaten at time zero, 4, and 10 hours. BG levels were measured on a OneTouch Profile meter, which measures whole blood. Triglyceride levels were measured on a BioScanner 2000 meter (now sold as CardioChek).

Second, the low-carbohydrate diet resulted in lower fasting triglyceride levels but much higher postprandial triglyceride levels. Which are more dangerous? I'm afraid I don't know, but abnormally high postprandial triglyceride levels have been associated with heart disease. However, high BG levels have also been associated with heart disease, and especially fluctuating BG levels as occurred after the high-carbohydrate breakfast. On caveat is that I had been on a low-carbohydrate diet for a long time before doing this test and didn't want to eat a lot of carbohydrate for three days before the test, as you're supposed to do before a glucose tolerance test, and the BG levels might not have been quite so high if I had.

You should also note that the high-fat, low-carbohydrate breakfast was *extremely* high in fat, including a lot of saturated fat. I don't normally eat that much fat but wanted to test extremes. However, it was equivalent to the amount of fat in a couple of slices of sausage pizza, which contain a lot of carbohydrate as well. Hence a person eating the standard American diet would probably be eating that much fat, and even more, every day.

Third, although the low-fat diet didn't produce the very high postprandial triglyceride levels that the high-fat diet did, it produced high BG levels that persisted for hours. Some people think that oxidized and glycated lipids are the dangerous ones, so high BG levels and lower postprandial triglyceride levels might be more dangerous than very high triglyceride levels and normal BG levels. High BG levels also contribute to oxidation.

Finally, these graphs should be interpreted with caution, as they show the results of one experiment with a sample size of one and a home meter, and I didn't keep careful records of the exact amounts of the food I ate, as I wasn't planning to publish the results. My physiology might not be typical. If you want to know how your own body's lipids respond to different types of diets, you should get a lipid meter and test yourself. Unfortunately, your insurance is unlikely to want to pay for this, so it will be an expensive experiment.

The main point of this is that the results of different diets are complex. We have to eat. And what we eat can affect many different systems in our bodies. Finding the ideal diet that matches our own physiology and results in the best lipid levels as well as BG levels is a real challenge.

What does it all mean?

All this means that when you're trying to decide which diet will be best for your diabetes, you shouldn't just read one popular diet book and think that it's the only possible way. No one diet is best for every person with diabetes. Try to understand the science behind the diets and figure out which one would work best for your own particular flavor of diabetes, lifestyle, and reasons for eating. Then try it, test your BG levels, your lipid levels, and your weight before you decide which one is for you.

Ask yourself a lot of questions:

- Does this diet keep my BG levels close to normal?

- What is the effect of this diet on my lipid levels?

- Does this diet provide me with enough energy to do the activities I like to do?

- Am I losing weight on this diet?

- Does this diet include the kinds of foods I like best?

- Does this diet control my hunger?

- Could I stick with this diet for the rest of my life?

- Am I an active person who needs a lot of carbohydrate to burn for energy when I run or ski? A low-fat diet might work best if you could control your BG and triglyceride levels. Note that some professional athletes find they do fine on low-carbohydrate diets and have more endurance when they follow them.

- Am I a pretty sedentary person who nibbles a lot when I'm hungry? A hunger-controlling low-carbohydrate diet might be better for you.

- Can I face not eating a particular kind of food for the rest of my life? If not, a calorie-restricted diet that lets you eat a variety of foods might be best.

- Is IR my main problem? Some people with a lot of IR find that saturated fat (see Month 6) increases their BG levels. In that case, a low-fat diet might work for keeping your BG levels down. However, be aware that some people feel that *very low fat diets* increase cardiovascular risks in people with a lot of IR and recommend substituting monounsaturated fat for saturated fat instead.

- Do I think I don't have much IR but I just don't produce enough insulin? In that case, a low-carbohydrate diet might match your needs.

If you decide to try a low-fat diet, which means eating the bulk of your calories as carbohydrate, make sure to measure your BG levels one or two hours after meals. Physicians used to think that postprandial BG levels didn't make any difference as long as they came back to normal before the next meal, but more recent evidence has shown that postprandial BG levels are the most important factor in predicting your A1c levels and risks of complications. Also keep track of your triglyceride levels, as high-carbohydrate diets sometimes make triglyceride levels go up.

If you decide to try a low-carbohydrate diet, which usually means more saturated fat, make sure to keep track of your lipid levels. Most people on such diets see their lipid panels improve, even when they're eating a lot of saturated fat, but some find their cholesterol levels get worse. If you're in the latter group, substitute lean for fatty meats, and monounsaturated fats such as olive oil, avocado, and nuts for saturated fats like butter and cheese.

If you decide a more varied diet like one of the exchange diets is what you need, you should also measure postprandial BG levels and keep track of your lipids as well. Keeping records on each diet you try lets you decide if another one is working better or worse.

A good dietician will work with you to answer these questions and come up with a diet that satisfies your own particular needs. If the dietician simply hands you a prepared "diabetic diet" sheet or says only one kind of diet works for people with diabetes, say good-bye and try to find one who will treat you as the individual you are.

Understanding the effects of different diets on diabetes control is difficult. As Edd A. said, "So which road do we take? None of them seem safe. Unfortunately, we each have to choose a path even if none of them are adequately illuminated." Sometimes a dietary theory sounds great, but it doesn't work for you. The important thing is not to get caught up in the diet wars but to look beyond the diet rhetoric and try to find the truth behind all the hype.

Sometimes the simplest theory of all may be just what you need. Linda C.'s mantra is to simply "eat less and move more." In a more poetic mood she added, "As my Irish grandmother would say, 'If you dance with the devil then you have to pay the piper.' So I stopped dancing with french fries and chocolate bars, and now I just dance alone for movement."

IN A SENTENCE:

■ *You may have to do some experimenting to find out which diet works best for you, but you should believe your own results more than what anyone else tells you.*

living

Finding More Resources

You've come through almost a year with this blinking disease, and I hope you've learned enough that you're starting to feel comfortable taking charge of your diet, your exercise, and anything else you need to do to control your diabetes.

You should have a good idea of what style of medical care works best for *you*, whether it's a full-fledged health care team of specialists who communicate well with each other and with you, a diabetologist at a major university, or just an old-fashioned family physician whose style of medicine is just what you need.

Regardless of the type of diabetes care you're getting and no matter how much you've learned already, continuing to learn should be a part of your diabetes care for a long time to come. Type 2 diabetes is an incredibly complex disease, and research into its causes and treatment are going on at a furious pace. New drugs and new theories are announced almost every week, it seems. Only a couple of decades or so ago, doctors treating patients with type 2 diabetes had a choice of only insulin or first-generation sulfonylurea drugs, in addition to diet and exercise. Today, there is a plethora of drugs, working in many different ways. Many more are working their way through the long process of testing by the pharmaceutical companies in an effort to receive approval by the Food and Drug Administration.

You'll probably want to keep up with these advances as they occur. And you may want to delve deeper into the science behind the disease and its treatment, subjects I could only summarize briefly in this book. Where should you go to look?

Magazines are useful

Newspapers and TV, radio, and Internet news programs usually announce major advances in diabetes research as they occur, but news stories are necessarily brief. Furthermore, the job of the news media is to present an interesting story, so they tend to overplay the importance of each tiny step that is made in solving the diabetes puzzle. They'll tell you that a new drug or a new way of administering insulin has been found and then rehash a description of what diabetes is and the difference between types 1 and 2, with a few statistics thrown in to fill the space. The headline often implies that the problem of diabetes has been solved.

To get more information than this, there are several popular diabetes magazines you might want to try. *Diabetes Forecast* is the magazine of the American Diabetes Association (ADA), and it's the best place to start. The ADA tries to have an upbeat tone and to provide basic diabetes education for people who know nothing about it, at a simple reading level.

Forecast also tries to have something for everyone. So you'll usually find inspirational stories of people who have triumphed over their diabetes, games for children, recipes, a feature article on some aspect of diabetes care such as foot care or kidneys or insulin pumps, and a short article describing some current research. The ADA also focuses on advocating for the rights of people with diabetes (as well as fund-raising), and every issue includes a report from its government affairs and advocacy department. Once a year it feature a buyer's guide to various diabetes products.

The problem is that by trying to have something for everyone, the ADA can't have a lot for any specific interest group. I also got tired of the continual upbeat tone. It's nice to hear about people with positive attitudes; this is especially important when you've just been diagnosed and for children, but after a while I wanted to hear someone say that diabetes stinks.

Another magazine, *Diabetes Self-Management*, as implied by the title, is geared to motivated patients who really want to take charge of their diabetes and want more in-depth information than *Forecast* is able to provide. Its articles are longer and less repetitive. Many of its articles are written by registered dieticians and certified diabetes educators, so the approach tends to be "party line." However, the magazine is also willing to tackle some controversial areas such as the use of herbal remedies, which are often frowned upon by official diabetes organizations and some physicians.

Many of the illustrations are trademarked cartoon-type drawings, which add a bit of humor and help keep the magazine free from (except in the ads) those unrealistic commercial photographs of slim couples jogging along a beach (to illustrate articles on exercise) or svelte middle-aged couples laughing as they prepare healthy salads (to illustrate articles on nutritious eating) that one often sees in other magazines.

One useful feature of this magazine when you get beyond the early learning stages is a section called "What Your Doctor Is Reading," in which recent diabetes research is described in a readable way. The definitions of diabetes terms are of differing complexity in each issue, which is useful to people who have already mastered the basics.

The magazine *Diabetes Health* (formerly *Diabetes Interview*) is difficult to characterize because it keeps changing. The editor seems to be very sensitive to reader input, and the format and content change from time to time. At one point the content seemed to be getting dumbed down. A lot of readers complained, and the next issues were quite different. If you want a magazine that cares about your input, this might be the one for you.

Diabetes Health has departments covering standard topics including research, exercise, diet (and here the slant keeps changing too), and charts summarizing the features of medications, meters, or pumps. But it also covers some alternative remedies and some patent medicines that might be considered taboo by the other magazines. It also carries ads for alternative treatments that aren't carried in other diabetes magazines.

The board and writers include those who support low-carbohydrate diets as well as those who support the ADA approach, and the magazine also uses freelance journalists. Hence the articles range from "party line" to alternative. But the articles are currently short, most often not more than a page.

The same company also publishes *Diabetes Professional*, a quarterly magazine that collects the product reference guides from *Diabetes Health* together in one issue, along with educational resources, research briefs, and articles of interest to health-care professionals.

All the magazines now have websites, so if you have access to a computer you can check out the table of contents for several issues and read a few of the articles to see which ones you like best. You can also read a comprehensive article by David Mendosa evaluating twenty-six diabetes magazines published in the United States as of 2013 (www.mendosa.com/magazines.htm).

Make use of libraries and bookstores

If you don't want to subscribe to diabetes magazines, check with your local library. Many libraries carry *Forecast*, and they might have the others as well.

If you want to go to the next level and take a look at some of the professional diabetes magazines, ask if your local hospital has a medical library. Most do, and most of these libraries are open to the public, although you might not be able to check out books unless you're a member of the staff.

The local hospital library probably carries major journals such as the *New England Journal of Medicine*, and it may carry diabetes journals such as *Diabetes Care* and *Diabetes* as well, although today many small hospital libraries are canceling their expensive journal subscriptions and using online sources instead. Ask if you can use their computers for your research.

If you live in a city with a medical school, check with the school to see if they have a library that is open to the public. If they say you have to be on staff, explain your need to get information and see if you can get special permission at least to read books and journals in the library. If you live near Bethesda, Maryland, you can use the National Library of Medicine, although I understand you need to take a wheelbarrow full of quarters to be able to pay the parking fees.

If you can't find a specialized medical library near you but you're close to a college or university, see if you can use the libraries there. They may not have as many specialized medical journals, but they may actually have more journals of basic science such as *Nature* and *Science*.

If you want more general information on a specific aspect of diabetes care, there are popular diabetes books that focus on particular areas, for example, books for diabetic men, diabetic women, diabetic African Americans, and diabetic children, books focusing on sports, complications, diabetic burnout, and different types of diabetic diets.

When you're ready to start delving into textbooks, you might want to start with a medical physiology text. They usually have a chapter or two on the control of carbohydrate metabolism in nondiabetic people as well as a discussion of diabetes. Another good source is endocrinology textbooks. They usually go into a little more detail. Even if it's more than you want to know at the time, there are often useful figures and tables. You can always go back to them later.

If you don't want to read that much background science, look for textbooks on diabetes and thumb through them until you come on a topic that interests you. Sometimes just seeing color illustrations of what can happen to your feet if you ignore your control is enough to inspire you to stick with your diet for another month.

Other things you might want to check out would include books on nutrition, books on exercise physiology, or, if you're really dedicated, biochemistry books. Books written for nursing students are usually a little easier going than more comprehensive texts.

If you just won the lottery, you might want to buy some of these books yourself, but be warned: they *are* expensive. Some of the major tomes on diabetes cost $200 or more. One two-volume set cost $380 in 2015. If you live near a medical school, there's undoubtedly a medical bookstore somewhere on the campus or nearby, and the stores should be open to the public. That lets you at least scan any books before you decide to buy.

You can often get deep discounts on the previous edition of a science textbook when the new edition comes out, for example, $17 for a textbook that costs $200 in the latest edition. Some aspects of science change quickly, but others don't, and some chapters don't change much from edition to edition, so you can learn a lot from the older books. In fact, most science textbooks were written at least a year before their publication date, sometimes more, and stay in print for several years after that, so by the time you buy even the current edition of a professional book, some of the information may be out of date.

If you have access to a computer (and if you don't have one at home, you can usually find one at your local library), you can easily see what's available at online bookstores. Amazon.com often has reviews by both professional reviewers and customers who bought the books.

The Internet offers breaking news

I find books and magazines much more efficient than computers for getting background information about the science of diabetes. I prefer reading curled up in a comfortable chair to staring at a screen, and I can read a page in a book faster than scrolling down a screen, especially when the webpage has a poorly chosen typeface or a background pattern that obscures the print. But if you have a computer and online access, the Internet is a good way to keep up to date with breaking news in the diabetes field. In the Learning section, David Mendosa, an Internet expert, will guide you through "surfing" the Internet for diabetes information.

Finding the truth takes work

When a book or journal cites another article to support a statement, you can usually assume the author has summarized the results of that article correctly. But if it's a crucial topic and you're especially interested in it, you're better off locating and reading the cited article yourself. When you do, there are a few things you should look for:

- What group was studied? Many papers refer simply to "diabetics." You know by now that this is a vague term that could mean different types of diabetes, different degrees of control, and different age groups. Sedentary, middle-aged type 2 subjects with A1c's of 10 might react differently from athletic, type 1 high-school students with A1c's of 7.

- Improved (worsened) control means improved (worsened) compared with what? The titles of many papers say that some treatment or other "improved control" without saying what they're comparing the treatment with. This is especially important in papers concerning diets.

- Is there interesting information here not mentioned in the title? Often a paper contains fascinating information that is not the central finding of the paper and hence is not mentioned in either the title or the abstract. For example, some of the studies done on alpha-lipoic acid were done with intravenous infusions, not oral pills, but this isn't mentioned in the title.

Sometimes it takes a long time to locate a paper, and when you find it, you discover it doesn't say very much. But sometimes it tells you just what you were looking for. It doesn't take a PhD to be able to get something out of most published papers. With a little work, you can learn a lot.

Keep learning

Today, opinions about the best way to treat type 2 diabetes can be very different. In the coming years, research into the causes and treatment of type 2 diabetes will continue to be intense. After the initial reports of the benefits of the adipokine *adiponectin* in 2001, more than a thousand papers on the topic were published in the next five years. For this reason, instead of just giving you "the answers," which of course would be *my answers*, I've tried to give you enough background information about the science of diabetes that you can make your own decisions about which treatments will be best *for you* and so you will also be able to understand the new developments as they occur.

Type 2 diabetes is a very complicated disease that can be very frustrating to understand. Sometimes you do exactly what you did yesterday, eat exactly the same foods, think you've had almost exactly the same emotions, and still your blood glucose levels after a meal are different. Don't despair. This is normal. But the more you understand about this disease, the more you will gradually learn to identify stresses, foods, or exercise patterns that affect you in a particular way. The best way to understand your diabetes is to keep on learning.

I've emphasized in this book that diabetes is not your fault. But taking control of your diabetes is your responsibility. Part of taking control means continuing to educate yourself.

After only a year with diabetes, no one expects you to know everything there is to know about this disease. But I hope you're well on your way to understanding what normal reactions to foods and physical and emotional stresses are, how to learn, where to get more information, when to seek help from professionals, and when to look for fellow patients with whom you can vent.

In type 2 diabetes care, knowledge is power. Seek it and use it. Then share it with others. Never stop seeking. Knowledge is the key to control.

IN A SENTENCE:

■ *There are many resources for learning more about diabetes, and you should learn to use them.*

Searching the Internet for Diabetes Information

by David Mendosa*

When you want to learn anything about diabetes beyond what you read here, the quickest and easiest way is to search the Internet. But the amount of information and misinformation there has grown so immense that the simplest search can seem like an impossible task.

In the past two decades or so, the Internet has become essentially the biggest library ever created. Consider that the British Library in London, which is the world's largest physical

---

*After earning a BA with honors from the University of California, Riverside, and an MA in government from Claremont Graduate University, David Mendosa went to work for the US government. During a fifteen-year career as a foreign service officer with the US foreign aid program, he served eleven years in Washington and four years in Africa. Subsequently, he became a journalist, initially specializing in writing about small business.

After he was diagnosed with type 2 diabetes in February 1994, he segued into writing about that condition. He started his www.mendosa.com website in February 1995, and only one other diabetes website is older. His website includes more than two thousand of his articles.

library, has about 170 million items, including some 14 million books. Nobody knows how many websites are out there, partly because that number changes so rapidly, but there are probably about one billion of them with well over four billion webpages.

Libraries use card catalogs, but the Internet has search engines and links to help you find your way around its vast resources. Compared to card catalogs, which index a library's holdings by author and title and may list only one or two subjects, the Internet's search tools take cross-referencing to a higher dimension.

Starting an Internet search is easy. You just enter the name of your search engine of choice in whatever browser you use. You can use one of many different browsers, like Chrome, Internet Explorer, or Firefox. But for search engines, two-thirds of all Internet searches use Google. So if you haven't used it, you might want to remember its Internet address: www.google.com.

It's stopping your search that's the challenge. No matter what you ask Google to search for, it will find dozens if not thousands of webpages. If you search for a big subject like *diabetes*, Google will likely locate one-quarter of a billion sites, and on almost all of those webpages will be many more links to related resources.

But searching the Internet effectively is more than simply clicking on Google. Even before you decide to search the Internet for something about diabetes or anything else, you have to take the first step. For most people this is the hardest one.

RAISE

To guide us through this maze I developed an acronym: RAISE.

Recognize

The R stands for *recognize,* as in recognizing that you need to know more about diabetes. The truly sad fact about diabetes is that when most people get a diagnosis of diabetes, they go into denial. Some other people panic when their doctors give them the verdict. It's only when you take the middle path of accepting that you have to deal with diabetes that you can begin to learn about it.

Accept

So, the second letter of the acronym is A, which is short for *accept.* Like the Apollo 13 astronauts who famously radioed to Mission Control in

Houston that they had a problem, no matter how hard it is, you have to face up to your diabetes diagnosis in order to manage it. Only then can you begin to investigate what you need to do.

Investigate

This brings us to the third letter of the acronym, I for *investigate*. When you are curious about the different means you can use to control your diabetes, you will begin to reach out to your doctors and other people you know, to books like this one, and finally to that huge thing we call by the little word *Internet*. It's at this point that you actually begin to search the Internet.

Search

The fourth letter of the acronym, S, stands, of course, for *search*. But searching on the Internet is not as simple as "seek, and ye shall find" because you will find too much unless you carefully formulate your search queries. Just as you have to know how a person's mind works when you ask someone a question, you have to know how computers think when you seek information from them. Of course, computers don't yet think, but what a computer program does is close enough for this analogy to work.

The Google search engine works so well that it actually seems to be intelligent. What sets it apart the most from other search engines is its PageRank software, which founders Larry Page and Sergey Brin developed when they were students at Stanford University. PageRank uses the web's link structure as an indicator of an individual page's value. In essence, Google interprets a link from page A to page B as a vote by page A for page B. But Google also analyzes the page that casts the vote. Votes cast by pages that themselves get a lot of votes help the pages they are linked to get more votes.

Then Google combines PageRank with sophisticated text-matching techniques to find pages that are both important and relevant to your search. This means that the first pages that Google returns are usually the best ones on that subject.

Internet search engines always let you use keywords, for example, *diabetes* and *complications,* to ask for what you wanted to know. But in 2013 Google's search took a big step forward by letting you do natural language searches. It now understands you when you ask a question like: How can I avoid the complications of diabetes?

You can narrow the search results when you put a phrase in quotation marks. The results will only include pages with the same words in the same order.

Google also has many special features. One that I use a lot is cached links, which is what the page looked like when Google found it most recently. If for any reason the page is unavailable when you find it listed through a Google search, all you need to do is click on the inverted triangle symbol just after the site's address. That brings up the word *cached,* which you can click on to see the page as it looked when Google most recently found it.

If a website is temporarily down, you can get the cached version. But what if it's down permanently? Even in this case you aren't out of luck thanks to Archive.org at https://archive.org (note that with most of today's search engines you don't need to type in the *http://* or *www* to reach the site), which keeps back issues of websites online. Its Wayback Machine has saved more than 400 billion pages for your viewing pleasure. All you need is a little time.

Another of my favorite tricks is to search a specific website for something I think is on the site but can't find because the site doesn't have a search tool or it doesn't work well. For example, if I wanted to find information on diabetes diets on my website, I would type in the following: site:mendosa.com diabetes diet. In place of mendosa.com, type in the name of the website that doesn't have a search tool and replace the words *diabetes diet* with what you are looking for. Please note that the site's name has to follow directly after the word *site,* with no space.

You can now also use Google to search the full text of many books or scholarly papers. Those addresses are http://books.google.com and http://scholar.google.com, but any results that Google finds from these sites will also be included in a regular search of www.google.com.

It doesn't matter whether you capitalize your search terms or not. And Google is remarkably tolerant of poor spelling, gently asking "did you mean" something else.

Evaluate

This brings us to the fifth letter of the acronym: E for *evaluate.* Choosing reliable diabetes websites is a lot trickier than picking the right browser or search engine. Be especially careful of those sites that want to sell you something. These are the hundreds or thousands of sites offering cures in exchange for your money.

Medical quacks have, of course, been buzzing around people with diseases even before the days of Hippocrates; the Internet simply makes their pitches easier. A famous *New Yorker* cartoon shows two dogs talking, as they do in cartoons. One dog sitting in front of the computer turns to the other and remarks, "On the Internet, nobody knows you're a dog."

That's all too true. A website costs very little and offers a forum for the most vicious animals to sell their wares. The real dogs of the Internet are the cyberquacks.

All of us have to understand the playing field and make our own evaluations. As in all research, the key is consistency. Is the information on the site internally consistent? Is it consistent with what you know of the world otherwise?

For example, you have to know that a site offering an eternal life device for $99.95 stretches credibility beyond reason. But even less outrageous claims should not pass your smell test.

Does the author of the webpage have some authority in the field? Here an endocrinologist can often be trusted but not necessarily a chiropractor or dentist, several of whom have diabetes websites.

Can you communicate with the site? Does it provide a physical address as well as email?

Is the information current? If there are a number of broken links or no news for several months, what does this say about the credibility of the information?

Remember as you read that if it sounds too good to be true, it probably is. If it claims to cure many diseases, it probably won't cure any. And if it claims to cure diabetes, it won't because no pill or supplement will do that.

Some websites are so important to people with diabetes that you shouldn't have to search for them. So let's discuss them now.

PubMed

When it comes to the science of diabetes, you have to recognize that not everything you believe is true. Not even everything that the scientists who investigate diabetes think they know will always stand the test of time. Science is a work in progress, and every one of us has to keep learning all the time.

The best studies are randomized, double-blind, placebo-controlled clinical trials reported in a high-quality peer-reviewed journal, with a large enough group of people over a long enough time to warrant generalizations. My friend Steven Bratman, MD, has a great article about these studies at www.mendosa.com/bratman.htm.

You will find all of these topnotch studies—and many inferior ones—online. In some cases the full text of the study is free online, although in most cases you will only be able to get the abstract. While a Google search will find many of these studies, usually it's more efficient to use PubMed.

PubMed provides free access to more than twenty-four million citations for biomedical literature from MEDLINE, life science journals, and online books. MEDLINE is the US National Library of Medicine's bibliographic database of studies reported since 1946 in more than five thousand journals worldwide in about sixty languages. The web address of PubMed is www.ncbi.nim.nih.gov/pubmed (you can also reach it with just pubmed.gov). Although a basic search with PubMed is straightforward, this website has some special tricks that you can learn there.

NIDDK

The website of the National Institute of Diabetes and Digestive and Kidney Diseases (NIDDK) at www.niddk.nih.gov was the first website to provide information about diabetes in 1994. It is still one of the most valuable for anyone with diabetes who is looking for basic information that is reliable. The NIDDK is part of the US National Institutes of Health, our leading medical research agency. It conducts and supports biomedical research and then makes research findings and health information available to the public.

CDC

Like PubMed and the NIDDK, the Centers for Disease Control and Prevention (CDC) is a part of the US government. The diabetes website of the CDC's Division of Diabetes Translation at www.cdc.gov/diabetes is the authoritative source of diabetes data, statistics, and trends in the United States. The name of the division refers to translating science into practice, not words from one language to another.

Nutrition Data

The most comprehensive source of quality nutrition data that I am aware of is the appropriately named website Nutrition Data at http://nutrition-data.self.com. Nutrition Data's website supplements the government's database with listings provided by restaurants and food manufacturers. In addition to food composition data, Nutrition Data also has several tools to analyze and interpret that data. CondéNet, a digital subsidiary of Condé

Nast Publications, which owns such publications as *Bon Appétit, Epicurious*, and *The New Yorker*, also owns Nutrition Data.

Calculators and Converters

The most important numbers that people with diabetes need to watch are blood glucose (BG) and weight levels.

People with diabetes check BG levels with a meter that in the United States reports the level in milligrams per deciliter (mg/dL). They also check the average BG level over the previous two or three months at a lab or with a home A1c meter. Because these tests use different units, converting your results from one measure to the other isn't straightforward. You need a calculator to do this, and one of the major manufacturers of BG meters provides one at www.accu-chek.com/us/glucose-monitoring /a1c-calculator.html.

The United States and countries in continental Europe use mg/dL to measure BG levels. But the United Kingdom and many other countries use a different measure, millimols per liter (mmol/L). So a British diabetes website provides a conversion tool at www.diabetes.co.uk/blood-sugar -converter.html.

The other number that is important to people with diabetes is body mass index (BMI). Several BMI calculators, which measure the amount of body fat that adult men and women have, are available online, but I prefer the standard calculator that the US government provides at www .nhlbi.nih.gov/health/educational/lose_wt/BMI/bmicalc.htm (you can also type *BMI calculator* into Google, and this site should be at the top of the list). This calculator lets you enter your height in fractions of an inch and offers the choice of the standard measure used in the United States or the metric measure used elsewhere.

Diabetes News

If you remember, you can read the latest news about diabetes online on several websites. But Google again has the easiest way to get a summary of daily news reports. Start at http:// news.google.com and click on "Personalize." From there in the search block "Add any news topic" enter what aspects of diabetes interest you. Although I search for all of the news about diabetes, that returns far too many articles for most people. Google will email links and summaries of relevant items every day, every week, or as they go online, depending on what you choose.

Mendosa.com

I would be remiss if I failed to mention my website. You can find one or two new articles that I write about diabetes every week at www.mendosa .com/blog. You can easily search within the site too.

I also have a free *Diabetes Update* newsletter that I will deliver to your email inbox once a month after you subscribe. You can subscribe by sending an email message to www.mendosa.com/subscribe, and you can contact me directly at mendosa@mendosa.com for more information.

These are the tools that you need to start exploring the wealth of information about diabetes on the Internet. There's so much you can learn about diabetes and anything else that interests you there; the only limits are your time and imagination. Go to it.

Appendix 1:

Learning More About Testing: Hemoglobin A1c, Fructosamine, and Anhydroglucitol

Hemoglobin A1c

Today, glycohemoglobin testing has become more standard-ized, so you may not need to know details about this test. How-ever, for the curious, I offer this information

The A1c test measures only averages

The hemoglobin A1c test (or the related *glycohemoglobin* test, the A1 test [see Day 5]), measures your average blood glucose (BG) levels over the past few months. Red blood cells live an *average* of 120 days; then the elderly ones are broken down, primarily in the spleen, and their parts are recycled. How much glucose gets attached to the hemoglobin in the red blood cells during their 120-day lifetime depends on how high your BG was on *average* during those 120 days.

Note the use of the word *average*. Not everyone's red blood cells live exactly 120 days. Some life-span differences occur because people's physiological makeup differs. Other factors that can alter blood cell life span include temporary illnesses and drugs.

Anything that reduces the lifetime of a red blood cell decreases the measured A1c. Such factors include *hemolytic anemia* (anemia caused by breakdown of the red blood cells), losing a lot of blood either through an accident or by donating blood, *hemochromatosis* (see Month 2), prolonged fever, or genetic variations.

Conversely, anything that increases the lifetime of the red blood cell increases the measured A1c. One such factor is removal of the spleen, because the spleen is the primary site where the old, tired red blood cells get taken apart. Genetic variations could also increase the lifetime of the red blood cells. So if your A1c results don't seem to agree with your daily BG measurements, see if you and your doctor can figure out if there's any reason your red blood cells might live longer (your A1c is higher than you'd expect) or shorter (your A1c is lower than you'd expect) than average.

But wait! There's more involved with this average stuff. Remember that the A1c measures the average BG level during the past several months. An average says nothing about the highs and lows that you might have had. If you've had BG levels of 200 mg/dL for half the time and 50 half the time, you will have an average BG level of 125 (200 + 50 ÷ 2), and you'll have the same A1c result as someone who has kept the BG level at 125 most of the time (an unlikely situation, as BG levels fluctuate even in nondiabetic people, but it's an easy example to understand). But the consequences of roller-coaster BG levels, going high one hour and very low the next, are very different from the consequences of smaller fluctuations. Fluctuating BG levels can cause symptoms of hyperglycemia for one hour and hypoglycemia (see Month 2) for the following hour. They can cause the osmotic pressure in your lens to keep changing, resulting in changing vision (see Day 6). And some people find that fluctuating BG levels make them hungry.

Remember that your A1c results indicate only what your average BG levels have been for the past month or more. You still need to do daily BG checks to learn how your BG levels fluctuate with food and exercise.

There are different ways to measure A1c

There are many different ways to measure glycated hemoglobin. As I mentioned in Day 5, some laboratories used to measure all the glycated adult hemoglobin, which means the hemoglobin A1, usually called just *glycohemoglobin* on the lab report. However, today most use methods that separate the glycohemoglobin into its hemoglobin A1a, A1b, and A1c components and report only the results of the A1c, which is the fraction that contains the glucose. The other fractions contain different sugars.

Even when they're measuring the A1c, different technologies are used to do the tests. Some methods separate the A1c by its more negative charge, some by its structure. The different methods give slightly different results and are affected in different ways by various factors.

Most adults have primarily a form of hemoglobin called *hemoglobin A* (for *adult*). But some people have inherited variations of the hemoglobin molecule. One of the most common is *hemoglobin S*, which causes *sickle-cell anemia*. Several different mutations can cause different hemoglobins that cause *thalassemia*, another type of anemia found in people of Mediterranean descent. Many people with thalassemia retain a lot of hemoglobin F (for *fetal*), which normally is not produced by adults.

Some of these variations (and there are many different rare types) separate along with the A1c fraction in certain types of tests for A1c. For example, if you have thalassemia, your A1c results may be higher than they should be, because hemoglobin F moves along with the A1c in some of the tests. If you have sickle-cell anemia, your A1c results may be lower than expected, because the glycated hemoglobin S doesn't show up where the A1c is expected in some kinds of tests.

A newer test called the *total glycohemoglobin test* measures *all* the hemoglobin types (hemoglobin A, S, F, and other variants) that have glucose attached and may be able to give an idea of your control even if you have one of these unusual hemoglobin types. However, some of the unusual hemoglobins live for a shorter time than hemoglobin A, and this would also affect the results. If you're reading older books, note that in the past, some people used the term *total glycohemoglobin* to refer to hemoglobin A1 (A1a, A1b, and A1c), which can be confusing.

Some labs now measure the total glycohemoglobin, then use a formula to convert the results to an A1c, and report it as hemoglobin A1c. In this case, the A1c results would usually reflect your average BG levels even if you had one of the hemoglobin variants.

If your A1c results don't seem to be what they should be, ask your doctor about the possibility that you may have an unusual type of hemoglobin. Then try to find out what kind of test the lab used to measure the A1c, and see if it's one of the ones that is affected by hemoglobin variants. If it is, you might want to have a fructosamine test (see later in this appendix), which isn't affected by variations in hemoglobin types.

Several other factors that have been reported to cause falsely elevated A1c's include kidney failure, chronic alcohol intake, and high triglyceride (fat) levels. When the glycohemoglobin test for all the hemoglobin A1 fractions is being used, factors that have been reported to cause false results include opiate addiction, lead poisoning, kidney failure, and alcoholism.

Because of all the different methods and ways of reporting results, people are trying to standardize the results so that you can compare your results from one lab with the results from another lab without worrying about different methods and normal ranges. The goal is to standardize all the tests so the results can be compared directly with those of the DCCT (see Day 6). To this end, the National Glycohemoglobin Standardization Program (NGSP) has begun certifying methods and labs that satisfy these standards. However, not all are certified yet, and even with NGSP certification, some hemoglobin variants could give erroneous results.

Glycation occurs in several steps

Nothing is ever simple when it comes to diabetes. This includes the process of glycation, or the addition of glucose to the hemoglobin molecule. This process occurs in several steps, and the first two are reversible.

What happens is this: when the BG level in the blood is high, the glucose first fairly quickly (over a period of several hours) attaches itself to the hemoglobin by a very labile bond (for scientists, it's a Schiff base). Some people call this temporary compound *pre-A1c*. You may also see it referred to as the *aldimine* form. This reaction occurs fairly rapidly, but if the BG level then goes down again, the glucose can come off. It's like suddenly having a high level of cash and quickly putting it into a bank. It's not a permanent situation. When your cash level goes down, you take the money out of the bank again.

But if your BG levels stay high, the glucose doesn't come off the hemoglobin molecule. In fact, it is slowly, over a period of several weeks, converted (for scientists, by an Amadori rearrangement) to a second compound, the hemoglobin A1c (you'll sometimes see this referred to as the *ketoamine* form) that is measured in the tests. This reaction is also reversible. It can revert to the pre-A1c again. But it takes a long time, several weeks, to go from A1c back to pre-A1c, so for the purposes of the testing, the A1c is pretty stable.

However, because the first step in this process happens fairly quickly and is a function of the current level of glucose in the blood, if your BG levels had been very good for several months but for the past two days you'd let them get very high, you could have very high levels of pre-A1c, the stuff that has "temporary glucose" that can come off again if your BG levels go low. If the lab uses a test that measures both the temporary pre-A1c and the permanent A1c, your results might reflect your control in the previous days instead of over the past month or so.

This is also a good reason to be fasting when you have the A1c test done, even though the instructions for the test say that's not necessary. An extremely high BG level could cause an increase in this temporary pre-A1c, especially if the blood sat around for a long time before it was tested.

Some labs control for this by doing a first step that removes the pre-A1c. Others don't. In most cases it probably won't make much difference. But if your results don't seem to reflect your home testing, this is yet another factor that you might want to consider.

The A1c is a weighted average

Older books about diabetes may say that the A1c measures your average BG level over the past two to four months. In a sense it does. A few of your red blood cells are always close to 120 days old. But not many. In fact, mathematical analyses of the A1c can show that it is heavily *weighted* to the past two or three weeks. The American Diabetes Association estimates that if your daily control suddenly got better or worse, 50 percent of the change in A1c would occur in one month. Another person estimates that 50 percent of the change would occur in only seven days, about 75 percent after two weeks, and 94 percent after four weeks. These analyses depend on assumptions about the speed with which glucose goes on and comes off hemoglobin, and different people using different assumptions have calculated different values for this weighting.

Because you'll always have some red blood cells that are older than others, if you've had terrible control and suddenly decide to get your act together and your BG levels fall to close to normal levels, your A1c may begin to go down a little in a few days, but it will take a few weeks before you see a significant change and at least a month before the A1c reflects your current control. The same is true if you've had good control and suddenly let it slip. So if your daily control has changed significantly shortly before you get an A1c, don't be surprised if the result isn't what you'd expect from your BG readings in the past week or so.

Check the normal range

Everyone has glucose in the blood, so everyone has some glycation of proteins like hemoglobin, even people who are not diabetic. Hence no one will have an A1c of zero. What you want to know when you have the test done is how you compare with people who are not diabetic.

In order to do this, the laboratory will tell you what the range of nondiabetic A1c's is. There's one problem with this. A lot of people who have diabetes don't know it, and their labs don't know it either. For example, someone with a fasting BG level in the normal range might go very high after meals, which would increase the A1c, but no one would know about it because they wouldn't think to measure. This person's blood would be classified as nondiabetic and would affect the so-called normal range in that area.

Many labs use local blood samples to determine their normal ranges. If you live in an area where the incidence of diabetes is unusually high, there are also probably a lot more undiagnosed diabetic people than in other parts of the country where diabetes is less common, and hence the normal ranges in that area might not really be normal.

For all these reasons, some people feel that the low end of the "normal range" is really the normal value. In most cases, people with diabetes are not apt to achieve A1c's that low, and if you can't, you certainly shouldn't feel bad about it. Just keeping your BG levels close to the normal range is an achievement in itself.

Don't blame yourself

Many books on diabetes tell physicians in training that when the patient's A1c doesn't agree with the home BG tests, the patient probably doesn't know how to use a meter properly or is fudging the data. Another suggestion is that perhaps the patient measures only before meals, and not after meals, when the readings could be high.

All these factors are, of course, possible. Teenagers especially, who think no harm will ever come to them, have been known to make up good BG readings to gain the approval of their physicians. However, it is also possible that either the home meter readings or the A1c tests are being affected by some other unknown factors.

I once had an A1c test done at my local hospital and got a result of 5.6, which was well below the top of the normal range for that lab (4.4 to 6.4). The very same morning, I mailed off a fasting sample to a research lab that was supposed to do very accurate testing. That lab gave a result of 7.1, which was clearly above the top of their normal range (4.2 to 6.1).

Remember, the A1c is simply one *estimate* we have of average BG levels. Because it's a pretty complicated test, small variations in the numbers don't mean very much. If your A1c was 7.1 last time and it's 7.3 this time, that doesn't necessarily mean that you're doing worse even if the test was done at the same lab. Maybe a few red blood cells lived longer this time. Or maybe something else interfered with the tests. Sometimes labs even make errors. Remember, the tests are usually run by human beings. It's only a major or consistent increase that is something to worry about, say 7.1, then 7.3, then 7.5, and 7.8.

Also, the A1c is not an absolute number. It's especially important to remember this when someone tries to tell you that a particular level of the A1c means your BG levels have averaged some number, or it means you won't have or will have complications. An A1c of 6 at one lab could be an A1c of 7 at another. When NGSP certification is universal, this won't be a problem, but universal certification hasn't yet been achieved.

The important thing is to use the A1c to see if your control is better or worse than it was three months ago, or last year. The best way to do this is to stick with one method done by the same lab. Then if you have some unusual condition that might affect one testing method but not another, you won't think your control has changed when in fact it's just a result of a different method. Unfortunately, you're not likely to have control over the methods used. Your doctor may start using a different lab, and this could result in a different A1c when your control was exactly the same.

Advanced glycation end products may cause aging

Glucose gets added to many different proteins in the body by a mechanism similar to that described for the hemoglobin A1c. First comes a fast reaction and then a slow reaction, both reversible if the conditions are right, that is, if the BG levels approach normal. However, the second form, the ketoamine form, can form permanent compounds called *AGEs* (*advanced glycation end products*). In other words, glucose attaches to a protein molecule, and then a lot of other, often unidentified, chemical reactions change the protein from its normal form into an abnormal form that is harmful to your body. These changes are not easily reversible. In the analogy used when discussing the several steps of glycation, this would be like depositing your money in a bank that wouldn't give it back to you instead of in a bank where you could get it out again.

These AGEs may form cross-links between protein molecules. When glucose reacts with the protein *collagen*, which is an important component of your connective tissue, the cross-linked AGEs that result may contribute to the loss of elasticity that comes with age, including aging of the arteries. Letting your BG levels stay higher than normal would thus accelerate this aging process. Glycation of red blood cell membranes may make them stiffer and less able to pass through tiny capillaries. When glucose reacts with various enzymes in the body, it could also modify their effectiveness and cause numerous problems.

AGEs are thought to be responsible for some of the complications from diabetes (see Month 10). Because the AGEs are permanent, sometimes the complications continue to progress even when the BG level is brought back to normal. This is another reason to get your BG levels under control as quickly as possible. Early complications, like the aldimine and ketoamine forms, can sometimes be reversed. At this time, AGEs cannot.

There are tools that can measure the level of AGEs in your arm or your eyes. The former is currently available in Europe but has not yet been approved by the FDA for use in the United States.

Fructose can also attach to proteins, and it is estimated that it does so about seven times faster than glucose. Thus, although fructose (and the fructose in sucrose, table sugar) won't raise your BG levels as fast as glucose, it is not completely benign.

Fructosamine and anhydroglucitol

Fructosamine measures medium-term excursions

If your A1c results don't jibe with your home BG testing, it's always possible you have some unusual kind of hemoglobin. If you know you do or think you might, it would make sense to have a *fructosamine* test done.

Glucose can react with many of the proteins in the fluid part of your blood. The fructosamine test measures the glycation of these proteins, primarily *albumin*, which is present in high concentrations.

Because these proteins turn over (the body breaks them down, recycles the components, and makes new proteins) faster than the hemoglobin in red blood cells, the fructosamine test is designed to measure your average BG level over the past two to three weeks.

Like the A1c test, the fructosamine test is not perfect. A lot of things can change the levels of proteins in your blood, including individual variation. The A1c test measures the *percentage* of glycated hemoglobin in your blood, so if you had more or less total hemoglobin, it wouldn't matter for the test. The fructosamine test measures only the *amount* of glycated serum proteins. So a low result can mean either your BG control has been good or your serum protein levels are down. Also, fructosamine results may vary inversely with body weight; the higher your weight, the lower the fructosamine level. High levels of vitamin C also interfere with the test, and people are sometimes told to abstain from vitamin C for twenty-four hours before a fructosamine test.

However, like the A1c, the fructosamine test is a good approximation of your control.

Anhydroglucitol test measures short-term excursions

The compound 1,5-anhydroglucitol (AG) is derived from glucose, and its concentration in plasma is normally pretty stable. When BG levels are higher than normal, AG levels are lower. A commercial test for AG is called Glycomark.

The lower AG levels when BG levels are high occur because AG and glucose compete for reabsorption from the kidney tubules. Many compounds are first excreted into the tubules by the kidney and then later reabsorbed. The normal reabsorption rate of AG is about 99 percent. In the presence of high levels of glucose, much less AG gets reabsorbed, and the rest is excreted in the urine, so blood levels are lower.

Thus, unlike hemoglobin A1 values, AG values will not revert toward normal if you have low BG levels for a while, and for this reason they can measure short-term BG excursions. The test is thought to estimate BG levels from about forty-eight hours to two weeks.

One advantage of this test is that it doesn't rely on the half-life of a blood protein like hemoglobin or albumin. However, it does have some limitations.

Because the test depends on high glucose levels in the urine, it will only register if your BG levels go high enough to spill glucose in the urine. This is normally about 180 mg/dL, but different people have different renal thresholds for glucose, and this can affect the test.

Most of the AG in the body comes from the diet, and although all foods contain some, the highest levels are found in carbohydrates, so it's possible that extremes of diet might affect the results.

With time, accurate and affordable home A1c, fructosamine, anhydroglucitol, and other tests meters may become commonplace. Until then, you must rely on labs to test your overall control. In general, they do a great job. Your job is to understand their limitations.

IN A SENTENCE:

▪ *The hemoglobin A1c, fructosamine, and anhydroglucitol tests can be affected by numerous factors, so if your results don't seem to match your daily blood glucose readings, see if any of these factors could explain the discrepancy.*

Appendix 2

How Did Diabetic Diet Recommendations Evolve?

Adapted from *The Four Corners Diet*

When you have diabetes, you can't produce enough insulin to keep your blood glucose (BG) levels normal, especially after you eat carbohydrate foods. So why, you may wonder, did many physicians and dieticians tell people with diabetes to eat a lot of carbohydrate foods? (In 2015, the tide is turning again, and more and more professionals support a low-carbohydrate diet for diabetes patients. But others, including the American Diabetes Association [ADA], still support a low-fat approach, which means lots of carbohydrate.) Why did the ADA tell people with diabetes to "make starch the star" and dieticians tell them to put raisins in their oatmeal and breadcrumbs in their meatloaf to "get the carb counts up"?

To answer this question, we have to go back a bit and look at the history of diabetic diets. Years ago, before anyone knew what caused diabetes, some people told those with the disease to eat a lot of starches, including candy. Their logic was that the patients were losing a lot of sugar in their urine, so it was important to replace that sugar by eating even more.

Others supported low-carbohydrate diets. One diet proposed in 1797 said people with diabetes should eat only blood pudding and old rancid meats.

In the early 1900s, just before the discovery of insulin, a standard diabetic diet was a very low carbohydrate diet, similar to low-carbohydrate diets today, and even a real starvation diet if the low-carbohydrate diet wasn't enough. This diet helped people with type 2 diabetes keep their BG levels down. It also helped people with type 1 diabetes, who produce almost no insulin at all, stay alive longer. But no diet was able to keep them alive for very long, and type 1 diabetes was always fatal.

Then in the 1920s, insulin was discovered, and some people thought that diabetes had been cured. People with type 1 diabetes who looked like walking skeletons and were close to death started regaining weight. They started living lives that were close to normal. However, most of them continued to follow the then-standard low-carbohydrate, high-fat diets of the time.

Although the type 1 diabetic children survived childhood and grew into adults, many of them eventually died of heart disease at a relatively young age. In the 1950s, attention was being paid to studies that showed that heart disease rates increased in people who followed a diet high in saturated fat. Hence in 1979, it was decided to reduce the amount of fat in the diet of people with type 1 diabetes and to increase the carbohydrate content to between 55 and 60 percent of total calories, also increasing the amount of insulin they injected to cover the extra carbohydrates they ate.

Eight years later, because people with type 2 diabetes also usually die from heart disease, these recommendations were made for people with type 2 diabetes as well, even though most of them weren't able to cover the extra carbohydrate with insulin. At the time, it was believed that the high BG levels they had after such meals weren't harmful. In fact, at the time, there were no studies showing that high BG levels caused the many complications of both types of diabetes, and doctors were more worried about having their patients avoid low blood sugar reactions than having BG levels that were too high.

During this period, studies showed that a diet high in carbohydrates *and fiber* resulted in lower insulin resistance and lower postprandial BG levels than the standard American diet or the high-glycemic-index ADA exchange diet, which didn't tell you what kind of carbohydrate you should eat as long as you ate the amount specified in the diet.

Finally, in 1994, the ADA decided that perhaps a high-carbohydrate diet wasn't best for everyone with type 2 diabetes and suggested individualizing diabetic diets and sometimes substituting *monounsaturated fat* for some of the carbohydrate. Current ADA guidelines recommend whole foods.

Unfortunately, some physicians and dieticians apparently didn't get the word and continued to prescribe lots of starches to all their patients.

Some dieticians also seemed to have forgotten that the original studies emphasized *high-fiber* carbohydrates, and they urged their clients to eat a lot of breakfast cereals, sweet fruits, bread, and rice, all foods that cause a rapid increase in BG levels.

Also seemingly forgotten was that the famous Seven Countries Study, which studied the relation between fat intake and heart disease rates, had focused on countries that ate high amounts of *saturated* fat. In Greece, where people ate a lot of *monounsaturated* olive oil, rates of heart disease were low. It's also important to note that the populations that ate a lot of saturated fat were also eating a lot of carbohydrate at the same time.

Thus studies suggesting that the best diet would be high in fiber and monounsaturated fat became misinterpreted to mean that the best diet would be high in starch and low in all kinds of fat.

Recently, studies have shown that two-hour postprandial BG levels are the best predictors of future problems. People with lower levels had fewer cardiac deaths. The old days when it was thought that postprandial BG levels don't matter are gone.

If you are taking insulin shots, of course, you can cover any carbohydrates with insulin. However, it is very difficult to use insulin injections to mimic the exquisite control of BG levels that occurs in nondiabetic people. Your injections have to match your intake exactly and account for other factors, such as exercise, stress, and the rate at which your stomach empties. When you eat a lot of carbohydrates, you're more likely to "roller coaster" from highs to lows and back to highs again. Limiting your carbohydrate intakes will smooth out these peaks and valleys.

Fashions in diets swing like a pendulum. Not long ago, some people were recommending diets of 60 percent and even 70 percent carbohydrate for people with diabetes. Today, the pendulum seems to be reversing. The Joslin Diabetes Center in Boston has reduced their recommended amount of carbohydrate to 40 percent, and more and more physicians and diabetes educators are becoming willing to consider prescribing diets with lower amounts of carbohydrate and more protein and fat (especially monounsaturated fat).

We are all individuals, with individual physiologies. Many people with type 2 diabetes do well with a low-carbohydrate diet. Others find that fat of any kind, even monounsaturated fat, causes problems for them and that they can control their BG levels better on a high-fiber, low-fat diet.

The important thing is to find out what works for *you*. Monitor your BG levels (including postprandial, or postmeal, BG levels), your lipid levels, your blood pressure, and any other parameters your doctor thinks are important for you. Then, after a few weeks or months, take a look at the results and see if the diet you're on is the best for you. If you think you would do better on another one, try that for a while, monitor your lab results, and then decide.

No matter which approach you choose, try to stick to a few principles. Try to make the fat you eat the healthy monounsaturated kind. Eat a lot of fiber. Eat probiotics such as yogurt and kefir and eat foods with health-promoting factors such as antioxidants and other natural disease-preventing compounds. Examples include cruciferous vegetables (broccoli, cauliflower, and brussels sprouts), tomatoes (they help prevent prostate cancer), and greens and berries (loaded with antioxidants). The Four Corners Diet calls these *pharmafoods*. Avoid fast-acting sugars and starches. Avoid processed foods. Eat as many of your carbohydrates as possible in the form of high-fiber vegetables.

Stay healthy—and enjoy your food.

Glossary

A1c: See **hemoglobin A1c**

ACE inhibitor: Angiotensin-converting **enzyme** inhibitor. The **hormone** *angiotensin* constricts blood vessels. By inhibiting the formation of the active form of angiotensin, ACE inhibitors reduce blood pressure. They also help prevent kidney complications, may improve insulin sensitivity, and may even slow down the appearance of **type 2 diabetes** in prediabetic people.

ADA: American Diabetes Association.

ADA diet: An old term referring to a low-fat **exchange diet**. The **ADA** now says that no one diet is good for everyone with diabetes, so this term should be avoided.

adipokine: A **hormone** secreted by adipose tissue (fat).

adiponectin: A beneficial **adipokine**. Low levels of adiponectin are associated with **insulin resistance**.

adrenaline: A **counterregulatory hormone** that is secreted by the adrenal glands and raises **BG** levels by increasing **insulin resistance**. Adrenaline contributes to the **fight-or-flight response** in several ways and also helps prevent **hypoglycemia**. It is also called *epinephrine*. One trade name is Adrenalin.

aerobic exercise: Exercise that requires oxygen and increases your heart rate, for example, running more than a quick dash. Aerobic exercise is good for your **cardiovascular** health.

AGE: Advanced glycation end product. These are substances, usually **proteins**, that have been modified by the addition of **sugar** molecules, making them not work as well as they should. AGEs are thought to be one cause of aging.

AHA: American Heart Association.

albumin: The major **protein** in your blood. It is used to transport other molecules, for example, **fatty acids**. The **fructosamine test** measures how much **glucose** is attached to albumin. When your kidneys are beginning to fail, they may allow albumin to leak into the urine.

alcohol: Usually refers to *ethyl alcohol*, or what is sometimes called *booze*. May also refer to *isopropyl alcohol*, which is used as *rubbing alcohol*. It is also the name of a type of chemical with a hydroxyl group, as in **sugar alcohol**.

aldose reductase: An **enzyme** that converts **glucose** to **sorbitol**. The *aldose reductase inhibitors* are a class of drugs that inhibit this enzyme and may prevent diabetic complications caused by sorbitol.

alpha cells: The cells in the **pancreas** that produce **glucagon**.

amino acids: The building blocks for **protein**.

analog: A compound that is similar in *structure* to another compound. See **mimetic**.

anaerobic exercise: Exercise that can be done in the absence of oxygen, for short periods of time. Examples are weight lifting and a 100-yard dash. Anaerobic exercise causes short-term increases in blood pressure and long-term increases in muscle strength.

antibody: A **protein** produced by the body's immune system to help get rid of infections or other substances it thinks don't belong there.

anticoagulant: A substance that keeps your blood from clotting, popularly called a *blood thinner*.

antioxidant: A substance that neutralizes free radicals.

ARB: Angiotensin receptor blocker. A drug that has the same effect as an **ACE inhibitor** but works in a different way, blocking the receptor for the active form of angiotensin instead of blocking its synthesis.

arteries: The blood vessels that bring oxygenated blood from the heart out to the rest of the body.

arteriosclerosis: Thickening and stiffening of the walls of **arteries**, regardless of the cause. Popularly known as *hardening of the arteries*. See also **atherosclerosis**.

atherosclerosis: Thickening of the walls of **arteries** as a result of the formation of fatty **plaques**. See also **arteriosclerosis**.

ATP: Adenosine triphosphate. It is the "energy currency" of cells.

autoantibody: An **antibody** produced against your own tissues.

autoimmune disease: A disease in which your immune system mistakenly attacks your own tissues. **Type 1 diabetes** is thought to be an autoimmune disease. Rheumatoid arthritis is another.

autonomic nerve: A nerve controlling an "automatic" function you don't have to think about in order to perform, for example, breathing or the beating of your heart.

autonomic neuropathy: A form of **neuropathy** that affects your **autonomic nerves**.

basal insulin: Insulin taken to maintain steady levels of **BG** in the absence of food.

beta cells: The cells in your **pancreas** that produce **insulin**.

BG: Blood glucose. Usually means the concentration of **glucose** in the blood in milligrams per deciliter (mg/dL) (usual American system) or millimols per liter.

blood thinner: See **anticoagulant**.

bolus insulin: Insulin taken to cover the **BG** rise caused by eating. Sometimes called *mealtime* or *prandial* insulin.

borderline diabetes: An old term referring to the early stages of diabetes. The term is misleading, can delay treatment, and should not be used.

capillary: A tiny, thin-walled blood vessel that allows nutrients, waste products, and gases to be exchanged with the surrounding tissue.

carbohydrate: A type of food consisting of **sugar** units, from one (**monosaccharide**) to many (**polysaccharide**). Carbohydrate has the greatest effect on your **BG** levels. It contains four calories per gram.

carbohydrate counting: A dietary approach in which you calculate the amount of **carbohydrate** you eat at every meal and don't keep track of calories, **protein**, or **fat**.

cardiovascular: Referring to your heart or blood vessels. A *cardiovascular event* is an incident involving your heart or blood vessels, for example a heart attack or a stroke

certified diabetes educator (CDE): A health-care professional who has received special training and passed an examination on educating people with diabetes.

cholesterol: A **lipid** that is a building block for cell membranes and a precursor for certain **hormones**. Too much of certain types of cholesterol, for example, **LDL**, in the circulation can contribute to the formation of **plaques**.

continuous glucose monitor (meter): A monitoring device that measures your **BG** level every few minutes without requiring you to get a sample of blood.

controlled trial: A way of testing a new treatment by comparing one group of people who get the treatment with a matched group who do not.

cortisol: A **counterregulatory hormone** released from the adrenal glands when you are stressed. It can raise **BG** levels by increasing **insulin resistance**.

cortisone: A synthetic hormone used as an anti-inflammatory agent. The body converts it to **cortisol**.

counterregulatory hormone: A **hormone** that opposes the action of **insulin**, causing **insulin resistance**.

C-peptide test: A test that measures the approximate amount of **insulin** that you are producing.

C-reactive protein (CRP): A protein whose levels increase with **inflammation**.

dawn effect or phenomenon: The normal rise in **BG** levels that occurs in the morning, often before rising.

depot: A reservoir of **insulin** in the tissues.

dextrose: Another name for **glucose**, often used in food labels.

Diabetes Control and Complications Trial (DCCT): An important study that proved that high **BG** levels increase the risk of complications.

diabetic ketoacidosis (DKA): A serious short-term complication that occurs mostly in people with **type 1 diabetes** when their insulin levels get extremely low. See also **ketosis**.

diabetologist: A physician, usually an **endocrinologist**, who specializes in diabetes.

dialysis: A method of artificially removing waste products from the blood, a job normally performed by the kidney.

dietician: A person trained to devise nutritionally balanced meals. A *registered dietician (RD)* is a dietician who has a specified amount of training and has passed a special examination. See also **nutritionist**.

dipstick: A chemically treated strip of material that changes color when it is dipped into a solution containing a particular substance. Different dipsticks detect different substances, for example, **glucose** or **ketones**.

disaccharide: A **carbohydrate** containing two **sugar** units.

diuretic: A drug that increases elimination of fluids from the body.

DKA: See **diabetic ketoacidosis**.

double-blind: Referring to a study in which neither the patient nor the medical people involved with the study know which patients have received the study drug.

eAG: Estimated average glucose. Your average **BG** level calculated on the basis of your A1c.

effective carbohydrate: The amount of **carbohydrate** that is digested and can raise your **BG** levels, that is, the total carbohydrate minus the indigestible **fiber**.

effective insulin: The amount of **insulin** that would have the same effect if you had no **insulin resistance**. You might produce 30 units but it might be equivalent to only 10 units because of insulin resistance. This is a concept only, as one can't actually measure it directly. You can measure insulin resistance in research labs.

-emia: A suffix meaning "in the blood." For example, *glycemia* means "glucose in the blood."

endocrinologist: A medical doctor specializing in disorders of endocrine (hormone-releasing) glands, including diabetes.

enzyme: A **protein** that makes a chemical reaction go much faster. Many of the body's control systems involve increasing or decreasing the levels or activities of enzymes.

exchange diet: A type of diet in which each food is assigned to a category, the amount of each food that represents one exchange is specified, and you are allowed a certain number of exchanges in each category. Within each category, you can choose between different foods, as they all have *approximately* the same amount of **protein**, **fat**, and **carbohydrate**.

fasting test: A test done in the morning before eating any food. Sometimes defined as after eating no food for at least six to fourteen hours.

fat: A type of food consisting primarily of **triglycerides**. It contains nine calories per gram. By itself, fat will not raise your **BG** levels, but it may cause **insulin resistance**. The body uses its own fat for long-term energy storage.

fatty acids: The building blocks of fats. Fatty acids are long, acidic molecules, mostly insoluble in water. Like **glucose**, they can be burned for energy.

FDA: Food and Drug Adminstration.

fiber: A **carbohydrate** that is not broken down by human **enzymes**. Fiber is classified as both **soluble fiber** and **insoluble fiber**.

fight-or-flight response: A complex response to stress that activates all the bodily systems that would help a person react in a stressful situation, for example, releasing extra **glucose** into the blood for energy. It also suppresses systems that aren't needed, for example, the digestion of food.

food pyramid: A former general guideline for eating developed by the US Department of Agriculture that put **carbohydrate** foods at the base of a pyramid, **fats** and sweets at the top, and other foods between. You were supposed to eat foods in amounts relative to their position in the pyramid, that is, lots of carbohydrate and relatively little fat and sweets. Today, the USDA uses **MyPlate**.

free radical: A chemical with an unpaired electron that is extremely reactive and can cause damage to cells. Free radicals can be neutralized by **antioxidants**, which are usually found in fruits and vegetables. See **reactive oxygen species (ROS)**.

fructosamine test: The name of a test that measures your average **BG** level for the past two weeks.

fructose: A **monosaccharide** found especially in fruits that does not raise your **BG** level as fast as **glucose** does. However, it can be converted to glucose in the liver and contains the same number of calories.

galactose: A **monosaccharide** that is part of the milk sugar **lactose**. It can be converted to glucose in the liver and contains about the same number of calories.

gastroparesis: A form of **autonomic neuropathy** that causes the stomach to empty slowly and sporadically, resulting in unpredictable **BG** levels and nausea or bloating.

gestational diabetes: A form of diabetes that can occur during pregnancy and usually goes away after the baby is born.

GIP: Glucose-dependent insulinotropic peptide, formerly called *gastric inhibitory peptide*. A gut **hormone** that stimulates **beta cells** to produce more **insulin**.

GLP-1: Glucagonlike peptide-1. A gut **hormone** that stimulates **beta cells** to produce more **insulin** after meals, inhibits the production of **glucagon** by the liver, delays gastric emtying, and reduces appetite.

glucagon: A hormone produced by the **alpha cells** in the pancreas that makes **BG** levels increase.

gluconeogenesis: The formation of **glucose** from nonglucose substances, especially **protein**.

glucose: A **monosaccharide** that is the main source of energy for most cells. The **BG** levels are normally kept within a small range. When this control is lost, you have diabetes.

glucose tolerance test (GTT): A test of your ability to keep **BG** levels in normal ranges after being given a large dose of **glucose** on an empty stomach.

glucose transporter: An apparatus in the membrane of most cells that "ferries" **glucose** into the cell. The number of glucose transporters in the membrane increases when **insulin** levels are high, or when you exercise.

glucotoxicity: A reduction in the production of **insulin** by the **beta cells** and an increase in **insulin resistance**, both caused by high **BG** levels.

glycated hemoglobin: A form of **hemoglobin** to which a **sugar** molecule has become attached. This is the substance measured in the **hemoglobin A1c** test. Also called *glycohemoglobin*. Sometimes the term *glycosylated hemoglobin* is used interchangeably with *glycated hemoglobin*, although some people define the terms slightly differently.

glycemic index: A measure of how quickly a **carbohydrate**-containing substance will raise your **BG** level.

glycerol: A small E-shaped **sugar alcohol** to which **fatty acids** can become attached, forming **fats**. Glycerol can be converted to **glucose** in the liver. Also called *glycerin*.

glycohemoglobin: See **glycated hemoglobin**.

glycohemoglobin test: A test that measures the amount of **glucose** attached to the **hemoglobin** in your blood.

glycogen: Long chains of **glucose** that are used for medium-term storage of energy in liver and muscle.

glycogenolysis: The breakdown of **glycogen** to form **glucose**.

grehlin: A **hormone** secreted by the stomach that causes hunger. See **obestatin**.

growth hormone: A **counterregulatory hormone**.

GTT: See **glucose tolerance test**.

HDL: High-density lipoprotein. The "good" cholesterol that takes extra cholesterol from the bloodstream and returns it to the liver.

hemoglobin: The protein in **red blood cells** that transports oxygen from your lungs to your tissues.

hemoglobin A1c: The fraction of **hemoglobin** that contains most of the **glucose** that has been attached to hemoglobin.

high-carbohydrate diet: A term often used for **low-fat diets**. Depending on your caloric intake, a low-fat diet does not necessarily have a large *amount* of carbohydrate.

high-carbohydrate, high-fiber diet: A diet that emphasizes carbohydrate foods that are high in fiber and minimizes fats.

high-protein diet: A term often used for **low-carbohydrate diets**. Depending on your caloric intake and whether you replace **carbohydrate** with **fat** or **protein**, a low-carbohydrate diet does not necessarily have a large *amount* of protein.

hormone: A substance produced in one part of the body that can act in another. **Insulin** is a hormone produced in the **beta cells** of the **pancreas** that acts throughout the body.

hyper-: A prefix meaning "more than normal."

hyperglycemia: A higher-than-normal amount of **glucose** in the blood.

hyperinsulinemia: A higher-than-normal amount of **insulin** in the blood.

hypo-: A prefix meaning "less than normal."

hypoglycemia: Less than normal amounts of **glucose** in the blood, popularly called *low blood sugar*.

IDDM: *Insulin-dependent diabetes mellitus*. An older name for **type 1 diabetes**. A person with **type 2 diabetes** may become insulin dependent but will still not have type 1 diabetes, which is **autoimmune**.

impaired glucose tolerance: A condition in which your **BG** levels are normal when fasting and are between 140 and 199 **mg/dL** at the two-hour point in a **glucose tolerance test**. Now usually called **prediabetes**.

incretin: A **hormone** that increases the production of **insulin** by the **beta cells**.

inflammation: A physiological state that helps fight infection and is hence beneficial in the short term. Chronic low-grade inflammation is associated with heart disease and diabetes.

insoluble fiber: **Fiber** that is not soluble in water, for example, cellulose. There is a lot of insoluble fiber in fruits, vegetables, and whole grains, especially wheat bran, rice bran, and corn bran.

insulin: A **hormone** produced by the **beta cells** of the **pancreas** that has many actions, including helping cells take up **glucose** and thus reducing **BG** levels.

insulin-dependent diabetes mellitus. See **IDDM**.

insulin receptor: A structure in the membrane of cells that binds **insulin** and triggers a cascade of events leading to an increase in the number of **glucose transporters** in the membrane. The net result is that more **glucose** can get into the cell. Not all types of tissue need insulin to take up glucose. The brain and liver do not.

insulin resistance (IR): A condition in which, for an as yet unknown reason, cells don't respond to **insulin**.

interstitial fluid: The nonblood fluids that are between your cells.

IR: See **insulin resistance**.

islet cells: The cells in the **pancreas** that produce **insulin** (the **beta cells**) and **glucagon** (the **alpha cells**). The full name for the islet cells is the *islets of Langerhans*.

ketoacidosis: See **diabetic ketoacidosis**.

ketone: A breakdown product of **fat** that can be burned for energy by some types of cells.

ketosis: A condition in which the level of **ketones** in the blood is higher than normal. This can be the result of very low **insulin** levels or a very high **fat** intake.

lactose: Milk sugar, consisting of **glucose** and **galactose**.

lancet: The needle used to draw blood for home **BG** testing.

LDL: Low-density lipoprotein. The "bad" cholesterol that can contribute to **plaques** in the walls of the **arteries**.

lipid: A general term for fatty substances that are not soluble in water. It includes **triglycerides** and **cholesterol**.

lipid panel: A series of tests for various **lipid**s in your blood, usually including total **cholesterol, LDL, HDL**, and **triglycerides**.

lipotoxicity: A reduction in the production of **insulin** by the **beta cells** and an increase in **insulin resistance**, both caused by high **lipid** levels.

low-carbohydrate diet: A diet that limits the amount of **carbohydrate** you eat and allows increased levels of **fat** or **protein**, or both.

low-fat diet: A diet that limits the amount of **fat** and fatty meats and emphasizes **carbohydrates**. Such a diet may or may not emphasize the **glycemic index**.

low-glycemic-index diet: A diet emphasizing **carbohydrate** foods that have low **glycemic index** values. It is similar to the **high-carbohydrate, high-fiber diet**, but some foods such as potatoes and beets that would be considered good choices on that diet have high glycemic index values and would be avoided on the low-glycemic-index diet.

macrovascular: Referring to the large blood vessels. *Macrovascular complications* are those resulting from damage to the **arteries**, for example, heart attacks, strokes, and **peripheral vascular disease**.

maltitol: A **sugar alcohol** that raises **BG** levels almost as much as **sucrose**. Maltitol is a common sweetener in "sugar-free" candies.

metabolic syndrome: A syndrome of symptoms including high **insulin** levels, high blood pressure, high **triglyceride** levels, low **HDL** levels, and **impaired glucose tolerance**. Also called *Syndrome X*.

metabolize: Convert into something else. *Catabolism* means breaking something down into smaller parts, and *anabolism* means building something up, as with *anabolic steroids*. *Metabolism* is the sum of the anabolic and catabolic processes in your body.

mg/dL (milligrams per deciliter): The units usually used in America when measuring **BG** levels.

microvascular: Referring to the small blood vessels. *Microvascular complications* are complications result from damage to the **capillaries**, for example, **retinopathy, nephropathy**, and **neuropathy**.

mimetic: A compound that mimics the action of another compound. A mimetic does not have to be an **analog**, but it can be.

MODY: Maturity-onset diabetes of the young.

monosaccharide: A **carbohydrate** containing one **sugar** unit.

monounsaturated fat: **Fat** containing one double bond. Monounsaturated fat is considered a "good fat" that does not increase **cholesterol** levels.

MyPlate: Current US Department of Agriculture dietary recommendations depicted as a plate divided according to recommended amounts of fruits, vegetables, grains, and protein.

nephropathy: Damage to the kidneys.

neuropathy: Damage to nerves.

NIDDM: *Non-insulin-dependent diabetes mellitus.* An old term for **type 2 diabetes**. Some forms of diabetes, for example, **gestational diabetes**, may not require you to use **insulin**, but they are no longer classified as type 2 diabetes.

nutritionist: A general term for someone specializing in nutrition. A nutritionist can be a registered **dietician** or a self-educated person.

obestatin: A **hormone** secreted by the stomach that opposes the actions of **grehlin**.

ophthalmologist: A medical doctor who specializes in eye diseases.

pancreas: An organ behind the stomach that contains the **beta cells** that produce **insulin**. It also contains **alpha cells** that produce **glucagon** and several other types of cells that produce other **hormones**. The pancreas also produces digestive **enzymes**.

PCP: See **primary care provider**.

peripheral neuropathy: The **neuropathy** that occurs in your hands and legs.

peripheral vascular disease: Clogging of the **arteries** in your hands and legs.

physical therapist: A person who has a degree in physical therapy and has passed national and state examinations.

plaque: A deposit of fatty substances including **cholesterol** in the wall of an **artery**, resulting in narrowing of the arterial cavity.

plasma: The part of blood that remains after you've removed all the blood cells and **platelets**.

platelet: Small disk-shaped structures in the blood that are required for clotting.

polysaccharide: A **carbohydrate** containing many **sugar** units.

polyunsaturated fat: A type of **fat** containing more than one double bond. Polyunsaturated fats are found in vegetable oils and tend to lower the "bad" **LDL** levels but may lower beneficial **HDL** levels as well.

postprandial: After a meal.

prediabetes: A condition in which your fasting **BG** level is 100 to 125 mg/dL (formerly called *impaired fasting glucose*) or your fasting **BG** levels are normal but they increase to between 140 and 199 mg/dL in a **glucose tolerance test** (formerly called **impaired glucose tolerance**), or both.

preprandial: Before a meal.

primary care provider (PCP): The physician who oversees all your care. This can be an internist, a family physician, or an **endocrinologist** or other type of specialist, depending on your needs.

processed carbohydrate: A **carbohydrate** that has been finely milled or otherwise separated from its natural **fiber**, resulting in faster digestion and a higher **glycemic index**.

protein: A type of food made of **amino acid** building blocks. By itself, protein contains 4 calories per gram, but most protein foods such as meat also contain **fat**. Protein may or may not raise your **BG** levels.

reactive oxygen species (ROS): Oxygen-containing compounds that are highly reactive, mostly oxygen-containing **free radicals**. ROS can damage healthy molecules in your body, but they can also be used to destroy bacteria, viruses, and cancer cells.

red blood cell: A type of cell in the blood that contains **hemoglobin**, the compound that transports oxygen.

registered dietician: See **dietician**.

retinopathy: Disease of the retina, the back part of the eye that senses light.

ROS: See **reactive oxygen species**.

saturated fat: **Fat** containing no double bonds, usually solid at room temperature. Saturated fat is thought to increase **cholesterol** levels and **insulin resistance**. Saturated fats are found in animal products and tropical oils.

SGLT: Sodium-glucose transporter. SGLT-2 inhibitors help control BG levels.

small, dense LDL: A type of **LDL** that is supposed to be more apt to cause arterial **plaques**.

soluble fiber: The kind of **fiber** that forms a gummy solution in water. It can delay the emptying of the stomach and slow digestion, resulting in smaller increases in **BG** levels after a meal. It is also thought to lower **lipid** levels. Soluble fiber occurs in fruits, beans, and oat bran.

sorbitol: A **sugar alcohol** often used to replace table sugar in diet desserts. When **glucose** is converted to sorbitol within cells, this may contribute to complications.

starch: A **carbohydrate** food consisting of long chains of **glucose**. There are different types of starches, and some have higher **glycemic index** values than others

steroid: A class of compounds derived from **cholesterol** and including the sex hormones *estrogen* and *testosterone* as well as anti-inflammatory drugs such as **cortisone** and *prednisone*.

stress hormone: A hormone released when you're stressed, for example, **cortisol** and **adrenaline**.

sucrose: Table sugar, a **disaccharide** consisting of **glucose** and **fructose**.

sugar: Any of a **carbohydrate** class of sweet, water-soluble compounds. The degree of sweetness depends on the particular sugar. The term is often used to mean **sucrose.** A "simple sugar" is a **monosaccharide,** but the term is often used loosely.

sugar alcohols: Derivatives of sugars that don't raise **BG** levels as much but contain almost as many calories and can cause diarrhea.

sulfonylureas: A class of compounds that reduce **BG** levels by increasing the output of **insulin** by the **beta cells.** They were the first oral drugs used to treat type 2 diabetes.

TAG: Used for both *triacylglycerol,* an alternative name for **triglyceride,** and *total available glucose.* The latter is a system of calculating insulin doses on the basis of the content of carbohydrate, protein, and fat in the meal.

thrifty genes: Genes that make you tend to gain weight when food is plentiful.

trans fat: A type of **fat** produced by the industrial treatment of oils to make them solid at room temperature. The trans fats are supposed to be more detrimental to health than **saturated fat.** They are found in cookies, crackers, solid margarine, and some salad dressings.

triglyceride: A type of **fat** composed of a molecule of the E-shaped **glycerol** plus three **fatty acids.**

type 1 diabetes: An autoimmune disease in which the body, for unknown reasons, destroys the **beta cells,** resulting in a total or almost-total lack of **insulin.**

type 2 diabetes: A disease caused primarily by **insulin resistance,** in which a person may actually produce more **insulin** than normal but it doesn't respond to it.

UKPDS (UK Prospective Diabetes Study): A twenty-year study that showed that microvascular complication rates with **type 2 diabetes** decreased when **BG** levels were kept lower.

unsaturated fat: Fat containing double bonds, usually liquid at room temperature. Unsaturated fats either lower **cholesterol** levels or have no effect. They are found in plant oils.

veins: The blood vessels that bring carbon dioxide from the tissues to the lungs, where it is exchanged for oxygen.

vitamin: A carbon-containing substance present in food, or manufactured in the body, that is required in small amounts for good health.

VLDL: Very low density lipoprotein. The form in which the body ships **triglycerides** from the liver to the tissues to be burned for energy or stored as **fat.** When the VLDL has dropped off its fat, it turns into **LDL.**

white blood cells: Cells in the blood that fight infection and perform other useful chores.

YMMV: Your Mileage May Vary, meaning that what works for me might not work for you, and vice versa.

For Further Reading

Basic diabetes care

American Diabetes Association. *American Diabetes Association Complete Guide to Diabetes.* 5th ed. Alexandria, VA: American Diabetes Association, 2011. (The official ADA viewpoint.)

Beaser, Richard S., and Amy P. Campbell. *The Joslin Guide to Diabetes: A Program for Managing Your Treatment.* 2nd ed. New York: Touchstone, 2005. (Viewpoint of a leading diabetes center. Guide is in both English and Spanish.)

Bernstein, Richard K. *Dr. Bernstein's Diabetes Solution: The Complete Guide to Achieving Normal Blood Sugars.* 4th ed. New York: Little, Brown, 2007. (Low-carbohydrate approach, but also contains a lot of useful information of interest to anyone with diabetes.)

Hamdy, Osama, and Sheri R. Colberg. *The Diabetes Breakthrough: Based on a Scientifically Proven Plan to Lose Weight and Cut Medications.* Don Mills, Ontario: Harlequin, 2014. (Has a good chart of oral drugs as of 2013 with benefits and side effects.)

Mayo Clinic. *The Essential Diabetes Book.* 2nd ed. Birmingham, AL: Oxmoor House, 2014. (Mayo Clinic viewpoint.)

National Diabetes Information Clearinghouse (see Resources). They have a lot of information in both English and Spanish; most of their publications can be downloaded free.

Peters, Anne L. *Conquering Diabetes: A Cutting Edge, Comprehensive Program for Prevention and Treatment.* New York: Plume, 2006. (The viewpoint of an empathetic endocrinologist whose husband has prediabetes.)

Saudek, Christopher D., Richard R. Rubin, and Cynthia S. Shump. *The Johns Hopkins Guide to Diabetes: For Patients and Families*. 2nd ed. Baltimore, MD: Johns Hopkins University Press, 2014. (The viewpoint of an MD and two CDEs.)

In-depth reading about diabetes

These books are all dated but still contain good background information in detail. Your hospital library may have them.

Davidson, Mayer B., Anne Peters Harmel, and Ruchi Mathur. *Davidson's Diabetes Mellitus: Diagnosis and Treatment*. 5th ed. Philadelphia: WB Saunders, 2004.

Kahn, C. Ronald, Gordon C. Weir, George L. King, Alan C. Moses, Robert J. Smith, and Alan M. Jacobson. *Joslin's Diabetes Mellitus*. 14th ed. Philadelphia: Lippincott Williams & Wilkins, 2005.

Porte, Daniel Jr., Robert S. Sherwin, and Alain Baron, eds. *Ellenberg and Rifkin's Diabetes Mellitus: Theory and Practice*. 6th ed. New York: McGraw-Hill, 2003.

Using insulin

Scheiner, Gary. *Think Like a Pancreas: A Practical Guide to Managing Diabetes with Insulin*. 2nd ed. Boston: Da Capo Lifelong Books, 2012.

Walsh, John, Ruth Roberts, Varma Chandrasekhar, and Timothy Bailey. *Using Insulin: Everything You Need for Success with Insulin*. San Diego: Torrey Pines Press, 2003.

Diets

I don't agree with the philosophy of all these diets, but I offer a variety so you can find something that works for you.

Low-carbohydrate diets

Allan, Christian B., and Wolfgang Lutz. *Life Without Bread: How a Low-Carbohydrate Diet Can Save Your Life*. New York: McGraw-Hill, 2000.

Atkins, Robert C. *Dr. Atkins' New Diet Revolution*. Rev. ed. New York: Harper, 2009.

Bernstein, Richard K. *The Diabetes Diet: Dr. Bernstein's Low-Carbohydrate Solution*. New York: Little, Brown, 2005.

Bowden, Jonny. *Living Low Carb: Controlled-Carbohydrate Eating for Long-Term Weight Loss*. Rev. ed. New York: Sterling Publishing, 2013. (Includes Bowden's reviews of various low-carbohydrate diets.)

Eades, Michael R., and Mary Dan Eades. *Protein Power: The Metabolic Breakthrough*. New York: Bantam Books, 1999.

Ezrin, Calvin, and Robert E. Kowalski. *The Type 2 Diabetes Diet Book*. 4th ed. New York: McGraw-Hill, 2011.

Feinman, Richard D. *The World Turned Upside Down: The Second Low-Carbohydrate Revolution*. New York: NMS Press, 2014. (A good introduction to the biochemistry of low carbohydrate diets.)

Goldberg, Jack, and Karen O'Mara. *The Four Corners Diet: The Healthy Low-Carbohydrate Way of Eating for a Lifetime*. With Gretchen Becker. New York: Marlowe & Co., 2004.

Rosedale, Ron, and Carol Colman. *The Rosedale Diet*. Reprint. New York: William Morrow, 2005. (A bit dated, but has information on leptin and other hormones that isn't covered in other books.)

Thompson, R., and Dana Carpender. *The Glycemic Load Diabetes Solution: Six Steps to Optimal Control of Your Adult-Onset (Type 2) Diabetes*. 2nd ed. Chicago: McGraw-Hill, 2012.

Westman, Eric C., Stephen D. Phinney, and Jeff S. Volek. *The New Atkins for a New You: The Ultimate Diet for Shedding Weight and Feeling Great*. New York: Touchstone, 2010.

Low-fat, high-carbohydrate, and high-fiber diets

Fuhrman, Joel. *Eat to Live: The Amazing Nutrient-Rich Program for Fast and Sustained Weight Loss*. Rev. ed. Boston: Little, Brown, 2011.

Goor, Ron, and Nancy Goor. *Choose to Lose: A Food Lover's Guide to Permanent Weight Loss*. 3rd ed. Boston: Rux Martin, 1999.

McDougall, John A. *The Starch Solution*. Emmaus, PA: Rodale Books, 2012.

Ornish, Dean. *Eat More, Weigh Less: Dr. Dean Ornish's Program for Losing Weight Safely While Eating Abundantly*. Rev. ed. New York: HarperTorch, 2002.

Pritikin, Robert. *The Pritikin Principle: The Calorie Density Solution*. Alexandria, VA: Time Life Books, 2000.

Stone, Gene, ed. *Forks Over Knives: The Plant-Based Way to Health*. New York: The Experiment, 2011.

Low-glycemic-index diets

Brand-Miller, Jennie, Kay Foster-Powell, Stephen Colagiuri, and Alan W. Barclay. *Everything You Need to Know to Manage Type 2 Diabetes: Simple Steps for Surviving and Thriving with the Low GI Plan*. Boston: Da Capo Lifelong Books, 2015.

Steward, H. Leighton, Morrison C. Bethea, Sam S. Andrews, and Luis A. Balart. *The New Sugar Busters!: Cut Sugar to Trim Fat*. Rev. ed. New York: Ballantine Books, 2003.

Other diets

Cloutier, Marissa, and Eve Adamson. *The Mediterranean Diet*. Rev. ed. New York: Avon, 2004.

Cordain, Loren. *The Paleo Diet: Lose Weight and Get Healthy by Eating the Foods You Were Designed to Eat*. Rev. ed. Hoboken, NJ: John Wiley, 2011.

Davis, William. *Wheat Belly: Lose the Wheat, Lose the Weight, and Find Your Path Back to Health*. Reprint. Emmaus, PA: Rodale Books, 2014.

Gedgaudas, Nora T. *Primal Body, Primal Mind: Beyond the Paleo Diet for Total Health and a Longer Life*. 2nd ed. Rochester, VT: Healing Arts Press, 2011.

Hornick, Betsy A. *101 Best Diabetic Foods*. Lincolnwood, IL: Publications International, 2011. (Not a diet, but if you're newly diagnosed and want a simple guide to foods that are better than the standard American diet, this would be a place to start until you figure out what diet is best for you.)

Kresser, Chris. *The Paleo Cure: Eat Right for Your Genes, Body Type, and Personal Health Needs—Prevent and Reverse Disease, Lose Weight Effortlessly, and Look and Feel Better than Ever*. Reprint. Boston: Little, Brown, 2014. (Formerly called *Your Personal Paleo Code*.)

Mosley, Michael, and Mimi Spencer. *The Fast Diet: Lose Weight, Stay Healthy, and Live Longer with the Simple Secret of Intermittent Fasting*. Rev. ed. New York: Attria Press, 2015. (Intermittent fasting.)

Planck, Nina. *Real Food: What to Eat and Why*. New York: Bloomsbury USA, 2007.

Schwarzbein, Diana, and Nancy Deville. *The Schwarzbein Principle: The Truth About Losing Weight, Being Healthy, and Feeling Younger*. Deerfield Beach, FL: Health Communications, 1999. (The introduction describes how medical school teachings about diabetes diets don't always correspond to reality.)

Sears, Barry. *The Mediterranean Zone: Unleash the Power of the World's Healthiest Diet for Superior Weight Loss, Health, and Longevity*. New York: Zinc Ink, 2014.

Willett, Walter C. *Eat, Drink, and Be Healthy: The Harvard Medical School Guide to Healthy Eating*. With P. J. Skerrett. New York: Free Press, 2005.

Exchanges and carbohydrate counting

Franz, Marion J. *Exchanges for All Occasions with Carbohydrate Counting: Pocket Guide to Healthy Food Choices Anytime*. Minneapolis, MN: International Diabetes Center, 2000.

Calculating nutritional content

Pennington, Jean A. T. *Bowes & Church's Food Values of Portions Commonly Used*. 19th ed. Philadelphia: Lippincott Williams & Wilkins, 2010.

USDA Nutrient Database for Standard Reference online at http://ndb.nal.usda.gov /ndb

Measuring SGIs

Paice, Derek. *Diabetes and Diet: A Type 2 Patient's Efforts at Control*. Palm Harbor, FL: Paice & Associates, 1997. (Available from Paice & Associates, 114 Rosewood Court, Palm Harbor, FL 34685.)

Metabolic syndrome and insulin resistance

Challem, Jack, Burton Berkson, and Melissa Diane Smith. *Syndrome X: The Complete Nutritional Program to Prevent and Reverse Insulin Resistance*. New York: John Wiley, 2000.

Krentz, Andrew J. *Insulin Resistance: A Clinical Handbook*. Oxford, England: Blackwell Science, 2002.

Reaven, Gerald M., and Ami Laws, eds. *Insulin Resistance: The Metabolic Syndrome X*. Totowa, NJ: Humana Press, 1999. (Very technical.)

Reaven, Gerald M., Terry Kristen Strom, and Barry Fox. *Syndrome X: The Silent Killer; The New Heart Disease Risk*. New York: Simon & Schuster, 2001.

Herbal medicine

Your bookstore or health-food store should have a selection of popular books on herbs and supplements. The following books provide the medical community's views.

Baily, Clifford J., and Caroline Day. "Traditional Plant Medicines as Treatments for Diabetes." *Diabetes Care* 12, no. 553 (1989).

Blumenthal, Mark, ed. *The Complete German Commission E Monographs: Therapeutic Guide to Herbal Medicines*. Newton, MA: Integrative Medicine Communications, 1998.

Blumenthal, Mark, and Alicia Goldberg, eds. *Herbal Medicine: Expanded Commission E Monographs*. Newton, MA: Integrative Medicine Communication, 2000.

Physicians Desk Reference Staff. *PDR for Herbal Medicines*. 4th ed. Montvale, NJ: Thomson Healthcare, 2007. (Designed for physicians, includes references, and is limited to herbs.)

Physicians Desk Reference Staff. *The PDR Family Guide to Natural Medicines and Healing Therapies*. New York: Ballantine, 2000. (Includes information about nonherbal therapies; without supporting references.)

Exercise

Colberg, Sheri. *The Diabetic Athlete's Handbook*. Champaign, IL: Human Kinetics, 2008.

Colberg, Sheri. *The 7-Step Diabetes Fitness Plan· Living Well and Being Fit with Diabetes No Matter What Your Weight*. Boston: Da Capo Lifelong Books, 2006.

Kenney, W. Larry, Jack H. Wilmore, and David L. Costill. *Physiology of Sport and Exercise with Web Study Guide*. 5th ed. Champaign, IL: Human Kinetics, 2011.

Nelson, Miriam E. *Strong Women Stay Young*. With Sarah Wernick. Rev. ed. New York: Bantam Books, 2005.

Other special focus

Goldberg, Riva. *50 Diabetes Myths That Can Ruin Your Life: And the 50 Diabetes Truths That Can Save It*. Boston: Da Capo Lifelong Books, 2009.

Jovanovic-Peterson, Lois. *Managing Your Gestational Diabetes: A Guide for You and Your Baby's Good Health*. With Morton B. Stone. New York: John Wiley, 1994. (Not the most recent book on this topic, but the author is not only a well-known research scientist but also has diabetes herself.)

Levin, Marvin E., and Michael A. Pfeifer, eds. *The Uncomplicated Guide to Diabetes Complications*. 3rd ed. Alexandria, VA: American Diabetes Association, 2009.

Polonsky, William H. *Diabetes Burnout: What to Do When You Can't Take It Anymore*. Alexandria, VA: American Diabetes Association, 1999.

Vieira, Ginger. *Dealing with Diabetes Burnout: How to Recharge and Get Back on Track When You Feel Frustrated and Overwhelmed Living with Diabetes*. New York: Demos Medical Publishing, 2014.

Diabetes history

Cooper, Thea, and Arthur Ainsberg. *Breakthrough: Elizabeth Hughes, the Discovery of Insulin, and the Making of a Medical Miracle*. New York: St. Martin's Press, 2009.

Tattersall, Robert. *Diabetes: The Biography. Biographies of Diseases*, edited by William Bynum and Helen Bynum. New York: Oxford University Press, 2009.

In-depth background reading

Brody, Tom. *Nutritional Biochemistry*. 2nd ed. San Diego: Academic Press, 1999.

Guyton, Arthur C., and John E. Hall. *Textbook of Medical Physiology*. 13th ed. Philadelphia: Elsevier Saunders, 2015.

Diabetes blogs

There are many diabetes blogs on the Internet today. I read about seventy diabetes and nutrition blogs, too many to list here, and sites come and go, so your best bet is to do an Internet search on "diabetes blog" or your special interest. Some blogs are chatty, discussing the blogger's daily life and dealings with friends and family, and others focus more on information.

Resources

American Diabetes
  Association
1701 North Beauregard
  Street
Alexandria, VA 22311
800-342-2383
  (800-DIABETES)
www.diabetes.org

American Medical
  Identifications
949 Wakefield Drive,
  Suite 100
Houston, TX 77018
800-363-5985
www.americanmedical
  -id.com

Blood Sugar 101
(Lots of information
  including a tool to convert
  hemoglobin
  A1c into average blood
  glucose levels.)
www.phlaunt.com

Bureau of Primary Health
  Care
Health Resources and
  Services Administration
  (HRSA)
Parklawn Building
5600 Fishers Lane
Rockville, MD 20857
888-275-4772
  (888-ASK-HRSA)
www.hrsa.gov

Department of Veterans
  Affairs
810 Vermont Avenue, NW
Washington, DC 20420
800-827-1000 (connects to
  your nearest benefits
  office);
  TTY 800-829-4833
www.va.gov

Diabetes Forecast magazine
Magazine is included with
  ADA membership (see
  above)
www.diabetesforecast.org

Diabetes Health
PO Box 1199
Woodacre, CA 94973
415-488-4526
www.diabeteshealth.com

Diabetes Self-Management
150 West 22nd Street
New York, NY 10011
Subscriptions to
PO Box 889
Boulder, CO 80322-2890
800-234-0923
www.diabetesselfmanage
  ment.com

Equal Employment
  Opportunity Commission
131 M Street, NE
Washington, DC 20507
800-669-4000 (connects to
  your nearest EEO office);
  TTY 800-669-6820
www.eeoc.gov

Hill Burton Program
Health Resources and
   Services Administration
   (HRSA)
Parklawn Building
5600 Fishers Lane, Room
   10C-16
Rockville, MD 20857
800-638-0742 (requires
   touch-tone telephone to
   receive information);
   800-492-0359 in Maryland
www.hrsa.gov/gethealth
   care/affordable
   /hillburton

International Association for
   Medical Assistance to
   Travellers
1623 Military Road, No. 279
Niagara Falls, NY 14304-
   1745
716-754-4883
www.iamat.org

International Diabetes
   Federation
166 Chaussée de la Hulpe
B-1170 Brussels
Belgium
32-2/538 55 11
www.idf.org

Joslin Diabetes Center
One Joslin Place
Boston, MA 02115
800-567-5461;
   617-732-2400
www.joslin.org

Lions Clubs International
300 West 22nd Street
Oak Brook, IL 60523-8842
630-571-5466
www.lionsclubs.org

Lower Extremity
   Amputation Prevention
   (LEAP) Program
National Hansen's Disease
   Program
1770 Physicians Park Drive
Baton Rouge, LA 70816
800-642-2477
www.bphc.hrsa.gov/leap

MedicAlert
PO Box 21009
Lansing, MI 48909
888-525-5174
www.medicalert.org

Medicare
800-633-4227
   (800-MEDICAR) (connects
   to your nearest Medicare
   office and
   can provide the number
   of the appropriate
   Medicare claims office)
www.medicare.gov

National Center for
   Complementary
   and Integrative Health
9000 Rockville Pike
Bethseda, MD 20892
888-644-6226;
   outside the U.S.
   301-519-3153; TTY
   866-464-3615
https://nccih.nih.gov

National Diabetes
   Information
   Clearinghouse
1 Information Way
Bethesda, MD 20892-3560
800-860-8747;
301-654-3327;
   TTY 866-569-1162
www.diabetes.niddk
   .nih.gov

National Hemoglobin
   Standardization Program
Department of Pathology
   and Anatomical Sciences,
   Room M767
University of Missouri
   School of Medicine
1 Hospital Drive
Columbia, MO 65212
573-882-1257
www.ngsp.org

Native Seeds/SEARCH
3584 E River Road
Tucson, AZ 85718
520-622-0832
(Source of seeds and foods
   that were traditionally
   used by Native Americans
   in the Southwest. Many,
   such as tepary beans,
   are low on the glycemic
   index.)
www.nativeseeds.org

Partnership for Prescription
   Assistance
950 F Street, NW
Washington, DC 20004
888-477-2669;
   202-835-3400
www.pparx.org

Acknowledgments

I thank all those who helped me in this endeavor, directly or indirectly, especially my fellow diabetic "passengers" in this voyage of diabetes, who shared their knowledge, their experiences, their feelings, their failures, their successes, their hopes, and their fears, as well as their wit, which made me laugh. I especially thank those who allowed me to quote their thoughts in this book.

I also thank David Mendosa for putting me in touch with my first publisher, Marlowe & Company, and for his contribution to the Month 12 chapter of this book; Virginia Rose Page for her intelligent interpretation and precise rendition of the rough drawings that I sent to her; Elizabeth Smith for her magical camera work; and Steve West and Wayne Wells for wise computer advice when I thought my Big Black Box had gone south.

I also thank Marlboro College for allowing me to audit Todd Smith's biochemistry course; Derek Paice and David Mendosa for reading the entire manuscript of the first edition and offering useful suggestions; and Randie R. Little for clarifying some hemoglobin A1c terms for me. Any errors are, of course, my own.

I thank my mother, the late Ellen V. Becker, for her support; June Biermann and Barbara Toohey for their encouragement; Janet Ruhl for her thought-provoking email debates; and Nancy Humeniuk and Nora Midlash for listening to my cyberspace whining when I was feeling overworked.

In addition, I thank Dr. Allison Goldfine for her caring treatment of patients (and research subjects), for devoting her keen mind to the study of diabetes, and for taking time from her busy research and teaching career to write the foreword to this book.

I thank everyone involved in the design and production of this book, including Alex Camlin for his striking cover design, Cynthia Young for her elegant interior page design, as well as Kate Mueller and Stephen Wagley.

Finally, I thank my first editor, Matthew Lore, who has the gift of guiding with a gentle nudge. The overall shaping of this book is his.

Figure Credits

Figure 1 (page 74) adapted from Tasaka Y., M. Sekine, M. Wakatsuki, H. Ohgawara, and K. Shizume. "Levels of Pancreatic Glucagon, Insulin and Glucose during Twenty-Four Hours of the Day in Normal Subjects." *Hormone and Metabolic Research*, 1975: 7:205–206.

Figure 2 (page 109) adapted from DeFronzo, R. A., R. C. Bonadonna, and E. Ferrannini. "Pathogenesis of NIDDM." *Diabetes Care*, 1992: 15:318.

Figure 3 (page 242) adapted from Grodsky G. M., H. Landahl, D. Curry, et al: In Faulkner S., Hellman B., Taljedal I-B (eds). *The Structure and Metabolism of the Pancreatic Islets*. Wenner-Gren Center International Symposium Series. Oxford, Pergamon Press, 1970, pp 409–422.

Figure 4 (page 257) adapted from Wilmore J. H., D. L. Costill. *Physiology of Sport and Exercise*. 2nd ed. Champaign, IL, Human Kinetics, 1994, p 353.

Index